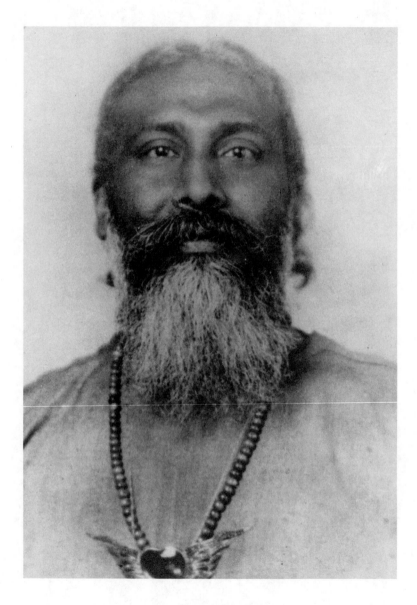

Hazrat Pir-o-Murshid Inayat Khan

The Sufi Message of Hazrat Inayat Khan

Centennial Edition

Volume IV
Healing and the Mind World

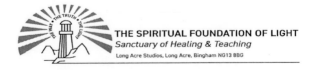

The Sufi Message of Hazrat Inayat Khan

Centennial Edition

Volume IV
Healing and the Mind World

HEALTH
HEALING
MENTAL PURIFICATION
THE MIND WORLD

Sulūk Press
Richmond, Virginia

Published by Sulūk Press
an imprint of Omega Publications, Inc.
Richmond, Virginia
www.omegapub.com

Cover background and ornament from Shutterstock.com
Cover design by Sandra Lillydahl

This edition is printed on acid-free paper
that meets ANSI standard X39-48.

Author: Inayat Khan (1882–1927)
Title: The Sufi Message of Hazrat Inayat Khan
Centennial Edition
Volume IV: Healing and the Mind World
Health, Healing,
Mental Purification, The Mind World
Includes introduction by Pir Zia Inayat-Khan,
biographical notes, glossary, index.
Subjects: Sufism; Spiritual healing; Sufism—psychology

Library of Congress Control Number: 2019948407

Printed and bound by Sheridan Books Inc.
in the United States of America

ISBN 978-1-941810-309 paper
ISBN 978-1-941810-316 hardcase

Contents

Contents

Contents

Contents

ACKNOWLEDGMENTS

Many thanks are due to Anne Louise Wirgman, Director, Nekbakht Foundation in Suresnes, France, who provided invaluable assistance with providing authentic source material. Additional skilled editorial assistance was provided by Cannon Labrie.

Sandra Lillydahl, editor

INTRODUCTION

Purification (*tazkiya*) is a central theme of Sufism. The goal of the process is to lay bare the primal nature (*fitra*) of the human being. In Hazrat Inayat Khan's teachings, the purification of the body leads to the purification of the breath, the purification of the breath leads to the purification of the mind, and the purification of the mind leads to the purification of the heart. The teachings in this volume touch on all four stages, with a primary focus on the purification of the mind.

Hazrat's discussion of the mind sheds illuminating light on the nature of consciousness, cognition, and mental habits. Reading these lectures, the reader's mind is drawn to reflect on its own inner workings. Hazrat's lectures are not, however, merely descriptive; they are also prescriptive in the sense that they trace, in outline, the path of "mystic relaxation" that leads ultimately to the experience of pure, unconditioned consciousness.

Alongside Hazrat's teachings on the mind, the volume contains extensive lectures on the subjects of health and healing, lectures which anticipate the findings of contemporary mind-body medicine. Taken together, these chapters constitute a comprehensive overview of the fundamental principles of Sufi healing. It bears emphasizing that Hazrat was an accomplished practitioner of the art of which he speaks. An account of his power as a spiritual healer may be found in the recollections of Sophia Saintsbury-Green:

The disciple who paints these pictures is able to give personal testimony to the great blessing received from the healing of the Master after having suffered from a serious internal complaint which had caused eleven months to be passed in bed. During this time four doctors gave it as their verdict that without an operation no cure was possible, but that the condition of the heart prevented one being attempted. The Master, who was staying near the disciple's house, hearing of the illness, came instantly, and by the bedside gave the healing blessing of the Laying on of Hands, an immediate cure resulting and no symptoms of the illness having recurred during the ten years which have passed since that day.[1]

The lectures assembled in this volume were given in various cities in Europe and the United States between the years of 1919 and 1924. Two sections of the book, *Health* and *The Mind World*, consist of lectures from the Suresnes Summer School of 1924. A century has since passed, but Hazrat Inayat Khan's teachings remain as vitally relevant as ever.

Pir Zia Inayat-Khan

---

1 Sophia Saintsbury-Green, *Images of Inayat* (New Lebanon, NY: Sulūk Press, 2014), 28. Cf. Sirkar van Stolk and Daphne Dunlop, *Memories of a Sufi Sage: Hazrat Inayat Khan* (The Hague: East-West Publications, 1975), 18–20.

HEALTH

The contents of "Health" were compiled from lectures given by Inayat Khan during the Summer School in Suresnes, France, from June 16 to September 8, 1924.

HEALTH 1

Illness from the Sufi point of view is an inharmony, either physical inharmony or mental inharmony. One acts upon the other. What causes inharmony? The lack of tone and the lack of rhythm. How can it be interpreted in physical terminology? Prana or life or energy is the tone. Circulation regulation is the rhythm—regulation in the beatings of the heart, of the pulse, and circulation of the blood through the tubes or veins of the body. In physical terms the lack of circulation means congestion, and the lack of prana or life or energy means weakness. These two things attract illness and are the cause of illness. In mental terms the rhythm is the action of the mind: whether the mind is active in harmonious thoughts or inharmonious thoughts; if the mind is strong, firm, and steady or if the mind is weak. If one continues to think harmonious thoughts, it is just like the regular beating of the pulse and good circulation of the blood. If this harmony of thought is broken, then congestion comes in the mind. Then a person loses memory, and depression comes as a result; what one sees is nothing but darkness. Doubt, suspicions, distrust, and all manner of distress and despair come when the mind is congested in this way.

The prana, life, or energy of the mind is when the mind can be steady on thoughts of harmony, when the mind can balance its thoughts, when it cannot be easily shaken, when doubts and confusions cannot easily overpower it. Whether it is nerve illness, whether it is mental disorder, whether it is physical illness,

3

all different aspects of illness have at the root of them only one cause, and that cause is inharmony. The body which becomes once inharmonious turns into a receptacle of inharmonious influences, of inharmonious atoms. It partakes of them without knowing, and so does the mind. Therefore, the body which is already lacking health is more susceptible to catching an illness than the body which is perfectly healthy. And so the mind which already has in it a disorder is more susceptible to taking every suggestion of disorder, and in this way it becomes worse.

It is experienced by the physicians of all ages that an element attracts the same element. And so it is natural that illness attracts illness, but in plain words, inharmony attracts inharmony, whereas harmony attracts harmony. Ordinarily we see in our everyday life that a person who has nothing the matter and is only weak physically, or whose life is not regular, is always susceptible to catching illnesses. Then we see those who ponder often upon inharmonious thoughts are very easily offended. It does not take long for them to get offended; a little thing here and there makes them feel irritated because the irritation is already there. It wants just a little touch to make it a deeper irritation.

Besides this, the harmony of the body and mind depends upon one's external life: the food one eats, the way one lives, the people one meets, the work one does, the climate in which one lives. No doubt, under the same conditions one person may be ill, and another person may be well. The reason is that one is in harmony with the food one eats, with the weather one lives in, with the people with whom one meets, with conditions that are around one. There are others who revolt against the food they eat, against people they meet, against conditions that are before them, against the weather. The outcome is that they are not in harmony, and they perceive and experience the same result in their lives. Illness is the result; disorder is the result.

This idea can be very well demonstrated by the present method that the physicians have adopted: to inject the same element in one which makes one ill. There is no better demonstration of this idea, that this makes one in harmony with a thing which is opposed to one's nature. If one only understood that one can inject oneself with all the opposing influences which come, and put oneself in harmony with them, and then see what result one experiences. The woodcutters do not get sunstroke. The sailors do not get cold. The reason is that they have injected themselves with the element which they have to meet in life, the element which will oppose their system, their nature. Therefore, in short, the first lesson in health is the understanding of this principle that illness is nothing but inharmony, and the secret of health lies in harmony.

* * *

Question: *What is the best way for a physician to heal?*

Answer: Where there is a need of manipulation, but in cases when it is not needed one can heal without it. The healing with manipulation is a different kind of healing. It is between the work of a physician and healer. One who manipulates is not necessarily a healer but is a masseur. A healer's work is with thought, with prayer. If one has an extra magnetism with which one manipulates, one will have more success, but that is a different thing. Healing is quite a different work.

Question: *The power of thought . . . they bring a better vibration to the person who is inharmonious?*

Answer: The power of thought comes from the healer, and a different vibration comes also from the manipulator. Of course, thought has vibrations also. They are more subtle than the vibrations that are given in massage; therefore, the thought vibration can do much more work than the vibration from the massage. No doubt there are certain cases in which massage is very necessary, and, together with healing, this can help. But when one sees the work of healing distinctly, it is apart, different.

Question: *Would you approve of inoculation for diseases?*

Answer: I approve of everything that cures.

Question: *How can you make yourself more in harmony in order to be stronger against illness, not to catch influenza?¹*

Answer: In the first place to keep the tone of the mind and body in order, and that is to nourish the body and to exercise it, together with harmonizing one's thoughts and feelings. And even then, if the germs of influenza came, to fight with them, to get rid of them.

Question: *Can mental healing cure faulty bones and wrong structure?*

Answer: Yes, there is nothing that healing cannot cure if the healer knew how to heal and if the one to be healed knew how to respond to that healing.

Question: *Why is it that when we hear music from a distance and it is only an indistinct mass of sound, the general impression is always minor harmony?*

Answer: You could have just as well have written "inner harmony." The sum total of all things is beautiful. As we read in the Qur'an, "God is beautiful, and loves beauty."² And when we compare things, one thing is more beautiful than another. But when we take in the glance of the whole, as one perfect whole, then we get that beauty which is the essence of beauty, which is at the back of it. So also with music. When we listen to music, close to it, we hear the faults that come to our ears, but from a distance what comes to us is a sum total. The inharmony is dropped; only the harmony comes to our ears, refined. So we enjoy the beauty which is at the back of everything and all things. This question on music we can turn into a picture of life

1 The Spanish flu pandemic of 1918, the deadliest in history, infected an estimated 500 million people worldwide—about one-third of the planet's population—and killed somewhere between 20 and 40 million. It was implicated in the outbreak of *Encephalitis lethargica* in the 1920s.
2 Hadith.

and look at life in the same way. The faults and shortcomings and the lack of beauty that we see all sums up if we do not take note of it so closely as we do. If we stand at a distance and look at it as one sum total of all things, then we get the essence of it; all the useless parts are left out.

Question: *How is it possible to inoculate yourself with inharmonious thoughts when . . . ?*

Answer: If you think them wrong, you need not think of them. You naturally do not eat anything you dislike. If that is so, the thought which you do not like, you should not think upon it. It is natural that the mind should not reflect it if you do not like it. But if unconsciously a part of your mind likes it and a part dislikes it, then a part holds the thought. Many people say, "I hate to think about it," but they think about it just the same; and they think about it more by repeating "I hate it." It is nothing: if one does not like any thought, one is the master of one's mind, so put it out. If one has no possession over one's mind, then what else can one possess? There is nothing else one can call one's own in this world. The only domain one has is one's mind. If one has no power over one's own domain, then what is one here for? The inoculating resistance must be understood in a different way, for it is what comes from the others. That is the thing one must get inoculated with, and this inoculation is tolerance to forgive, to endure; that is inoculating. One meets with a thousand experiences a day when one lives in the world. One must either oppose experiences or assimilate them, or one must become ill. Either one or the other. When the conditions are inharmonious, attack you from all around, and there is no other way to escape, then inject yourself. Be able to tolerate it, able to assimilate it, to meet it, to face it, and in this way to be done with it.

Question: *Do you think it wrong to allow a person to die if suffering from a hopeless disease?*

Answer: I would not advise a doctor or a relation or anyone to kill that person who was suffering very much with disease in order to save the person from pain. For nature is wise, and every moment that one passes on this physical plane has its purpose. We human beings are too limited to judge and to decide for ourselves to put an end to a person's life who is suffering. Yes, we must try to make less suffering for that person, do everything in our power to make this person feel better. Of course that artificial means of keeping a person alive for hours or days is not the right thing to do, for that is going against nature's wisdom and against its divine plan. It is as bad as killing a person; the tendency is that we always go further than we ought to, and that is where we make a mistake.

HEALTH 2

The disorder in the tone of the body and irregularity in the rhythm are the principal causes of every illness. This disorder of tone may be explained thus, that there is a certain tone that the breath is vibrating throughout the body, through every channel of the body, and this tone is a particular tone continually vibrating in every person. And when the mystics have said that every person has a note, it is not necessarily the note of the piano; it is the note which is going on as a tone, as a breath. Now, if one does not take care of oneself and allows oneself to be influenced by every wind that blows, like the water in the sea, one goes up and down, disturbed by the air. One who is susceptible to rejoicing in a moment and to becoming depressed in a moment, changes one's moods. One cannot keep that tone which gives equilibrium and which is the secret of health.

How few know that it is not pleasures and merrymaking that give one good health. In the club life, as it is known today, there is dinner and merrymaking one day and ten days of being ill, for people do not take care of their equilibrium.

Besides, for a person who becomes sensitive to every little thing that comes along, it changes the rhythm of that tone, the note of that tone. It becomes a different note to which one's body is not accustomed, and that causes all illness. Too much despair or too much joy—everything that is too much—must be avoided. There are natures who always seek extremity: they must have a joy and amusement, so much that they are tired of

9

it; or then they must have a collapse with sorrow and despair. And it is among these people that you will find an illness always continues. But besides this, if an instrument is not kept in a proper tune, if it is knocked by everyone who comes and handled by everyone, then the instrument goes out of order. The body is an instrument, the most sacred instrument, an instrument which God has made for God's own divine purpose. If it is kept in tune, the strings not allowed to come loose, then this instrument becomes the means for that harmony for which God created humanity.

How must this instrument be kept in tune? In the first place, the strings of gut or the wires of steel both require cleaning. The lungs and veins of the body also require cleaning; it is that which keeps them ready for their work. And how to clean them? By carefulness in diet, by sobriety, and by breathing correctly, because it is not only the water and earth which are used for cleansing. The best means of cleansing is the air and the property which is in the air, the property which we breathe in; and if we knew how, by the help of breath, to keep these channels clean, then this secures health. It is this which maintains the tone, the proper note of each person without being disturbed. When one is vibrating one's own note, which is according to one's particular evolution, then one is oneself. Then one is tuned to the pitch for which one is made, the pitch where one ought to be, and one naturally feels comfortable.

And now, coming to the rhythm: There is a rhythm of pulsation, the beating of the pulse in the head and in the heart. And whenever the rhythm of this beating is disturbed, it causes all illness because it disturbs the whole mechanism which is going on, the order of which depends upon the regularity of rhythm. If a person suddenly hears of something fearful, the rhythm is broken. If a person is hurt by having heard something which disturbs, the rhythm is broken, the pulsation changes. Every shock given to one breaks one's rhythm. One very often notices that however successful an operation, it leaves a mark even for the whole life. Once the rhythm is broken, it is most difficult to get it aright. Gentleness which is taught morally is one thing, but gentleness in action and movement is also necessary. In every move one makes, every step one takes, there must be rhythm. For instance, you will find many examples, if you will look for them, of the odd movements a person makes, and that person can never keep well because the rhythm is not right. That is why illness continues. Maybe there is no illness that one can trace in that person, and yet the very fact of the movements not being in rhythm will keep that person out of order. Regularity in habits, in action, in repose, in eating, in drinking, in sitting, in walking—in everything—gives one that rhythm which is necessary and which completes the music of life. Someone asked Babur, the Mughal emperor who ruled for a hundred years, what was the secret of his long life in the midst of the turmoil that he lived in. And he said, "Regularity of life."

And when we come to the mental part of our being, that mechanism is still more delicate than our body. There is a tone also, and every being has a different tone according to that being's particular evolution, and everyone feels in a good health when one's own tone is vibrating. But if that tone does not come to its proper pitch, then a person feels lack of comfort, with all illness arising from it. Every expression of passion, joy, anger, fear which breaks the continuity of this tone interferes with one's health. Behind the thought there is feeling, and it is the feeling which sustains that tone; the thought is on the surface. The mystics work especially at keeping the continuity of that tone.

There used to be a custom in ancient times that, instead of using an organ in churches, they used to keep one tone: four or five persons together, with their lips closed, all of them humming that one tone. This custom still exists in some places. I was most impressed by it to hear it again, after having come from India, when I heard it in Russia in a church. The secret of keeping that continual ringing of the bell, that the churches

11

did at all times. And even now it exists. It was not only a bell to call people, it was to tune them up to their tone. It was to suggest that there is one tone going on in you; get yourself tuned to it. And if that tuning is not done, and a person has gotten the better of an illness, still weakness remains. External cure is no cure if mentally a person is not cured. If one's spirit is not cured, the mark of illness remains there. And the rhythm of mind is broken when the mind is going at a speed which is faster or at a speed which is slower than it ought to be. A person who goes on thinking one thought after another thought, and so goes on thinking a thousand things in one minute, however intelligent, cannot be normal.

A person who holds on to one thought and lingers there instead of making any progress, also clings to depressions, fears, disappointments, and that makes the person ill. I do not mean to say that the rhythm of the mind of every person must be like the mind of another person. No, each one's rhythm is peculiar to oneself. But if one can sustain the proper rhythm of one's mind, that is sufficient to keep oneself really healthy. Mental illnesses are more subtle than physical illnesses, though till now mental illnesses have not been thoroughly discovered. And when a thorough discovery will be made of mental illnesses, we shall find that all external illnesses have some connection with them.

The mind and body both stand face-to-face. The body reflects the order and disorder of the mind, the mind reflecting at the same time the harmony and inharmony of the body. Therefore if the body is ill, there is some part of that illness that reflects upon the mind. If the mind is ill, there is something of it that reflects upon the body. And this is the reason that you will find many who are ill outwardly also have some illness of mind. Does it not show us that the human being is music, that life is music, that this whole creation is a symphony, that this whole universe is music?

In order to play our part best, the only thing we can do is to keep our tone and rhythm in a proper condition, in which is the fulfillment of our life's purpose.

* * *

Question: *How to bring back the rhythm if it is once lost?*

Answer: It must be brought back with great wisdom, because a sudden effort to gain the rhythm may make one lose it worse. If the rhythm is gone too low or too fast, by trying to bring it to its regular condition, one may break the rhythm, and by breaking the rhythm one may break oneself. This is a gradual process; it must be wisely done. If the rhythm has gone too fast, it must be brought gradually to its proper condition. If it is too slow, it must be gradually increased to its proper speed. It requires patience and strength to do it. For instance, someone who tunes a violin wisely does not at once move the peg and bring it to the tone, because in the first place it is impossible and always risks breaking the string; and however minute may be the difference in the tone, one can bring it to its proper place by careful tuning, by which effort is spared and the thing is accomplished to perfection.

Question: *Must church bells strike some special note in order to create the desired effect? Why are old bells more impressive?*

Answer: It is not necessary that the church bells should strike a special note, and if they did only a mystic would know which note will be harmonious to all people. Nevertheless, everyone who hears the church bells is responsive. One forgets one's note and attaches one's soul to that note with all others, and in that way one can receive through that bell a universal harmony and can tune oneself with it. But as I always say, the blessed one will receive blessings in all things. Those who are not ready close themselves off from that blessing, wherever it may be.

Question: *Why are old bells more impressive?*

Answer: They tell us the old tale.

Question: *Can a mother help her suffering baby to find back its tone and rhythm by her thought of love?*

Answer: Certainly, the healing that a mother gives, very often unconsciously, to the child, the physician cannot give in a thousand years. The song she sings, however much inefficient, it comes from the profound depth of her being. It brings with it the healing power; it tunes the child in a moment. The caressing, the petting of the mother does more good than a medicine to the child. When it is out of harmony, when its rhythm is disturbed, when the tone is not in its proper place, the child feels more than a grown-up person. The mother, even without knowing, instinctually feels like petting the child when it feels out of rhythm, singing to the child when it feels out of tone.

Question: *How is one to find out which is one's proper tone and rhythm, physically and mentally?*

Answer: In answer to this I happened to think of an amusing instance when a friend accompanying me, with all his pleasure and kindness to accompany me, felt a great discomfort at times because he could not walk as slow as I did. Being simple and frank he expressed it to me. I saw it too. But in answer to it, I said, "It is a majestic walk." The reason was that his rhythm was different. He cannot feel comfortable in some other rhythm. He must be trotting along in order to feel comfortable. And so one can feel the tone and rhythm in oneself. One can feel what gives one a comfort and what gives one a discomfort in everything one does. If one does not feel it, that shows that one does not give attention to it. The wisdom is to understand oneself.

Question: *How can one control the heart that beats too violently, causing constant interruptions in rhythm through fear, shyness, anxiety?*

Answer: It comes by a kind of abnormal condition. It is not a normal condition. Normal condition is to be able to stand firm through fear, joy, and anxiety; not to let every wind blow one hither and thither like a scrap of paper, but to endure it all and to stand firm and steady through all such influences. One might say that: Is not water subject to the rock? I will say in answer to this, "A human being is made to be neither water nor a rock. A human being has all within." A human being is the fruit of the whole creation; one ought to be able to show one's evolution in one's balance.

Question: *How is it that often when people are out of their minds, their physical health is perfect? Is there any general cause for mental disorder causing great suffering?*

Answer: Very seldom you will find a case where a person is mentally ill and physically perfectly well. Such a person may be seemingly well. Once I happened to go to see the insane asylum in New York, and the physicians very kindly brought before me the different skulls showing how the different cavities in the brain, in the spots of decay, have caused that insanity, and the life of the person. This gives an answer to this question. There is always on the physical body a sign of it. It may be an apparent suffering, something at the back of it, yet not known. I asked him, "I would like to know if this cavity has brought about insanity, or if insanity has brought about the cavity?" His idea was that this cavity has brought about insanity. It is not always that the mental brings a physical illness. Sometimes, from a physical body, the illness goes to the mental plane. Sometimes, from mental plane, it goes to the physical body.

Question: *Is there any general mental cause?*

Answer: There are many causes, but if there is a general cause, it is the lack of that music which we call order.

HEALTH 3

Movement is life, and stillness is death. For in movement there is the significance of life, and in stillness we see the sign of death. One might ask from a metaphysical point of view if there is such a thing as stillness. I will answer no. But what we call movement is perceptible to us in some form, whether it is visible or audible or in the form of sensation or vibration; the movement which is not perceptible to us we name stillness. The word *life* we only use in connection with that perceptible existence, the movement of which we perceive. Therefore, with regard to our physical health, movement is the principal thing: the regularity of movement, of its rhythm, in pulsation and in the circulation of the blood—all. All death and decay can be traced in the lack of movement. All different aspects of diseases are to be traced in congestion; every decay is caused by congestion, and congestion is caused by the lack of movement.

There are parts of the body where the veins, the nerves, are stuck to the skin and there is no free circulation. There arise all diseases. Outward diseases of that manner we call skin diseases; when it works inwardly it manifests in the form of certain pain. A physician may bring to us a thousand different reasons as the causes of different diseases, but this is the one and central cause of each disease, and of all diseases: lack of movement; in other words, the lack of life.

This mechanism of the body is made to work according to a certain rhythm and is maintained by a perpetual rhythmic movement. The center of that perpetual current of life is the breath. The different remedies that humanity has found in all ages often brought an immediate cure to the sufferers. But they are not always cured, for the cause of the disease remains unexplored. At the back of every illness the cause is some irregular, unnatural living in the way of food or drink or action or repose.

If I were to define death, it is a change that comes by the inability of the body to hold what we call the soul. The body has a certain amount of magnetism, and that is the sign of its perfect running order. When, owing to the illness, whether suddenly or gradually, the body has lost that magnetism by the power of which it holds the soul, it, so to speak, helplessly loses its grip upon something that it was holding; and this losing of the grip is known by us as death. Generally it is a gradual process. A little pain, a little illness, a little discomfort first manifest. One does not take note of it, which in time grows to become an illness. Very often diseases are maintained by the patients, not knowing that they are maintaining them just by their ignorance of their condition, by their neglect of themselves. There are a larger number of patients who leave their condition to be studied by the doctor; they do not know what is the matter with them from the beginning to the end of illness. As in ancient times the simple believers trusted the priest to send them to heaven or to the other plane, so today patients give themselves into the hands of the doctor. Can anyone with a keen observation imagine that there is anyone besides oneself who is capable of knowing as much as one can know about one's own self if one did wish to know about oneself? Is it a fault? No, it is the habit. It is a kind of neglect of oneself that one does not think about one's own condition and wants the physician to say what is the matter. The pain is in oneself.

One can be the best judge of one's own life; it is the self who can find out the cause of an illness because the self knows its life best. Numberless souls today live in this way: ignorant of their own condition of life, dependent upon someone who has studied science outwardly. Even the physician cannot properly help if one does not know one's own condition clearly. It is that clear knowledge of the complaint that enables one to give the physician a correct idea. In the cloth where there is a little hole, if one does not see to it, it will tear easily and become a larger hole; so it is with health. If there is something a little wrong with it, we neglect it, absorbed in the life as we are; and so it is allowed to become worse every day, nearing thereby the death which could have been avoided otherwise. The question is, "But is it necessary that we must think of our body and our condition of health?" Yes, so long as we do not become obsessed by ourselves. If one thinks about one's health so much that one becomes obsessed by it, it is certainly wrong, because it is not helping, it is working against one. If one pities oneself and says, "Oh, how ill I am, and how terrible it is, and if only I should be well," then the impression becomes a kind of fuel to the fire. That person is continually adding, feeding the illness by the thought of it. But on the other hand, if one became so neglectful of oneself that one says, "Oh, it does not matter; it is, after all, an illusion," that person will not be able to keep that thought. Then the pain will increase.

It is as necessary to take care of oneself as it is necessary to forget about one's illness. For an illness comes to a person hiding, as a thief enters the house quietly, works without the knowledge of the dwellers in it and robs them of their best treasures. If one keeps a guard against it, it is not a wrong thing as long as one does not contemplate upon one's illness. One might ask, "Is it worthwhile to live long? Why must we all not end life? What is it after all?" But this is an abnormal thought. A person with a normal body and mind will not think in this way. When this abnormal thought grows it culminates in insanity, which brings many people to suicide. The natural tendency of every soul is to desire to live a life of perfect health, to make the best of its coming into the world. Neither God nor the soul is pleased with the desire for death, for death does not belong to the soul. It is a kind of agitation, a revolt that comes in the mind of someone who then says, "I prefer death to life." To have a desire to live and yet to live a life of suffering is also not a wise thing. And if wisdom is anything, one must spare no effort to come to the proper condition of health.

HEALTH 4

In ancient times people attributed to every illness a spirit of illness as its cause. There was a spirit known for every kind of illness, and they believed that particular spirit brought that illness. The healers made attempts to cure every patient that came with that illness, and they were successful in making the patient well. Today that spirit of illness has come to a material manifestation, when the physicians now declare that every illness has a germ or a microbe. Every day a new invention brings to their eyes a new microbe, and if every day a new microbe were discovered till the end of the world, numberless microbes would be discovered and numberless diseases.

In the end it will be very difficult to find one healthy person, for there must be some microbe—even if it is not of a recognized disease—of a disease which is not yet discovered. If it is a world of innumerable lives, it will always show innumerable lives. Each life having its purpose, constructive or destructive, will show that purpose even in a microbe. And so this discovery of microbes of diseases will go on with the increase of diseases, for to prevent microbes from existing is not always in the power of human beings. Sometimes they will destroy the microbes, but in turn they will find that each microbe destroyed will, in turn, produce many more microbes.

What is life? Every atom of it is living; call it radium or electron or atom or germ or microbe. The people of old thought that they were spirits, living beings, in the absence of the tools which today distinguish these spirits in the form of microbes. And yet it seems that the ancient healers had a greater grip upon the illness, for the reason that they did not see the outer microbe only, but the microbe in its spirit. In destroying the microbe they did not only destroy the outer microbe but the inner microbe, in the form of the spirit of the germ. And the most interesting thing is that in order to drive away that spirit which they thought had possessed the patient, they burned or they placed before them certain chemicals, which even now can prove to be destructive of the germs of diseases.

Now we come to the idea that, with every measure that physicians will take to prevent the germs of diseases from coming, in spite of all the success they will have, there will be greater failures. For even if the germ is destroyed, it exists; its family exists somewhere. Besides, the body which has once become the abode of that particular germ has become a receptacle of the same germ. If the physician will destroy the germ of disease from the body of an individual, that does not mean that the physician will destroy it from the universe. This problem, therefore, must be looked at from another point of view: that everything that exists in the objective world has its living and more important part existing in the subjective, and that part which is in the subjective is held by the belief of the patient.

As long as patients believe that they are ill, they are giving sustenance to that part of the disease which is in the subjective. If not only once but even a thousand times, the germs of the diseases were destroyed from a patient's body, these will be created in the subjective sphere, because the same source from where the germs spring is in one's belief, not in one's body, as the source of the whole creation is within, not without. The outer treatment of several of such diseases is just like cutting the plant from its stem; the root remains there in the ground. The root of every illness, being in the subjective part of one's being, in order to drive away that illness, one must dig out the root by taking away the belief in illness even before the outer germ was destroyed. The germ of illness cannot exist without the force, the breath, which it receives from the subjective part of one's being. And if the source of its sustenance was once destroyed, then the cure is sure.

Very few can hold a thought, but many are held by a thought. If such a simple thing as holding a thought were mastered, the whole life would be mastered. When once a person gets into the head that "I am ill," and when it is confirmed by a physician, then the belief becomes watered like a plant. Then the person's continual reflection of it, falling upon the illness like the sun, makes the plant of illness grow. And therefore it would not be an exaggeration if one might say that, consciously or unconsciously, the patient is the gardener of the patient's own illness.

Now, the question is: Is it, then, a right thing not to trouble about microbes? If a physician has found it, and shows it to us, must we not believe it? You cannot help believing it if you have gone so far as to let the physician show it to you. You have helped the physician to believe it. And now you must believe, you cannot help believing something which has been shown to you, which is before you.

Of course, if you rise above this, then you have touched the truth. For when you rise above facts, you touch reality. One might ask, is it not deluding oneself to deny facts? It is no more deluding than one is already deluded. Facts themselves are delusions. It is the rising above this illusion that enables one to touch reality. As long as the brain is muddled with fact, it will be more absorbed every day in the puzzle of life, making life far more confused than ever before. It is therefore that the Master has taught, "Seek ye the kingdom of God first."[1] That itself means to rise above facts first, and with the light that you gain from there, throwing it upon facts, you will see the facts in a clear light. By this it is not meant at all that you should close your eyes to facts. It is only meant to look up first, and when

---

1 Matthew 6:33.

your eyes are once charged with divine light, then when you cast your glance, your eyes, on the world of fact, you will have a more and more clear vision, the vision of reality. There is no lack of honesty if you deny the fact of illness. It is no hypocrisy if you deny it to yourself first; it is only a help. For there are many things in life which exist, being sustained by your acknowledging their existence. Fear, confusion, depression, pain, even your success and failure, these all are sustained by your acknowledging their existence. Deluded by the outwardly appearing facts, one holds them in thought as a belief. But by denying them, one roots them out; and they cannot exist, starved by the sustenance for which they depended upon you.

* * *

Question: *How to equilibrate inner and outer power?*

Answer: By balance.

Question: *Have not the great prophets, in spite of their great God-realization, been limited in the power they had at their command?*

Answer: The life of the prophets is not to be envied. Though their realization was of God, their life was to be among the crowd. It is being in the world which does not belong to them, a world of limitations with the thought of perfection. Therefore, although in many things they showed perfection, still the limitation has always been there. The very fact that they had to live in the midst of the world, in the midst of people, made them limited; it could not be otherwise.

Question: *Please explain closely the difference between this merging in God as a conscious force and the medium?*

Answer: In the first place it starts as the medium. The sunglass[2] shows the quality of sun, although it is not sun. It is exposed to the sun, yet begins to show the quality of sun. It partakes in itself

---

2 A sunglass is a convex lens.

of the sun, whereas other objects do not partake of the sun as the glass does. So it is with the souls who focus their heart to God: then God becomes reflected in their heart. And the beauty and power which is to be found in God as perfection, that beauty and power begins to show among the souls who partake of it, just like the sunglass does with the sun, and they express it in their lives. There is a term used among Sufis: *akhlaq Allah*, which means "the divine manner." Divine manner is not refinement nor politeness, nor a put-up manner of pleasing persons. It is a divine impulse which expresses itself in the form of a manner which not only wins the friend, but impresses even the foe. Are there not in this world people of good manner? Many. But this outward refinement in the end proves to be empty. But the manner of the great souls such as Buddha and Krishna, Moses and Muhammad, and a great many other souls who have shone in their times, has not only won the persons before whom it was shown, it has left its impression for centuries to come. A manner which has won the whole universe, so to speak, that is God's manner expressed through a human being. One cannot teach this manner, but it comes when the heart is focused to God. Not only manner but inspiration, power, all that is in God becomes manifested through a human being. Then a human being is not a superman. That is a small word for such a person. That person is the God-realized one.

Question: *Does not this question mean the complete recognition of the God within?*

Answer: Certainly. But when this realization comes, then there is no more God within. There is God within and without. As soon as God is realized, then God does not remain within. It is before realization that God within is found, and it is God within which will help to find the perfect God. But once God is realized, God is within and without, in all.

Question: *What have we to do when we begin to feel ill?*

Answer: This is a very nice question, because you may not lose time. That is the time, as I say, to pull oneself together, because illness is falling, falling into pieces, and against it must be the different action to pull oneself together.

Question: *Where is the role of the microbes limited?*

Answer: We realize that there is one life, then there are forces, there are influences which are working toward destruction. There are other influences which are working toward construction. Influences which are working toward destruction have manifested in all form towards destruction, as the animals with poison, as the human being with revenge, spite, and bitterness, with destructive thoughts and tendencies. Do we not see among human beings the desire to hurt or harm another, and the delight in it? For them it is a game, it is their play; they are not wakened to the feeling of doing harm to another. It is just for them an amusement, a pastime, a trying of their power. So if among human beings who have now come to the point of God-evolution, if a destructive element exists among the majority, then it is natural among germs and worms. They must be the destructive element which comes in some form or other. With all this destruction and destructive activity, if there is anything a person can do, it is to do the reverse of it, contrary to it. That is the only way of going above destruction and causing less destruction. But if one saw that this is destructive and answered it with destruction, that would be worse and worse. There would be no end to it. If one follows the theory of "tooth"[3] it could continue forever till both have no teeth left in their mouths. If there is a destruction on one side, there must be on the other side compassion. That is the only way of going above it. But very often people think, "Is it not a weakness?" Yes, apparently, but it is a strength just the same. But if your compassion has made you so weak that you are eaten up? I will answer, "Can compassion be eaten away? Is it such a small

_____
3 "An eye for an eye, and a tooth for a tooth." See Matthew 5:38–42.

thing that it can be eaten up?" The good has a greater power than evil. Compassion is more powerful than revenge. Even an apparent loss will prove to be a gain in the end. If a dreadful dragon has swallowed a pill of compassion, do you think the pill is lost? No, it will turn the dragon into compassion.

HEALTH 5

I do not mean to say that the fact of germs should altogether be ignored, for it is not possible to ignore something which you see. Besides, I do not mean to say that the discovery of microbes has not been of some use for the physician to attend to the patient better. But at the same time, one can be too sensitive. One can exaggerate the idea of germs to more than what really exists. But there is one person who is susceptible to taking these germs and being their victim, and there is another person who assimilates these germs and, by this assimilation, destroys them. In other words, one is destroyed by germs, and one destroys germs. Then the key must be found, the key to rising above the susceptibility of being given to germs.

It is not only germs but the climate. Has weather not an effect upon a person, more or less? One is more susceptible to it, another is less susceptible to it. And the one who is more susceptible to it is not necessarily delicately weak. Very often a person may be bodily strong and yet most conscientious about exposure to the weather. I have seen singers who take the most care of their throat everyday get a cold on the day of their concert by fearing the effect of weather, by being too conscientious about it. They unconsciously cultivate in themselves the idea of its effect. They say contagious diseases are taken by taking the microbes from one person to another. In breath, in air, in everything, they fly and they go from one person to another.

But it is not always the microbes; it is very often the impression. When a person has seen a friend having caught cold and thought, "I fear I will catch it," certainly that person has got it; by being afraid and impressed by it, the person has caught it.

It is not always necessary that the germs of a cold have gone from one person to another by the way of breath. The impression that a person has taken can create the cold. For behind the whole creation there is thought power. We often see that the more one is afraid of a thing, the more one is pursued by it, for unconsciously one concentrates upon it. There are germs and impurities, but then there are elements to purify them. These five elements—earth, water, fire, air, and ether, as spoken of by the mystics—do not only compose germs but also destroy them, if one only knows how to make use of these five elements in order to purify one's body with them and also one's mind. As there is the need of sun and water for the plants to grow, so there is need of the five elements for the person to keep in perfect health. These five elements one breathes according to one's capacity of breath. But by breath every person does not attract the same properties, for everyone attracts from the breath elements according to one's particular constitution. One attracts more fire element in the breath, another one attracts the water element more, another one attracts the earth element more. Sometimes one receives an element which one does not require.

Besides, the sun currents have the greatest healing power, more than anything else. A person who can breathe well, who knows how to breathe perfectly, who can attract sun currents in the body, can keep the body pure from every kind of influence. No microbes of destruction can exist if the sun currents can touch every part of the body which is within, and that is done by the breath. The Sufis in the East have shown this in their lives, living a long and perfectly healthy life. Emperor Babur, with his responsibilities and being an emperor at a difficult time, was able to live more than a hundred years. It is natural that the parts of the earth which are hidden from the sun—which are not touched by the air—became damp, and there several little lives are created; and the germs of destruction are born there, the air in that place becomes dense. If that is true, then the body needs it too. The body needs the sun and the air. Every particle within the lungs and intestines and veins and tubes of the body all need the sun and the air, and it is taken in by the perfect way of breathing. And the benefit of this is even derived by the mind, for even the mind is composed of five elements, the elements in their most fine condition. Rest and repose, as well as action and movement must have a certain balance and certain rhythm. If there is no balance between activity and repose, then health is also not secure. Our great mistake is that with every little complaint the first thing we think of is the doctor. We never stop to think, "What has been the cause in myself? Have I been too active? Too lazy? Have I not been careful about my diet, about my sleep? Have I not breathed in all the elements which are necessary to keep this mechanism of body and mind going?"

Frightened by every illness, we first turn to the doctor. As long as the illness has not appeared before us, we do not mind if it is growing inwardly in us, without our having noticed it. It may continue to grow for a long time, for years. Absorbed in our outward activities, we never think that we are giving a home to our worst adversary in our body. Therefore, very often illness is caused by negligence. Then there are others who become too careful; they think of nothing else except of their illness. That is the first question before them, "How shall I be well?" Pondering upon the illness, they give a kind of fuel to that fire of illness from their thought, keeping it burning without knowing that it is by their unconscious effort the illness is kept alive. In order to keep health in perfect order, one must keep a balance between body and mind, between action and repose, and it is the psychological outlook on one's health which helps more than any medicines.

I remember an instance when I was seeing a patient who was suffering from an illness for more than twenty years and had lost every hope of getting better. Several physicians had been consulted; many different treatments had been experienced. I told this patient a simple thing to do. I did not teach any special practices, but just an ordinary little thing to do in the morning and in the evening. And to the great surprise of those at home, this patient began to move her hands and legs, which was first thought to be impossible, and it gave them great hope that someone who had always been in bed could do this. And to the patient it was such a great surprise. I went to see them after a few days and I asked those around the patient, "How is the patient progressing?" They said, "The patient is progressing very well. We could have never thought that this person could move her hands and legs. That is the most wonderful thing, but we cannot make this patient believe now, after twenty years' suffering, that she could ever be well. This illness has become such an impression upon her that she thinks that this is a natural thing for her, and that to be well is a dream—it is an unreality." This gave me the idea that when a person lives in a certain condition, after a long, long time that condition becomes a friend, unconsciously. One does not know it. One may think that one wants to get out of it, yet there is some part of one's being that is holding it in one's hand. Even if outwardly one says that one does not want to be ill, unconsciously one is holding the illness just the same.

One day, in order to see a peculiarity of human nature, I asked a person who was brought to me to be cured of an obsession how long this obsession had been. That person explained to me how horrible the obsession was, how terrible life was. I heard for half an hour everything that the person said against the obsession. But in order to see an amusing part of human nature, I asked this person, "You do not really mean to say that you want to get rid of this spirit? If I had this spirit I would keep it. After all these years that you have had it, it seems unjust, too cruel for this spirit. If this spirit had not cared for you, it would not be with you all these years. In this world, is it easy for a person to be so long with one? This spirit is most faithful." Then the person was saying, "I do not really want to get rid of it." I was very amused how at the back of it this person wanted sympathy and help and assistance, but did not want to give up the spirit. It was not that the spirit was obsessing this person, but that the person was obsessing the spirit.

* * *

Question: *Would you tell the students how necessary it is to understand the psychic impression of an illness?*

Answer: A psychic nature is more susceptible to gross vibrations, and especially those inclined to spiritualistic séances. Their body becomes so susceptible to any kind of nervous illnesses, also to obsessions, that they, really speaking, prepare themselves to welcome any other spirit.

HEALTH 6

As medical science has advanced during this modern time, the different diseases and complaints that one feels are more distinguished and very fine. Each such complaint has been given a certain name, and in that way, even if a person had a little complaint, after an examination by a physician that person is told the name of the complaint. The complaint may be as small as a molehill, but it is turned into a mountain. There is no greater misfortune than hearing from a doctor that one has taken on an illness which is dangerous, the name of which is frightening. What then happens? That name, being impressed in the heart, creates the same element; and in the end one sees the truth of something that was told to one by the physician.

If this is true, then the impression the words of a fortune-teller makes upon one, in many cases, makes the fortune-telling realized in the end. The fortune-teller is not always a saint, not always a clairvoyant who has seen it. The fortune-teller may be an imaginative person who has said something. And that impression has gone with the person, and yet the fortune-teller realizes in the end that it comes true. Among a hundred physicians authorized by the medical authorities in whom one immediately lays one's trust, there is hardly one who has insight into the real nature and character of a disease, and it is only after seeing a hundred patients that one can correctly say the nature and the character of the complaint. Then what a great danger there is for a person to be impressed at the beginning of an illness by a right or wrong remark made by a physician as to that illness.

Among ancient people the physicians only knew the names of diseases, but the physician was not allowed to say to the patient what the complaint was, because from a psychological point of view it would be doing wrong. For there was not only a material medical science, but there was a psychological idea attached to it.

I have seen numberless cases having come to me frightened by something that a physician has said to them. Perhaps there is nothing the matter with them, only a little illness. Perhaps they have not yet realized what it is, but they are frightened just the same. And if there is an imaginative patient, then that one has a wide scope of imagination. Everything that goes wrong is attributed to something the patient has heard from the physician. One relates every condition of one's life to that particular remark. In the life such as we live in the world, with so many things to do, so many responsibilities resting upon us at home and in the outside world, with the strife that is inflicted upon us by our life in this world, we naturally have ups and downs physically. Sometimes one is tired, sometimes one needs a rest; sometimes one must fast one day, there is no inclination for food. If one attributes all these little things to an illness that a physician has once said, then one is certainly making one's illness stronger. For the root of illness is in the mind, and when that illness is watered all the time by that feeling and thought, then illness is realized in the end.

Now when thinking of the surgical world, there is no doubt that wonderful operations are being done, and humanity has experienced great help by surgical operations. And yet it is still experimental, and it will perhaps take one century more or longer for surgery to mature. It is in its infancy just now. No doubt, the first impulse of a surgeon is to look at a case and only look from that one point of view, and that is how that person can be cured by surgery. The surgeon has no other thought in mind. The surgeon has not the spare time to think that there is another possibility. A wise surgeon gives you confidence, yet knows that it is an experiment. It is a person, it is not wood or a stone that can be carved and engraved upon. It is a person with feeling, it is a soul which is experiencing life through its every atom, a soul which is not made for a knife. Now a person has to go through this experience, fearing death, preferring life to death. Very often what happens is that what was considered wrong before operation is thought right after the operation. Of course, some wrong is to be proved because an operation has been performed. And it is not something that is finished, but it is something which has its action upon nerves and then upon the human spirit, and then its reaction upon life again. Do we not see that after one operation a person's whole life has become impressed with it? A certain strain on nerves, a certain upset in the spirit has been caused. The care of the surgeon continues only till the patient is apparently well, outwardly well. But what about the aftereffect of it on the spirit of the person, on the mind of the person, and its reaction on the person's life? The surgeon does not know it, is not concerned with it. Cure means absolute cure, within and without. By this I do not mean to say that surgery has no place. I say it is a most important part of medical work, but at the same time it must be avoided when it can be avoided. One must not readily jump into it. A young person with strength and energy thinks, "What is it? I can go through it." But once done, there remains an impression for the whole life.

Humanity is given intuition as its heritage, and it is intuition which is the bottom of every science. At this time when science is taken as a book study, it takes away that part that intuition must perform. If in the medical world there was an intuitive development introduced, I am sure if many physicians were occupied in finding remedies that can avoid operation, a very great work could be accomplished. It is amusing that once the operation of appendicitis began to be known in the United

States, it was a fashion among rich people to have that operation, because of a few days at home. And then the physicians
began to choose the appendicitis patients among those who
have the means to stay at home for some time. It was the fashion. One asked, "Did you have it?" "Yes, I have had it." It was
a kind of duel playing out; then one has to say, "I have gone
through it."

And now, coming to the use of drugs, any physicians, after a lifelong experience, will find out that at some time they
had prescribed drugs and yet, whatever the result they had got
of curing for that time, it was not done right. The aftereffect
of drugs is sometimes so depleting, and what it creates in the
brain and the mind so confusing, that it ruins a person's life. I
have seen many persons after medical treatment. Their illness,
once accustomed to drugs, has made the body a kind of receptacle for drugs: the body lives upon drugs and cannot live
without them. In order to digest their food they must have
something, in order to sleep they must have something, in order to feel cheerful they must take some drug. Now, as these
natural things such as digesting one's food, such as feeling joyful or cheerful, such as sleep, which are natural blessings—if
these blessings depend upon outer, material things, then how
can that person be called healthy? In order to make the best of
today they take it, and then tomorrow it becomes worse.

When one considers that the human body is an instrument
which God created for God's own experience, then what a mistake it must be to allow this body, by drugs and medicines,
to become unfit for the use of divine spirit. I do not mean by
this that medicine is not necessary; medicine has its place, even
drugs are needed when there is that necessity. But when for every little thing that can be cured by some other means, a drug is
given, then in the end health goes out of one's hands, and even
drugs cannot give a person rest. The best medicine is a pure
diet, nourishing food, fresh air, regularity in action and repose,
cleanness of thought, pureness of feeling, and confidence in the

perfect being with whom we are linked and whose expression we are. That is the essence of health. The more one realizes this, the more secure will be one's health.

* * *

Question: *I asked a modern operator what the reaction of X-rays is upon the patient three or four years afterwards. He said we do not know. We only know the immediate result. Even that is in its infancy.*

Answer: There is a case. Once a person came to me with a complaint about kidneys, and the doctors had warned this person that if the operation did not take place in one week's time, then they were not sure about the life of this person. They had given up hope for the life of this person. This person was told by everyone who cared for her, her relatives and friends, that she must have an operation. But I did not advise it. I said it must be avoided if it can be avoided. And this person now was going to the clinic for the operation, reading *The Rose Garden* on the way, and she read in *The Rose Garden* the address on faith.[1] This person said, "I am not going to the clinic, I have changed my mind, I am going to Murshid." And this person, instead of going to the clinic, came to see me in Switzerland. I also told this person to have another X-ray examination, to see what they say about this examination. Now what opinion will these others form? The same opinion or something else? However, whether the opinions came together I do not know, but I have doubts. But the result was that this person did not go for the operation, and the result was a marvelous cure.

I know another person whom a physician had examined and said the person must die within three months. If that person was impressionable, he would have taken that impression. But he came before me and said, "What nonsense! Die in three months—I am not going to die in three hundred years!" And to our great surprise the doctor died within three months and

---

1 *The Rose Garden* (*Gulistan*) by the Persian poet Sa'di.

this man brought us the news. He was quite unaware of his own death. The whole thing is that what we must learn is to respect the human being, that a human being is beyond birth and death, that a human being has a divine spirit within, that all illnesses and pains and sufferings are only trials and tests. We are above them, and we must try to raise ourselves above illnesses.

Question: *When matter is the outcome of vibration, how have we to think about vibration in modern science? Is the idea of vibration being taken as a certain movement of particles of matter?*

Answer: Yes, but what causes the certain movement of matter, of a vibration, is felt by us. Vibration is realized by our sense in this form, a certain movement of the particles of matter. But vibration itself is a movement. It is therefore that the power of the word is sometimes greater than any medicine or any other treatment or operation, because the words cause certain vibrations in one's own being, in the atmosphere, in one's environment, bringing about thereby a cure which nothing else can bring about. When we see a healthy person and a person suffering by some illness, and we take the condition of their pulsation and of the circulation of the blood, we shall find that behind it all, there is a movement, there is a vibration which is going on. In one person in its proper condition, there is health. In the other person the vibration is not in its right condition, therefore there is illness. It is a physician in America who happened to think of it, only the difficulty is that when a scientist thinks of such a thing, even if it comes by intuition, the scientist pursues it by going from the bottom of the mountain to the top. And it is very difficult to climb the mountain; and very often, before the scientist climbs the mountain, the scientist's life has ended. I have now heard that physician is dead. His was a very good idea, although he had not yet come to the secret of it. Yet, as an idea it inspired many physicians in the United States and in the world, and it created a great excitement in the medical world. But as the mystics say, "Seek ye the kingdom of God first and all will be added."[2] That is another way. That is not going from the bottom to the top, which is so difficult; it is climbing. It is reaching the top first, and then all is easy. For the one who is on the top of the mountain, it is easy to move anywhere one likes from the top. It does not take that energy, it does not weigh one down. Avicenna, the great physician of ancient times, on whose discoveries medical science was based, was a Sufi who used to sit in meditation, and through intuition he used to give his prescription. Just now a physician in England has discovered the great treasure that this man has given to medical science, and he is now writing a book to interpret, in modern language, the ideas of Avicenna.[3]

Question: *How do you explain the cure by faith in certain cases?*

Answer: Cure by faith in all cases, certain cases, or whatever may be the nature or character of any case, is the first thing. No treatment or anything can bring a better result if faith was lacking. Faith is the first remedy, all else comes afterward.

Question: *Remedies are to be given, but faith is not to be given to a person.*

Answer: That is why faith is so sacred. It cannot be given; it must be discovered within oneself. But there is no one in the world without faith, only it is covered for a time being. What covers it? It is a kind of pessimistic attitude towards life. There are people who are pessimistic outwardly, there are others who are pessimistic unconsciously; they themselves do not know that they are pessimistic. One can fight with the whole world, but cannot fight with one's own doubts. And the one who can break the clouds of doubts has accomplished everything in the world.

---

2 Matthew 6:33.
3 Inayat Khan refers here to the work of Dr. Otto C. Gruner, whose commentary on Avicenna was published in 1930.

HEALTH 7

Most of the cases of physical and mental illnesses come from the exhaustion of nerves. Not everyone knows to what extent to use nerve force in everyday life and to what extent to control it. Very often a good person, a kind, loving, affectionate person, gives out energy at every call from every side and so, continually giving energy, in the end finds the nerves troubled and weakened. In the end the same person who was once kind and nice and polite cannot keep up that niceness, because when the funds of energy are expired, then there is no control. There is no power of endurance. There is no patience to take things easily. Then one becomes irritated and troublesome and tired and disgusted with things—the same person who has once proven to be good and kind. Very often it may be called abuse of goodness, for it is not always giving out that answers the demands of everyday life. It is the balanced condition of one's body and mind which answers the demands of life to satisfaction.

And sometimes it becomes a passion for one to waste energy either in doing something or in speaking continually. And this passion can grow to such an extent that even when one has lost a great deal of energy, then also one will find satisfaction in giving out still more. In that one's presence others will feel depleted, because one who has no energy left is trying to give out what little one has, and this irritation and strain falling upon the others makes them nervous also. The weakness of nerves is not only the cause of physical diseases, but it leads to insanity.

There is one main cause of physical diseases as well as of mental diseases: overstrained nerves, exhausted nerves. And in spite of all virtues and goodness, goodwill and desire to do right, one will prove to be doing wrong, to one's own surprise, because one has lost self-discipline. One's high ideals are of no use, for one has not oneself in hand. One's qualification, knowledge, attainments, morals—they will all prove to be futile in the absence of that nervous force which keeps one fit and capable of doing all that is proper for one to do in the world.

The lack of soberness also causes the nerves' exhaustion, because all things made of alcohol and things that intoxicate consume the energy of the nerves, eat the energy of the nerves. One might ask why a person takes a delight in such things? And the answer is that it is again a passion. It is an excitement of nerves for the moment. Anything that gives an intoxication excites nerves for the moment. And one feels, so to speak, more cheerful for that moment but is dependent upon something outside. Then the reaction comes, when the effect of that intoxicant has left. Then one feels twice as weak and exhausted than before, and then needs twice the amount of drug or alcohol in order to feel as cheerful as one once felt for a few hours. And so one goes on and on until one has no power over mind or body; one becomes a slave to something one takes. That is the only time when one thinks one lives, and at other times, when it is not there, one feels miserable. That becomes one's world, one's heaven, one's paradise, one's life.

All manner of excess in passion, in anger, all manner of sensual life and rejoicing in it makes one robbed of the energy and power and vitality of nerves. Besides, every effect that is created in voice, in word, in singing, is created by the nerves' power. The whole secret of magnetism is in nerves. The sign of a person with health, physically and mentally, is that a person develops that influence which is expressed by the nerves' power, and it has its influence upon all things. Strength gives one more power; weakness causes a greater weakness. And today's system of keeping patients closed in the hospitals and in asylums is just like making them captives to the disease. The atmosphere of the place and the very thought of being in the hospital makes one feel ill. And so is the life in asylums: however efficient the treatment may be, it gives one an impression that one is out of one's mind, there is something wrong with one's mind, and the atmosphere all around suggests the same thing. Besides, it would be kinder on the part of the society, on the part of the family, if patients could be taken in hand by friends and relations in their difficult times. They can be helped much more than by putting them in places where they can think of nothing but of their illness. I have seen myself many cases which relations and friends have taken in their hands, and they have been helped much more than with the help that one receives in the hospital. One might say that modern treatments require a certain place prepared for such things, and there they have everything, besides the physician to look after them, and that is the only way in large cities that such cases can be looked after. Yes, it is true, and one cannot help where the situation is difficult; still, where someone can be helped, one must try to help.

Nervous diseases are very often treated by physicians by giving medicines. There is no medicine in the world which can do good to nerves, for nerves are the most natural part of one's being, the part of one's being which is linked with the physical world and the mental world. The nervous system is the central part of one's being, and there is no better remedy for one's nerves than nature, a life of rest and repose, quiet, proper breathing, proper nourishment, and someone to treat this patient with wisdom. It is the knowledge of psychology of human nature that is necessary, more than medical knowledge, to treat nervous patients. By understanding the law of environments and climatic influences, by understanding what influences other people make upon such a patient, one can cure the person.

* * *

Question: *Are the nerves the storehouse of vital energies or only conductors? What role do they play in the process of thinking?*

Answer: A nervous system is a kind of battery for the whole mechanism of the mind and body, for the mechanism of mind, because it is the clearness of nervous mechanism and good working of nervous mechanism which enables us to make our thought paths clear to us or to imagine or think or memorize. And when the nervous system is not clear, then one cannot keep things in memory. One cannot hold thought. One cannot concentrate. One cannot think very much. One cannot keep on one thought, and all different conditions of mental disorder begin to show. In the body, the nervous system is called centers by Yogis. The different centers are the parts of the nervous system, centers through which one experiences intuition, one feels, one observes keenly. Besides, this proper condition of nerves enables one to impress. A person nervously depleted, even if that person were in the right, cannot impress it upon another because there is no strength behind it. And so, even if one may be in the right, one will have to say, "What am I to do?" There is no power to go forward, no power to stand for one's own right.

Besides, in everything one does, acts or plays or sings or speaks, it is nervous energy that is necessary. The whole secret of success of one who is public on the stage of a concert hall is nervous power. The success of the lawyer, the barrister, is nervous power. You will always find that a good barrister who has made a name has that power, and that is a magnetism. Now, you may ask where to get it and how to get it? But our body and mind is a receptacle of that power, it is made for it. We are that power. The magnetism of a human being is much greater than anything else in the world. No flower, fruit, gem, or jewel has such magnetism as humankind has, if one knows how to retain it, how to keep oneself in that condition. Because with all the scientific discoveries of radium, electrons, and all different atoms, there is no atom in the world which is more radiant than the atoms with which the human body is composed, an atom which is not only attractive to the human eye, but it attracts the whole creation to a human being. The tigers surrender to human beings. The elephants work by human command. But when human beings lose their proper spirit, then it is just like losing the salt. As it is said in the Bible, "You are the salt of the earth, and when you have lost the salt there is nothing else to give savor to it."[1] When one's own being and spirit is more radiant than anything else, then there is nothing else that can give one more spirit, because one is the spirit. Within one is the spirit.

---

1 See Matthew 5:13.

HEALTH 8

One often wonders to what extent spirit has power over matter. And the answer is that as matter is the outcome of spirit, spirit has all the power over matter. One becomes pessimistic after having tried the power of thought to cure oneself or to cure others and failed, and then one begins to think that perhaps it is not the spirit that can help, it is something outside. I do not mean for one moment that the things outside cannot help, but I shall repeat just the same that spirit has all the power to cure a person from every malady. No doubt, in order to cure every malady the spirit must reach to that state so as to cure it perfectly. At the present age a person realizes that intelligence is born of matter. By a study of biology one begins to realize that first there was matter, and then it evolved, and then in humanity it developed and sprung up as intelligence, as human intelligence. But according to the mystic, the whole thing is a play of intelligence: in the rock, in the tree, in the plant, in the animal and human beings, intelligence has gone all along and developed itself, and through humanity it comes to its pure essence. And it is coming to the pure essence that makes us become aware of our origin.

In Christian Science they teach that matter does not exist. Even if they do not explain it fully, nevertheless there is one life, it is that one aspect that we call matter and spirit. And the motive behind it is that we must realize that there is one life, and that is all spirit. Even matter, which is a passing state, is a passing state of spirit. And spirit is intelligent, intelligence itself, besides powerful and free from death and decay. As it is free from death and decay, it is capable of giving its life even to the dense substance which has been made out of itself, and that is matter. And therefore it is beyond words to tell to what extent thought, feeling, and attitude help one to become cured.

There are many illnesses, but hopelessness is the first illness. When a person has lost hope, this illness cannot be cured. And hope is part of intelligence, hope is the strength of intelligence. If intelligence worked against all disorder, whether physical or mental or moral disorder, certainly a cure can be obtained.

The mystics have always known and practiced in a most perfect way the idea which is coming out in its most elementary way in the thought preached by Coué, that by repeating to oneself that, "I am well, I am better, I am better," one becomes better.[1] There are many who do not see the reason of it, but you will see that, as days will pass, the most material people will begin to realize the truth of it, that it is the attitude of the mind. It is the willingness to be cured, it is desire to get above an illness, it is an inclination to fight against disorder which helps one to health.

There is a difference between belief and thought. One might say, "I am thinking every day of becoming well, but that does not do me any good." The idea is that, yes, thinking is one thing, believing is another thing. When you compare belief with thinking, the one is automatic, the other is more living. And if one says, "I am thinking this," or "I am practicing this every day, but I do not get any benefit," it only means that one is practicing one thing and is believing some other thing. One is believing that "I will be well," and one is believing that "I am ill." It may be that one unconsciously believes, but there is a belief that "This does not cure me," "I shall continue to be ill." At the same time one will be repeating a thousand times a day, "I am well, I am well," but one does not believe it.

---

1 Émile Coué de la Châtaigneraie (1857–1926) used positive autosuggestion in his psychotherapy practice.

The way that mystical healers have brought about wonderful cures is beyond comprehension. What thought power can do is seen in their work. No doubt, if a person is a hindrance to healing influences then, of course, even healers cannot do their work properly. But if a person's attitude is right, if one believes that spirit has all the power to cure, certainly one can be cured. The mystics have proved in their lives that not only their power can cure, but even death stands before them as their obedient servant. Death for them is not a constable which arrests and takes a person when the time has come. Death for them is a porter that carries their baggage when traveling.

For a pessimistic person, healing apart, even medicine will not do any good. If one does not believe in it, it has no power over one. If belief makes the power of medicine perfect, then how much more can belief do if one believed in the power of the spirit upon matter. What generally happens is that one does not know if there is a spirit. Often one asks the question if there is any spirit, for what one knows is only matter, as a person once asked me. When traveling on a ship, a young Italian came to me and said, "I only believe in the eternal matter." I said, "Your belief is not very different from my belief." He was very surprised to see a priest—he thought that I was a priest—saying such a thing. He said, "What is your belief?" I said, "What you call eternal matter, I call eternal spirit. What does it matter? It is a difference of words, because one is eternal. You call it matter, I call it spirit." He became very interested from that time on. Before that he was very afraid.

The secret of healing is to rise by the power of belief above the limitations of this world of variety so that one may touch, by the power of intelligence, the oneness of the whole being. It is there that one becomes charged with the almighty power, and it is by the power of that attainment that one is able to help oneself and others in their pain and suffering. Verily, spirit has all the power there is.

* * *

Question: *In thinking of this oneness in the human being, where would one consider it as existing—as a force along the nerve channels, this divine essence of oneness of intelligence?*

Answer: Yes, through the nerve channels, through the veins and tubes, feeling that it is the divine blood circulating through one's veins, which is perfect, which is complete, which is pure. That helps one very much. In other words, what is illness? Illness is inharmony. And it is very often to be noticed that every illness follows an inharmony somewhere in one's life, outwardly or inwardly, as every failure follows inharmony somewhere. If one were to analyze one's life most minutely, one will find the cause of every illness and every failure in inharmony existing somewhere in one's mind or spirit or in one's life. If inharmony causes illness and failure, so harmony causes cure. If one can harmonize one's life in every way, in every form, certainly it must result in a perfect harmony, and this will manifest also as a cure from an illness.

Question: *What was first created: the ultimate atoms or the sun?*

Answer: What first existed was the motion, the movement, which the Vedantists call *nada*, and in the Bible it is called the word, the vibration.[2] It is the outcome of vibration which manifests in radiant atoms, not the atoms which are known to us just now, but atoms which existed before the sun. It is the centralizing of the all-pervading radiance that made the sun, and the atoms afterwards became different from the atoms which existed before.

Question: *If two people are inharmonious, is it necessarily the weaker one who falls ill? Why would one be ill, and the other feels no results?*

Answer: Perhaps the one is a little more harmonious, so one is waiting one's time.

Question: *Is it true that if one has a limb taken off, one can get it back through thinking?*

2 See John 1:1.

Answer: I have not said through thinking. It is Coué who said it. This question must be asked of Coué. I have said spirit. Before spirit there is nothing impossible. If there was something impossible we would not call God almighty.

Question: *What about young children?*

Answer: Young children are susceptible to the inharmonious vibrations of others, and it is that inharmony that causes them pain. It is wonderful to notice that with infants and with little children, every person they meet has a result. They can just be in the presence of a person, and you will see them cry all day long; or even to such an extent that, if the children are fine in spirit, an inharmonious person may come to your house and go, and the children may not see it. The children will be inharmonious all day long. Sometimes they are so sensitive that they can be mischievous, just because a shadow has fallen upon them. Therefore they are susceptible to influences.

Question: *Have all who are ill the strength to compel themselves to believe to become better, or must they be helped?*

Answer: As I have said that all the strength is in the spirit, everyone has the strength to the extent that one is close to the spirit. But everyone can trace a spark of that spirit in oneself, and everyone must know that there is a responsibility that one has for one's own health as a healer for oneself, that one has a part to play in one's own life that is not a physician's responsibility, or a healer's. Of course, if one cannot help oneself fully, one can ask another to help. One must be ready first to play a part as a physician and healer oneself, first to see what is lacking, what is the matter, how to heal. If one cannot do it, one can ask another. But one must be the first to desire it.

Question: *Suppose there was something organically wrong, would a time have to elapse?*

Answer: It is according to the faith.

Question: *Suppose that the faith was very great?*

Answer: No, the faith would speed the condition. As great the faith, so quick the time.

Question: *What is the working of curing illness by magnetism? Is that also a belief in the person to whom it is done?*

Answer: That is quite a different thing. It is only another form of prescription. When a prescription is given by a physician, a certain medicine is given to act or react on a certain condition. Well, so with the prana, which is the life energy that is given in a certain form in order to give patients what they are lacking. So it is not as material as an external remedy, but it is objective just the same.

Question: *So the person has to have faith?*

Answer: It is not only the magnetized person, but also the person who takes a medicine. If the patient has no faith, even medicine does not do the patient any good.

Question: *How is it that some feel everything spiritually? When they pass through spiritual difficulties, they feel ill. It reflects on their health. Other people do not feel it.*

Answer: It is only a question of temperament, of consciousness. There are those, if they have not said at a particular time one word just as they should have said, are feeling remorse about it for six months. There are others who have said a thousand things and fought and quarreled, and when they have gone out of the house, it is all gone. They are quite cured, because it is nothing to them. It has become their habit; they live in it. There are germs and worms who live in the mud, they are quite happy in it. It is their life, their being. But there is another person of delicate sense: if that person passes through there, it gives an unpleasant feeling. So it is the difference between people. There is such a vast variety among human beings and individual natures, as vast as there is variety between animals and birds. Sometimes there is such a difference in evolution that one cannot imagine what a gulf there is between one person and another.

There is a story told that four persons were brought before a wise king who was to judge them for the same crime. The king said for one that he must be sentenced to death. The other, he said, must be sentenced to prison for his whole life. For the third one he said he must be exiled. And for the fourth one he said, "Bring him to my chamber." And this fourth one was brought to his chamber. The king looked at him and said, "I did not anticipate such a thing being done by you. Do not show your face again to me." That is all. He gave him no other punishment. The ministers and everybody, they were all disturbed by the thought: "Why? It is one crime, and four different punishments?"

What was the result? The person who was exiled was quite happy, he thought, "So much the better! I got away from my belongings, from those near and dear to me, got rid of some responsibility in life." The one who was sentenced to prison for life became friends with the prisoners. He was enjoying life very well. But this fourth man went home, and he committed suicide. For the king did not see the law—he did not judge them according to the law of the book. He judged them according to the psychology of human nature. He saw the difference among the four.

HEALTH 9

The idea of calling certain diseases incurable diseases is a great mistake that people make today. It is only because they have not got the remedy of curing those diseases and call them incurable diseases. But by calling a certain disease an incurable disease we make that patient hopeless, not only in our help, but also in the help that one can get from above. Therefore, it cannot be a right idea to make a living being believe that there is no cure. If the source and goal is perfect, then perfection is possible to attain; and health is perfection, it can be attained. And what generally happens in the cases of what are called incurable diseases is that the impression that is made upon the patient of knowing and feeling that the disease cannot be cured becomes the root of the illness. And therefore, in the belief of the patient the illness becomes rooted, and then no remedy, no help can root it out. The best treatment that a healer, a physician, can give to a patient is to give first the belief that the patient can be cured; and then medicine, a healing treatment, or whatever method may be adopted to cure the patient.

We hear the accounts, the stories of the physicians of ancient times, of the mystics, of thinkers, that they used to find out a person's illness just by looking at that person. This comes by intuition, and if the people in the past ages were proficient in it, it does not mean that the soul has lost this quality. Even today, if one develops that quality in oneself, one can find out by the first glance all that is wrong with a person in that person's

51

body, mind, and spirit—all. For the outward expression of the person is the narrative of the inner condition. Any disorder in the mind or body is clearly manifest outwardly, and it is only a matter of developing that faculty in order to read it and to find it out. When this faculty is developed a little further it makes one know also what the reason is behind an illness that a person has, mentally or physically. If this faculty is developed still further, one can also find out what would be the best way, the best remedy to cure this person. Avicenna, the great mystic of Persia, was a physician and a healer at the same time. Mystics by nature are physicians, by nature are healers; but the attainment of the outer knowledge enables mystics to best use their faculties in the work of healing.

One might ask, "What must one do in order to develop this faculty, in order to find out this further, if one has it in oneself?" The answer is, as a mechanism wants a winding, as a musical instrument wants a tuning, so every person, whatever be one's life and occupation, wants a tuning every day. And what is this tuning? This tuning is to harmonize every action of the mechanism of the body, the harmonizing of pulsation, of the beating of the heart, of the beating of the head, of the circulation of the blood, and that can be done by the proper way of repose. When once that is done, then the next thing is to harmonize the condition of mind. Mind, which is constantly working, which is not under the control of will, which cannot be pulled together at a moment's call, which is restless, this mind should be harmonized. This can be harmonized first with the will. When there is a harmony between the will and mind, then the body and mind—so controlled and harmonized— become one harmonious mechanism working automatically. Merely bringing the mind and body in order allows every faculty which has not shown itself in its fullness to manifest, and a person begins to observe life more keenly, comprehend life more fully. And so perception becomes keen, and this faculty of knowing develops.

No doubt, the more spiritually one becomes evolved, the more one gets insight into the lives of things and beings. The first thing is to understand the condition of one's own body and health—of the physical health, of the mental condition. And when one can understand one's own condition better, then one begins to see the condition of the other person. Then intuition becomes born and active. As one develops intuitively, one begins to see the pains and sufferings of people. And if one's sympathy is growing and becoming vaster, one's sight becomes more keen, and one begins to observe the reason behind the complaint.

And if one goes still further in the path of intuition, one begins also to see what remedy would be the best remedy for the person who is suffering. Furthermore, there are some signs a seer sees, outward signs which explain the fundamental principle of health. Every person represents the sun: one's heart, one's spirit, one's body—all. And there are two actions of the sun: the sunrise and the sunset. There is a tendency of the body which draws it toward the earth and shows the sunset, because the soul is drawing itself toward the goal. And there is another tendency, which is like sunrise; the body naturally is inclined to raise itself. It seems that the earth is not drawing the body; it is something above which draws it. That is the sign of the sunrise, and it does not depend upon the age, it depends upon the condition, upon the harmony that is established by the spirit and the body. For a mystic it is a usual thing to find out if a person is going to die in three years' time, and easier still if a person is to die in one year's time. The inner spirit apart, even the tendency, the inclination of the body gives every sign.

* * *

Question: *Do the elements of fire, air, and water well balanced help one to a permanent cure?*

Answer: The knowledge of the elements is the most essential knowledge for understanding the law of nature. No doubt there are outer signs, but at the same time intuitive knowledge helps one to understand them. The examination that a physician makes, the analyzing of the blood and refuse and saliva, the examination of the skin, the tongue and lips, and the color of the eyes, in all this analyzing one sees the play of different elements, whether it is the fire element or water element or earth element. And it is either by remedies, by medicine, by thought power, by whatever way the patient is helped, the knowledge of the elements is most helpful. One can even go so far in understanding the secret of the elements that not only in the skin or in the body the elements show themselves, but even in the action of a person the elements show themselves. There is a person with a fire element predominant; this person is quite different from the person in whom the air element is predominant. The person with air element differs from the person with water. The likes, dislikes, things to which one has attraction are quite different and significant to the element which is predominant in one's nature. No doubt, a balance, an evenness of a right proportion of all the different elements which make the body is the ideal thing. And that can be brought about by harmonizing one's body, harmonizing the mind by meditation.

Question: *Can astrological determination help to find the cause of a disease? Is such a method recommended?*

Answer: Yes, astrological help can find out the cause, if it was right. But I would not recommend it. A person who looks at a condition before which one is helpless, in the case when it is favorable it is all right, but when it is not favorable then it works to one's disadvantage. For instance, if an astrologer says, "After three years you will become ill and you will die," even if the astrologer was mistaken in saying that, still the impression is that this will finish the person in three years. Why must one therefore depend upon such things? Why not depend upon the life and light of God, which is within? Why not say to oneself that life lives and death dies? And why not always hope for the best to come, and neither look at nor expect the worst to come? One might say that in order to be ready to face the worst, we must look at the black side. By looking at the dark side of things one focuses one's spirit on the dark side of things. And so one evolves into obscurity instead of rising above it and seeking for the light, hoping for the best to come; in this way one prepares oneself also to face the worst if it came.

Question: *It was said that the seer can see every inharmony in body, mind, and spirit; is there ever any inharmony in spirit?*
Answer: Yes. The spirit holds the inharmony of the body and mind in it. Inharmony does not belong to the spirit. It holds, while body and mind are reflected in it.

Question: *It is said that people mentally deranged are affected by the phases of the moon. Why is that?*
Answer: The moon is respondent to the sun, and so the mind is respondent to its impressions. The impressions which have deranged the mind, when they are more impressed by the response of mind, make a person worse. The effect of the moon is to make one responsive. If one is responsive to inspiration, one becomes more inspirational. For instance, a poet can write better in the waxing moon than waning moon.

Question: *Then would the mad person become more mad in the waxing moon?*
Answer: Yes. I have seen a bird in the Himalayas. That bird is called the lover of the moon. And during the rising moon this bird is happy, most joyous, singing and running in the moonlight, and it can walk with you miles at that time, when there the moon is rising. But in the waning moon it becomes sad, and it does not even eat for days. It seems as if it has lost all its joy and it awaits eagerly for the first moon, for the new moon. And that is the condition of the mind. Those who have mystical ideas begin every work, every enterprise they have in mind with the waxing moon.

Question: *Why is the river streaming from the perfect source to the perfect ocean through those bad and rocky mountains?*

Answer: That symbolizes life. Our soul, as a stream, comes from the perfect source and goes to the perfect source. And what we call life is going through the rocky mountains as we see. It is the same picture.

Question: *If one has, say, the earthly or watery elements predominant in one's nature, what is the most effective way to bring about the action of fire and air, which must be necessary for a perfect balance?*

Answer: By putting that person under a condition which will bring out the element which is wanted. For instance, with a person who likes to sleep, sending that person on an errand to Paris will bring about that balance which will [*text missing*].

Question: *Where does perfection exist if not in the spirit? And can the perfect hold or reflect the imperfect?*

Answer: Yes. The word *spirit* is used for two things. Divine spirit, the spirit of God, is a different thing. The individual spirit, the word which we use in spirit communication and for communicating with a person, that is quite a different meaning. And it is in that sense, if I have said that the spirit holds the condition of harmony of mind and body.

Question: *Is the state of consciousness of people reflected in the climate?*

Answer: Certainly. In the end of examination and analysis of cosmic life we shall come to find what Rumi has said: that the earth, water, fire, and air seem to everyone as objects, as something dead. Before God they are living beings; they are God's obedient servants. And where is God's intelligence to be found? In the human being. If a human being thinks and feels a certain thing it has its effect upon the whole cosmos. And if there is one thought held by a multitude, it has a still greater effect upon the cosmos, and therefore it is in the end we shall find, in spite of a human being's helplessness before natural law, that humanity as a collective being represents God, the creator who reigns and rules over nature.

HEALTH 10

There are different ways of looking at illness. One person looks at an illness as a punishment from above. There is another person who looks at an illness as a punishment brought about by one's own deeds. There is another way of looking at illness, and that is that it comes from the past karmas: that one has to pay back by illness the karmas of the past, the actions of the past. I have seen patients going through their illness with the thought that, as it is the debt of the past that one has to pay, it is just as well that it is paid back.

When we look at it critically, we find the person who thinks that it is a punishment that God sends upon a person, no doubt puts God in a serious light of making God a hard judge instead of a most merciful and compassionate father and mother, both in one. If the earthly father and mother would not like to inflict pain upon their child, it is hard to think that God—whose mercy and compassion is infinitely greater than that of earthly parents—could send upon a person illness as the punishment for that person's action. It seems to be more reasonable when a person says, "The illness is brought about by my own actions." But it is not always true; it is not true in every case. Very often the most innocent and the best souls who have nothing but a good wish and a kind thought will be found among sufferers. When one thinks that it is the debt for the past life, in that case it gives one the idea of fatalism: that there is a certain suffering through which one must pass, that there is no other way;

therefore, one must patiently endure something which is for the moment disagreeable. I have seen a young man suffering an illness who most contentedly told me, on my giving him advice on him doing this or that, "I understand that this is a debt for the past that I have to pay. I had just as well pay it." From a business point of view it is very just, but from a spiritual, psychological point of view, it can be looked at differently. What one does not wish for oneself is not for one, it is not one's portion. For in every soul there is the power of the Almighty. There is a spark of divine light, there is a spirit of the Creator. And therefore, all one wishes is one's birthright, all one wishes to have is one's birthright.

Naturally a soul does not wish to have an illness, except that it was unbalanced. If the soul knew the power of its natural inclination to enjoy health, it would experience health in life, in spite of all difficulties that conditions of life may present. No doubt, very often one's own self is the cause of the disorder of this physical mechanism. It is this disorder which one calls illness, whether it is physical or mental. Sometimes one neglects an unbalanced condition of the mind or body which causes it. Sometimes conditions around one cause an illness. Nevertheless, to have a yielding attitude toward illness is not the right thing. No doubt it is a good thing to look at the illness which has passed already, that "It was a trial, it was a test, an ordeal through which I was passing and which I have left behind. And it was for the better, that I am more purified. I have learned a lesson from it. I have become better, I have become more thoughtful and considerate toward my own being and toward others by an experience like this."

But to think that, "What I am going through is something that I must contentedly bear" is not the right attitude. The attitude must be, "No, this is not my portion in life, I will not have it, I must not have it, I must rise above it, I must forget it, I must do everything in my power to overcome it by a thought, by a feeling, by a belief, by a good action, by a prayer, by concentration, by a healing, by whatever method." There must be no limitation. Sometimes a person says, "I believe in healing, I will not touch a medicine; it is material." That is wrong also. Sometimes a person says, "I only believe in a medicine, I have no faith in healing." That is wrong, too. To yield a perfect health, to bring about a cure, one must heal oneself from morning till evening. In the sun one must think that, "Every ray of the sun cures me; the air heals me; the food I take has an effect upon me. With every breath I inhale something which is healing, purifying, bringing me to a perfect health." With a hopeful attitude toward cure, toward health, toward a perfect life, a person rises above disorders, which are nothing but inharmonious conditions of mind or body, and makes one more fit to accomplish one's life's purpose. It is not selfish to think about one's health. No doubt, it is undesirable to be thinking about one's illness, to worry about it or to be too anxious about it. But to take care of one's health is the most religious thing there is, because it is the health of the body and mind that enables one to do a service to God and to one's fellow human beings, by which one accomplishes one's life's purpose.

One must think that, "I am coming from a perfect source, and I am bound to a perfect goal. The light of the perfect being is kindled in my soul. I live, move, and make my being in God. And nothing in the world of the past or present has the power to touch me, for I rise above all." It is this thought which will make one rise above influences of inharmony and disorder, and will bring a person to enjoy the greatest bliss in life, which is health.

* * *

Question: *When a child is ill how can it be helped?*

Answer: By a helpful thought. Sometimes mother's healing thought, mother's sympathy works with a child more successfully than the medicine that is given to the child; and in this is the proof of the power of healing. There are numberless cases that can be observed in which, consciously or unconsciously, the desire of the mother becomes a healing influence for the child to recover. If the mother is anxious for and worried about a child, of course that has a contrary effect, because she unconsciously then holds an illness in her thought for the child.

Question: *When we see a babe born with a hereditary illness, can we say that its soul has been impressed by the idea of that illness in coming to the earth?*

Answer: Not at all. "Hereditary illness"—that explains it.

Question: *Can illness be caused by sorrow?*

Answer: But sorrow itself is the worst possible illness. No illness is worse than sorrow. Sorrow is the worst illness. No doubt, sorrow causes all illness because it makes mind and body both inharmonious, which then easily catch an illness. To me a real brave person is the one who says, "What has happened, has happened. What I am going through I shall rise above, and what will come I shall meet with courage." If one wants to be sorry, there are many things that can make one sorry. One need not wait for causes to arrive that make one shed tears. Every move one makes can make one shed tears, if one had that inclination. One should not look for ill luck. Ill luck can be found everywhere if one were pursuing it. Many unconsciously do so—they are looking for ill luck.

Question: *Please explain why a child of perfect parents should have been affected by an incurable illness from childhood, that child being a most noble character?*

Answer: There is an answer in the Bible when somebody asked the Master whether his parents sinned or he sinned that he was born blind, and the answer was, "Neither did this man sin nor his parents, but that the works of God may be made manifest in him."[1] But that is for us to understand, not for that person to think. There is another theory of understanding. This is the

1 John 9:1–12.

theory from which we understand how it is, but for a sufferer this is not the thing. For one who suffers the thing is that it must hold to one's birthright that one is coming from the perfect and that one is going to the perfect. One must hope for perfection, life is created for it. Life is evolving toward it. That must be one's desire and goal.

Question: *Is healing by hypnosis good practice?*

Answer: Now surgeons make use of ether or something else in order to perform operations although it is harmful for the person; but at the same time it is necessary. And so if this way is used to make a person better, and if it was necessary, it may be allowed. But at the same time everyone must be able to do for oneself, by prayer, by meditation, by silence, to cherish that belief in perfect health, and to root out the belief in illness.

Question: *Do not people lose their own free will if they have been hypnotized once.*

Answer: Yes. But only if they are in a condition where they cannot help themselves. It is very good if one walks oneself, to walk on one's own feet, but when there is a condition when a person cannot walk then, if another person gives a hand, it makes that person dependent but it gives a help.

For instance, there are some people who, after an operation, have taken a habit of taking a drug, for once it was necessary and now they continue to have to take it. At that time it was right to have it, but when it was continued it was wrong. I had seen a great power—of course it was spiritual healing power in a mystic—that was in the Nizam of Hyderabad. First he began by curing patients who were affected by serpent bite. They generally die, and he had given orders that at any time, even in the midst of the night, if a person was bitten by a serpent that person might be brought to him. He sacrificed his sleep for curing them. Then after three years' time he developed that power so that he used to say through the telephone, "It is all right, you are well," and the person got well immediately, instantly. I have seen also a person who used to cure people who had been stung by a scorpion. A person suffering in a great pain was brought before him, and the first thing he said was, "Now you have not got any pain, have you? It is not there." And it was gone instantly, at once. He did nothing but say, "It is not there." He did not give one moment for the person to think whether it is there or not. The secret is not only in the faith of the patient. The secret is in the power and belief of the healer. The idea is that, suppose ten persons repeat one phrase, and if that phrase was drawn on a paper by a seer, the seer would draw one line quite short, and the other line one inch and the other line one meter, and another line perhaps one mile long or longer still. The thing is, where the voice comes from is the question. If it comes from the mouth, it only reaches the ears of the hearer. If it comes from the heart, it penetrates the heart. If it comes from the soul, it penetrates the soul of a person. It cures the person entirely. It is not every person who can put power in a word, unless the soul was capable of doing it. In the Bible we read, "First was the Word and the Word was God."[2] This will always prove true in every sense. But when they do not see God in the word then it becomes hypnotism and mesmerism and everything else. When God is realized, then it is much greater than that, then it is divine will. It is how we look at things. And if God is left out, then the soul is left out. Many play with hypnotism and with its effects, and sometimes they find success. But the soul is not there. When God is not the ideal of the person, and when one is not doing it in God, with God, and for God, then it is only done mechanically. It has no life. A machine will only go without an engineer for some time, then it will go no longer. There ought to be an engineer. Therefore, to do the right thing there ought to be God.

---

2 See John 1:1.

HEALTH 11

There is a saying in the East that there is one illness for which there is no remedy. In the Arabic language that illness is called *wahm*, which means "imagination." With every illness the imagination plays its role; the greater the imagination, the greater becomes the illness. But illness apart, in every little thing in life, your imagination makes its mischief, exaggerates it, and makes it more difficult to bear. It is not seldom, it is often that you see that one feels tired—before one has worked—at the thought of the work. When working, that tiredness has increased still more, which was imagined before. Before the work is finished the person is done. This is often to be seen that a head of a factory is more tired after two hours' work than perhaps the workman who has worked all day long with engines. A superintendent of a garden has become much more tired than the gardener who has been working in the garden all day long. You will very often see that a person in the audience has become more tired than the singer who has sung the whole program of the evening. It is often one sees that before having walked so many miles a person has become tired at the thought of it.

Imagination always leads, illness follows. No doubt, the one who has control over imagination can master oneself and can rise above illness. It always amused me to see a lady who used to give lectures, that when the lecture was now at a fifteen days' distance, that lady began to be worried. And as the worry came, then some illness followed, and the doctors examined it, and so it went on. About the time when the day of the lecture came, the lady was quite finished. Healers had to see her, occultists had to advise her. Astrologers had to make her horoscope in order to tell her that she would be successful in her lecture before she was ready to give a lecture. It is not rare. Very often one finds that one exaggerates tiredness, confusion, pain, trouble, and makes a mountain out of a molehill, without knowing it. If that person were told, that person would not accept it, would not admit it; and at the same time it is so.

Out of a hundred persons who suffer from a certain illness, you will find ninety-five who can be cured if the imagination allowed them to be cured. Upon many a fear of illness comes, even before they have felt pain, if a physician has told them that there is something wrong with them. The physician may be mistaken, yet the fear of the pain that is anticipated takes the place of the disease. The body is constructed with a nervous system, which is the main mechanism of one's physical being; and this mechanism is most respondent to imagination when compared with flesh, bone, or skin. Nerves instantly respond to the thought, not skin, flesh, or bones—they partake of the influence coming from the nerves. Therefore, the nervous system stands between physical and mental aspects of being. Therefore, as imagination can cause an illness, can maintain an illness, so imagination can cure a person from illness also. Once illness is cured by imagination, what is left of that illness in the body has no sustenance to exist, and therefore it naturally dies out.

I have often seen, for an experiment, a person who said that, "I have got a very bad headache." I asked that person to sing, and in the end found that the person was cured. Anything that takes away from the mind the imagination of this illness cuts the arms of evil that holds that illness; then the illness cannot stand on its feet. There must be something to hold it, and that is imagination.

Self-pity is the worst enemy of humankind, although sometimes it gives a tender sensation in the heart to say, "Oh, how poorly I am," and it is soothing to hear from someone, "Oh, I am so sorry you are not well." But I could expect something else from someone, that is to say: "I am so happy to see you are so well." In order to create that tender sensation one need not be ill. What is needed is to be thankful. We can never be too thankful. If we can appreciate the privileges of life, there are endless gifts from above which we never think about, and we never value them. If we think of them thankfully, naturally a tenderness is felt, and it is that tenderness which is worth having.

By outward evidence very often a person builds a conception of an illness. For there are signs of illness, no doubt. But mind has such a great power that, if there is a sign of illness, the mind sees a thousand signs of illness. For instance, as soon as you begin to think that your friend is displeased with you, everything the friend does, either good or bad, for you it all seems that it is all going wrong. And if you think your friend is loving and kind to you, all that the friend does, it all shows as a support to your thought. When a person begins to think that, "I am under an unlucky star," everything that happens, good or bad, that person thinks, "It all brings bad luck to me. From everywhere there is bad luck, from every side bad luck is coming." Even if a good thing is coming, one thinks it is bad because one is looking at it from that way. And when a person is in the thought of, "Good luck is coming to me," everything that comes is in the form of good luck.

The more we study this question, the more we find that our mind is the master of life, and that we become the possessor of the kingdom of God as soon as we have realized the power of imagination upon our life. There is the absence of self-knowledge in that one does not value that divine spark which is within oneself. And by being unaware of it one goes down and down, till one reaches the deepest depth. No sooner does one realize this than one begins to respect oneself, and it is the self-respecting one who has respect for another. It is the one who helps oneself who is the one who will help another. It is those who will raise themselves, who will take another person also toward the heights. Once we have found the remedy to cure this incurable disease which comes out of imagination, then there is no other disease which we cannot manage to get above. We only have to realize the source of perfection within ourselves.

* * *

Question: *What is imagination?*

Answer: Imagination is an automatic working of mind.

Question: *What part does it play in the illness of children and the mentally deficient?*

Answer: Among children pain increases with imagination, and therefore the one who understands this can stop the pain of a child sooner than any other medicine. For the child is responsive to advice. A grown-up person who holds imagination in hand and does not let it loose is difficult to help. But a child can be helped in a moment. A child may be crying in pain, and in a moment's time, if you can get its imagination away from it, you can cure that child. As to the mentally deficient, imagination is the main reason at the back of their illness. It is irregularity in rhythm of mind which causes mental disorder. Physicians may give reasons for having cavities in the brain, but this disorder begins before the cavity in the brain. The cavity in the brain is caused by their mental disorder. Mental disorder is not always caused by a cavity in the brain, for the inner being has a greater influence on the physical being than what physical being has on the mental existence.

Question: *How can you train imagination?*

Answer: By training thought. We must make thoughts out of imaginations. There comes a development of mind that shows itself just like a muscular development of the physical body: that each muscle is distinct when a person has exercised one's body, and so every thought becomes distinct and clear before it is expressed. In that way imagination is developed, trained.

Question: *Thinking illness has mostly to do with imagination, is it not dangerous for the parents to overlook any real illness of the child?*

Answer: That is another thing. Parents must neither overlook the illness of a child, nor a person overlook the complaint that person has, for it is not always imagination. But at the same time, imagination plays a great role, and it is better for one to analyze to what extent imagination plays a part in one's complaint. And that one can analyze by trying to forget one's pain, to entirely forget by trying to deny facts which stand before one as evidence of illness. When a person is able to go even to that extent, then that person will be able to realize how much illness there is and how much there is of one's imagination. That person will also observe a phenomenon that, as soon as one will withdraw the imagination from the illness, one will starve the illness of the food which maintains it, and it is possible that by this starvation that illness will die. About children, one must not overlook their illness, but at the same time one must not exaggerate. One must not think too much about it, because imagination has a living effect. Imagination can create an illness in a person who has not got it in reality, and it would be a great mistake on the part of parents to worry over children's health when it is not necessary.

Question: *Is there a body between the mind and the physical body, such as Theosophists call an astral body?*

Answer: It is a question which must be gone through in detail. It evolves into a great many ideas which must be considered, and therefore this is not the time to go into it.

Question: *There is often much spoken about the imagination of a poet, but can it be said that all poems are written by a mechanical working of the mind?*

Answer: If they are made by the mechanical working of the mind, they are much better than by the effort of the brain of the poet. For in order to become a poet, a real poet, what is necessary? The mind must become music, the music which is expressed in language. Besides, a real poet is a spiritual medium. Inspiration comes from a higher source, and what the poet writes by inspiration, that is something worthwhile. At other times, when writing as a poet, it is nothing.

Question: *Is it possible after having avoided illness by* [text missing], *also to get strong, having a delicate body?*

Answer: No. There are other things also necessary. This physical body is subject to physical laws; one must observe them. In diet, in activity, in repose, and in all things of life there must be a rhythm, there must be a regularity. A consideration must be given to it in order to keep it in a right condition.

Question: *What is the difference between imagination and inspiration?*

Answer: The mind which is circling only in the earthly spheres is creating imagination. When the mind has become so widened that the bottom of the wheel touches the earth and the top touches the heavens, then there is inspiration brought from heaven to the earth. It depends upon the width of the circle, whether it is a large circle or a smaller circle. I have often said that evolution is largeness. Spirituality is a fullness of being.

HEALTH 12

A regular life, pure diet, good sleep, a balance between activity and repose, and right breathing all help one to health. But the best remedy for healing oneself of all illnesses and infirmities of mind is one, and that is belief. Many think that they believe, but very few are they who really believe. The belief of many is, as I heard someone say, "I believe, I believe. May God strengthen my belief." It is an affirmation which has no meaning. If a person says "I believe," that does not mean the person believes, for it is belief in its perfection which becomes faith. And what does Christ says about faith? He says, "Faith removes mountains."[1] Of course, the priest says faith in the church, the clergyman says faith in the book. But that is not the real meaning of faith. Faith is the culmination of belief. When belief is completed it turns into faith.

There are people who think that they will never give in to such an error of believing in something which has no evidence, and that, they think, is most clever. And when we search into the world of evidence, we shall find one deluding cover under another; and so one can go on, probing the depth of life, from one illusion to another, never arriving at the realization of truth. Evidence which is subject to change—how can you rely upon it? Therefore, if there is anything to rely upon, it is one thing and that is belief. It is not evidence which gives us belief. And if evidence gave belief, that belief would not last, for the

---

1 See Matthew 17:20.

evidence is not lasting. Belief which stands above evidence is that belief which, in the end, will culminate in faith.

It is people like Bayazid,[2] whom many people would consider to be in the clouds, who proved in their lives what belief means. Bayazid was going to Mecca for a pilgrimage. A dervish was sitting on the way of his journey. Thinking that it is nice to pay homage to a spiritual man, he went to that dervish and sat to receive his blessing. The dervish asked him, "Where are you going?" He said, "I am going to Mecca." "For any business?" "No." He [Bayazid] was astonished. "For business? No, for a pilgrimage." "For a pilgrimage? What are they doing in the pilgrimage?" "What do they do in pilgrimage?" This man [Bayazid] said, "They walk around the holy stone of Ka'ba." The dervish said, "You do not need to go so far for that pilgrimage. If you will take circles around me and go back, your pilgrimage is done." Bayazid said, "Yes, I believe it." He circled around the man, went back home, and when people asked, "Did you make a pilgrimage to Ka'ba?" "Yes," said he, "I made a pilgrimage to a living Ka'ba."

Belief is not an imagination. Belief is a miracle in itself, for belief is creative. If one believes what does not exist, the belief will make it existent. If there is a condition that one believes and that condition does not exist, it will be produced.

The difference between the mind of the believer and the mind of the unbeliever is this, that the mind of the believer is like a torch, the mind of the unbeliever is like a light which is covered under something, which does not spread its light. Very often people are afraid of losing common sense. They would rather like to be ordinary than to become extraordinary. They are afraid of losing themselves. But they do not know that losing themselves means gaining themselves. A person says, "To think about these things is like moving in the air." But if we would not be in the air, what would be of us? What would become of us? Air is the substance on which we live, more important for

2 Bayazid (Abu Yazid) Bistami (804–740), Persian Sufi.

us than the food we eat and the water we drink. Belief, there-fore, is the food of the believers. It is the sustenance of their faith. It is on the belief that the believers live, not on food and water.

What is this mortal world? What is this physical existence? What is this life of changes? If it were not for a belief, what use is it all? Something which is changing, something which is not reliable, and something which is liable to destruction. There-fore, it is not only for the sake of health but for life itself that one must find belief in oneself, develop it, nurture it, allow it to grow every moment of one's life, that it might culminate in faith. It is that faith which is the mystery of life and secret of salvation.

* * *

Question: *If faith is attained to a certain degree in us, will it always grow?*

Answer: Certainly, it will grow as a plant. All our failures, sor-rows, disappointments, difficulties in life, they all have as a cause our lack of belief.

Question: *Everything that one believes comes to reality. How can one attain this belief concerning one's illness?*

Answer: Illness means lack of belief. Beyond and above all other outer evidences, illness is the sign of lack of belief, and if one believed, certainly illness has no place. But illness takes the place of a belief. One cannot disbelieve in what one believes. Illness becomes one's belief; that is where the difficulty comes. When a person says, "I am fighting against my illness," that means "My imagination is fighting against my belief." That person af-firms that, "I am fighting against my illness," which means one establishes illness in oneself just the same. One fights against something which one affirms to be existing. Therefore, the first place in belief one gives to illness, the second place to one's imagination of curing it. Therefore, the power with which one wishes to remove one's illness is much smaller than the power already in one by illness.

Question: *Is faith a gift or attainable by perseverance, by belief?*

Answer: Things of heaven cannot be attained by persevering, they are the grace of God. No perseverance is required to ask for the grace of God, to believe in the grace of God, and to open oneself for the grace of God, to trust in it. It is this which strengthens belief to faith.

Question: *When belief is in creating, how is it possible that many persons who have no real belief, live?*

Answer: If they have no real belief, they have false belief. They have some belief just the same. Besides that, I have not said, "Believe in creating." I said, "Belief is creative." For instance, a person certainly believes that so many centimes he can get from a franc. And everyone believes it because there is evidence. A person has not far to go for the evidence. A person just has to go to the shop to find the centimes received for the franc. Belief is only difficult when there is no evidence. It is just like building a castle in the air. But then that castle becomes paradise.

Question: *What about the diseases of animals?*

Answer: The animal is more responsive to nature than humankind, and nature helps the animal to forget its illness more than it does to a human being because people are not respondent to nature. Everyone has one's little world. It may be so little sometimes that it is like a doll's house, and in this world a person lives. That person is not concerned with this wide world, or concerned with the universe. One just lives in one's small world, and that is the only world one knows, that is all one is concerned with, that is all one is interested in. And therefore, if one's world is full of misery and illness and ill-luck, one cannot come out of it, because one has made a kind of shell, like the insects in the water make a little shell to live and they live in it. The planet does not make misery for one. One has made misery for oneself, and one likes to hide in this shell; because one has made it, one likes to live in it. It is one's home even if it is a shell of weakness, of misery, of goodness, of piety—anything.

Question: *Are not some of us happy enough always to live by the grace of God? Why do we get this blessing?*

Answer: Everything belonging to the earth costs us, more or less. We purchase it. And there is only one thing which does not cost. It does not cost because we can never pay its price, and that is the grace of God. We cannot pay for it in any form, in any way—by our goodness, by our piety, by our great quality, merits or virtues, nothing. For what does our goodness amount to? Our lifelong goodness is nothing more than a drop of water compared with the sea. We as human beings are too poor to pay for the grace of God in order to purchase it. It is only given to us, for God is love. What do we expect from love? Grace.

Question: *One's illness has to be seen as the will of God? And if illness be not, how with death?*

Answer: Death is different from illness. For illness is worse than death. The sting of death is only momentary, that idea that one leaves one's surroundings. One moment's bitter experience, no longer. But illness is incompleteness, and that is not desired.

Question: *You speak of death as of a disagreeable experience, but it need not be so.*

Answer: It need not be so. If a person is awakened, certainly death is no longer bitter.

Question: *Will you give a definition of what is the grace of God?*

Answer: Grace of God is love of God, love of God manifesting in innumerable blessings, blessings which are known and unknown to us. Human beings live on earth, as I have already said, in their shells, mostly unaware of all privileges of life and so unthankful to the giver of them. In order to see the grace of God one must open one's eyes, raising one's head from the little world that we make around ourselves. And then to see up and down, right and left, before and behind, the grace of God reaching us from everywhere in abundance. If we can try to thank, we might thank for thousands of years and it will never be enough. But when one looks in one's own little shell, one does not find the grace of God. What one finds is miseries, troubles, difficulties, injustice, hard-heartedness, coldness of the world, all ugliness from everywhere. Of course, naturally, when one looks down, one sees mud. When one looks up, one sees beautiful stars and planets. It only depends which way we look. Do we look upward or downward?

HEALING

The contents of "Healing" are taken from esoteric papers given from 1919 to 1920.

THE MAIN ASPECTS OF HEALING

Balance 1

Health depends upon the balance of activity and repose of the five senses: sight, smell, hearing, taste, and touch; and every sense, in the normal condition of health, must be able to express itself and respond. More time is required for the repose of the senses than for their activity. Therefore, the mystics go into seclusion in order to give a chance for repose to the senses, which are different in every person.

Everyone passes every moment of the waking state in activity of the senses, partly by intention, partly accidentally. For instance, the eyes look at things when they are willed to do so, perhaps a hundred times a day, but nine hundred times they look at things without intention. This shows a waste of energy in an average person's life.

In order to develop healing power one must regulate control of the senses by regulating their activity and repose; and this, done with a spiritual thought, converts power of mind into divine power. A person can heal with power of mind alone, but the results will be limited. But a person with divine power can obtain through it unlimited results.

Balance 2

It depends on the condition of the health how much activity one can stand and how much repose is necessary; a general rule cannot be made for everyone. A normal amount of activity stimulates and strengthens the body. Therefore, physical exercises are given for physical development, and exercises of concentration and studies are given for development and repose of the mind. According to psychic law, the day is natural for activity and the night for repose, and when this is not carried out it naturally works against health. It is not necessary that after every little exertion one must take repose, but a degree of balance ought to be maintained. And it is advisable to manage to take repose in life without allowing it to develop into laziness.

Breath

Breath is the first essential power that can help in healing. There is a silent healing, and a healing by fixing the glance, by holding the painful part with the fingers, by rubbing the painful part, by waving the hand over the painful part, by touching and not touching the part. But behind these different ways there is one power working, and that is the power of the breath. This power can be developed by breathing practices, and when the breath is so developed that it creates an atmosphere around the healer, then the very presence of the healer heals. The power of the breath can be developed by physical exercises, by rhythmic exercises of the breath, by pure living, and by concentration.

The power of healing is greater than the power of the channels one uses to heal, such as the fingertips or eyes. The eyes have more power than the fingertips. They are finer, and the power that manifests through them is radiant, while it is not so radiant in the fingertips. But besides the power of healing one must have a clear idea of the complaint of another person and know what would be the best way to heal that person.

Healing with the Fingertips

Hygiene is the first subject to consider in healing with the tips of the fingers. Hands that have been engaged in any work or that are stained with any liquid must be washed; even after shaking hands they must be washed for healing. The healer must first observe the hygienic rules of keeping the healer's own body, as well as the healer's own clothes, pure and clean; especially at the time of healing the healer must be absolutely free from all that is unhygienic. The sleeves, at the time of healing, must be rolled back; and the fingernails must be properly trimmed and clean. After healing, one should wave the hand, as if shaking it, to shake off any fine atoms or even vibrations, so that a poison taken from the painful part of the patient may not be given to the patient again. At the end of the healing the hands must be washed again.

There are cases when the sensation of the body is deadened by the pain, and the pain has gone into the depth of the affected part of the body. In such cases waving the hand or touching is not enough. Rubbing is necessary. In cases of the effects of poison from the sting of a bee or a scorpion, or a snakebite or the bite of any other poisonous animal, a simple soft touch or stroking of the affected part is necessary. If the pain is more intense, touch is not necessary, simply the waving of the hand close to the affected part will do. In the case of the bite of a mad dog, one should put some lime mixed with water on a copper coin and tie it on the part that the teeth have touched, and the rest of the affected part must be healed by touching and stroking it with the tips of the fingers. Bites of mosquitoes and midges may be cured by applying butter that has been allowed to boil and cool again, and then waving the hand over the affected part. Rose water may be used for bites of all kinds in cases of severe inflammation.

The Tracing of Disease

The healer's work in tracing disease is subtler than healing, for in healing, power is necessary; but in tracing the disease—its nature, its cause, its secret—psychic power is of no use. There inspiration is needed, and a healer without it is an incomplete healer.

The patient generally does not know the real cause, nature, and secret of the complaint. The patient is not supposed to know, for the patient knows the effect of the pain, not its cause, nature, and secret. The healer must trace the patient's complaint from the patient's face, expression, voice, word, and movement; everything tells. Sometimes the healer must find out the cause by asking the patient the details about the pain and the situation of the patient's life, and by knowing the attitude that the patient takes to things, and by knowing the inclinations of the patient.

The secret of the disease can be traced also by seeing what a person desires in the way of food, and in what environments a person prefers to be, and what attitude a person has toward friends and foes, a person's choice of sweet and savory, and attraction to colors.

For instance, a person with a complaint that originates from melancholy will have a liking for purple. A person who has lost control of passions will have an inclination to red. A person, who is lifeless, with an inclination to emptiness, will have a tendency toward white, because no color will appeal to that person. A person who has gone through a sorrow and mourned over things and weakened the heart by it, will have an inclination toward black.

So it is with sweet and savory: the patient who shows an inclination to sweet shows weakness of heart and, by that, general weakness; and the patient who shows inclination toward savory lacks circulation.

There are many more things in the patient that one can perceive, not only from the patient's inclinations but also by noticing the patient's face and features, for in this way one reads more than anything else. The features tell the general characteristics, and therefore a person knows the weakness that may have been the origin of the complaint. And the general expression shows the thought behind it, since mind is the cause of all causes. The healer gets at the root of the complaint as soon as the healer touches the mind of the patient. How true is the saying that the face is the mirror of the heart.

The Chief Reason of Every Disease

According to the mystical point of view there is one chief reason, which can be called a common cause and from which all diseases are derived, and that is disorder of rhythm. The upset of the nerves is stated by scientists as the chief origin of all mental diseases, and their effect upon the body produces different diseases in the body. Religious people teach concentration and meditation, sitting in a prayerful attitude. The wisdom behind this is to bring the activity of mind and body to a normal condition. For it is the nature of activity to be active at every moment, for it is the activity itself that produces energy. And the consequence is that, by so producing energy, its own strength throws it out of its normal rhythm.

This one can see in the burning of a fire. The activity is little at the start, but at every moment its activity increases and culminates, in the end, in its utmost speed. And the speed of the beginning compared with the speed of the end will prove that it was the increase of speed of the fire which brought about the climax, when it has eaten itself.

In human nature we see the same tendency. When speaking one is inclined to speak more and more quickly until the speed is so increased that one leaves out several words of the sentence without any intention of doing so. So it is in walking: the speed of the walk increases with every step until one finds oneself almost running. So it is with the imagination, and perhaps one sees the same thing with the pulsation of the body and blood circulation. Uncontrolled increase of speed, in all its aspects, hastens the climax and, when unbalanced, culminates in disastrous results.

Healers without this knowledge are blind healers who do not know the cause of diseases; their healing is by chance. But those who know this are more than physicians and more than healers. They will control their own activity, and the power of control thus gained will enable them to control the activity of others in order to keep it normal, in which is the true health of mind and body.

The Reason for Tiredness

Tiredness is caused by three reasons. Loss of energy is the chief reason, but also excess of activity of mind and of body. One generally knows tiredness to be caused by excess of bodily activity, but one is apt to overlook the fact that excess of activity of mind also causes tiredness.

The activities that especially cause tiredness are worry, fear, anxiety, and pain. There is, however, besides these, one mental cause that still remains and is less observable, and that is the thought of being tired. Among a hundred cases of tired people you will find ninety cases of this particular kind of tiredness. When a person thinks, "I am tired," the very thought creates the feeling of tiredness in support of the thought, and reason brings forward a thousand reasons that seem to have caused the tiredness. There are some people who think that the presence of people or of some people, or the presence of a particular person tires them. Some think that their energy, their life, is eaten up by some people. Some think that a particular action takes away their energy. Some think that their strength is taken out of them by their everyday duty in life or the work they happen to do, such as singing, speaking, doing bodily or mental work; and of course, as they think, so they experience.

Coming to the truth of the matter, there is no doubt that every kind of activity must take away some energy, more or less, from a person. Thinking of the loss increases the loss, but by preserving the energy and using it economically, one saves it to a great extent. But there is one way, which is a spiritual way, by which one can give out energy with every activity that necessitates one's giving it out, and at the same time, one can absorb much more energy than one loses from the life within, without, around, and about one. It is for this reason that religion has given the conception of God being almighty. Those who consider God to be far away in heaven keep away from God, but those who realize the meaning of Christ's teaching that we live and move and have our being in God[1] feel God, at all times, by their side. When consciousness of wealth makes one feel rich, and when consciousness of strength makes one feel strong, how much stronger and richer should that one feel who is really God-conscious!

Balance 3

A healer often finds patients whose complaints may differ, and yet they may have originated in a lack of balance. Balance is the most difficult thing in life to keep for anybody and everybody. Many times a healer succeeds in curing a patient by just showing some practices by which the patient can attain balance. This, besides healing, brings about a most desirable effect.

Balance is gained in different ways, even in ordinary actions such as sitting, lying, standing, and walking; standing with even weight on both legs; sitting cross-legged or on the heels, each knee having an equal part of the weight of the body; as well as kneeling, walking rhythmically with an even force given to the swing of both arms. One also gets balance by regularity of eating and drinking, working and resting, sleeping and rising. And the first thing a healer should consider when treating a patient is that the healer must give the patient balance.

Pain

Pain has two origins: the mind and the body. Sometimes it is caused by the mind and held by the body, and sometimes it is caused by the body and held by the mind; and it is the harmony of both that sustains the pain. If one were absent or did not partake of the pain suggested by the other part of the being, the pain would not exist; and if it existed it would vanish. The body, being the servant of the mind, can never refuse to bear the pain given by the mind, having no free will of its own. It is only the mind that can refuse, if it were trained to do so.

---

1 Acts 17:28.

The doctrine that some people have, that there is no such thing as pain, is very helpful in the training of the mind, although its truth may be questioned. If it is true that there is no such thing as pain, it can only be true in the sense that everything in this world is an illusion and it has no existence of its own; it does not exist in reality compared with the ultimate reality. But if a person says that it is only pain that does not exist, and that joy exists and all other things exist, then that person is wrong.

Among the Sufis, dervishes have tried to become pain-proof by inflicting upon themselves cruel injuries, such as whipping the bare arms or cutting the muscles of the body or piercing the body with knives or taking the eyes out of their sockets and replacing them in their sockets again, which I have witnessed myself. By this they have discovered a truth and have given it to the thinking world: that the mind can refuse to partake of the bodily pain, and by so doing the bodily pain is felt much less than it would otherwise be. For when the mind goes forward to receive bodily pain out of fear or self-pity, it increases the pain and makes it much more than it would otherwise be. The proportion that fear or self-pity add to the pain is ninety-five percent. And the first thing that the healer must do in curing patients suffering pain is to erase the pain from the surface of the patient's mind by suggestion and also by healing power. In the absence of help on the part of the mind, the body must give up pain, for it has no power to hold it any longer without the mind.

Healing by Medicine

Very often it happens that a healer or believer in healing goes to such an extreme as to not accept medicine. In reality, the idea of being given medicine by a doctor and the thought of repeating the prescription so many times a day, apart from the medicinal influence, is psychically helpful. And the healers of the East, considering this, have in their lives played some of the part of a physician as well, [combining it] with other healing power: spiritual, psychic, and magnetic. With their magnetic suggestions and with their mesmeric influences, they gave the patient something to eat or to drink in the form of medicine. Sometimes they gave a charm to keep and sometimes magnetized water.

The idea is that a person is more conscious of the objective world and its activity than of any other plane of existence, and by eating or drinking, or by holding or possessing a certain thing, the impression becomes more real.

The thought of the healer that should ease the mind is often hindered when the external senses of the patient are not fully responsive to it. But when the patient eats or drinks something, or tastes something, or feels something applied to or touching the painful part, the patient's sense or senses become the mediums for the healer's thought to proceed through them and so reach the mind of the patient.

The knowledge of the physical medium is most essential for a healer, for every psychic operation requires a medium. And through a distinct and responsive medium every psychological work meets with success.

THE PSYCHOLOGICAL NATURE OF DISEASES

Causes of Diseases

The psychological nature of diseases can be explained in a few words as being the lack of life, either by the lack of sufficient matter in the body or by of excess of matter, which leaves no scope for the spirit. And it is the impression of pain which the mind holds. Pain is not always physical. There are physical causes, but as soon as the mind knows of discomfort, out of fear, it holds it; and this is called pain.

Disease is often caused by the lack of rhythm, be it in thought or feeling, in breath, in action, or in one's everyday life. For instance, keeping awake in the night when one is accustomed to sleep, changing the dinner hour, taking a nap when one is not accustomed to it, or doing anything that one is not accustomed to doing puts one out of rhythm. People who are accustomed to being angry or to quarreling would become ill if they were not allowed to do so. There is a story told in India about a person who could not keep a secret and who was compelled to keep quiet. In the end he was ill, and the doctor had to cure him by permitting him to give it out. All of this signifies rhythm. Every habit forms a rhythm.

The fear of catching a disease is also a cause of illness. There are people who wonder if they are ill and try to find out if there is something wrong with them. There are some who enjoy self-pity or sympathy from others; these invite disease. Some entertain disease when they are, to a certain extent, unwell. They wish to surround themselves with the environment of a patient or try to take a lazy life. By so doing the mind naturally holds the disease longer since it is allowed to do so.

There are many other causes of illness. Among them, the most unfortunate cause is the impression that: "I have an illness that can never be cured," for this impression is worse than a disease. In fact, the soul of every individual, healthy or ill, is pure from any pain or disease, and it constantly heals mind and body. And if it were not for the mind and body, which create illness, a person would always be well. It is natural to be healthy; and all illness, pain, and discomfort are unnatural.

Magnetic Power

The health of both mind and body depends upon a magnetic power, which may be called, in metaphysical terms, the power of affinity in elements and in atoms. It may be pictured as scattered grains of rice united by being attracted to one another, and it is this power which attracts them and shapes them into a certain form. Both mind and body are made of atoms, the former of mental atoms, the latter of physical atoms; and the power that gathers them and makes them into one body or one mind is magnetic power.

The lack of this power causes all pain, discomfort, and disease; and the development of this power secures health of body and mind. By physical practices the power in the body is developed, and by mental exercises the same power is improved in the mind. It is generally seen that the ill lose their magnetism to a certain extent. A healthy person often seeks to escape from the presence of the ill. It is natural because it is magnetism in a person to which people are attracted, and it is its lack which gives repulsion. This also explains the reason for the attraction of youth and childhood, although in childhood this magnetism is not fully developed. The lack of this is felt in age for the same reason.

In Sufi terms this magnetism is called *quwwat-i maknatis*; and it springs from every atom, physical or mental. It may be called strength or energy. It is a wealth, and just as one can enjoy wealth for a longer time if one is careful with it and another may spend it thoughtlessly following fancies, so can a person do with this magnetism. Either one attracts others or one is attracted to others. In one case one is better off, in the other case one is at a loss. A human being, of whatever evolution, whatever disposition, in whatever condition of life, needs this magnetism most of all things; for health, which is the greatest of all gifts in life, depends greatly on magnetism.

Breathing

In Sanskrit breath is called *prana*, which means "life." This prana, not only gives life to oneself, but it gives life to another person too. Sometimes the presence of someone fills you with life, and sometimes the presence of another, so to speak, takes your life away from you. One feels tired and depressed and eaten up by the presence of one person, and another person's presence gives one added strength, life, and vigor. This is all accounted for by reason of the breath. The one who has more life gives life, while the one who has less life takes it from the one who has more. But there is a contrary process too. Sometimes the stronger one takes away what little life is left in the weaker one, and sometimes the weaker one gives out life to the stronger one. A person who takes life away, in fact, absorbs the life from another. In the presence of that person even flowers fade sooner and plants die.

Many deaths occur and many lives are retained by the phenomenon of the breath. Therefore, for the healer there is no greater source of healing than by means of the breath. The healer can throw breath upon the affected part of the patient as easily as the healer can cast a glance upon a painful part. Even edibles and objects that a healer's breath has magnetized carry with them the power of healing. If touch makes certain marks through perspiration of the fingers upon a thing, why should not the breath, the very essence of life, live in an object and give the object some part of life which could produce in it an effect which may be a greater cure than medicine?

When the breath is developed and purified, it is not necessary for the healer even to make an effort to throw breath upon the patient. But the atmosphere that the healer's breath creates, the very presence of the healer brings about a cure, for the whole atmosphere becomes charged with magnetism.

Insanity

There are, no doubt, many physical causes for the various aspects of insanity, but a keen study of the subject will prove that insanity is mostly due to mental causes. Some lack of balance caused by the intensity or excess of a certain thought and feeling is found to be at the root of every case of insanity. Physicians fail to cure such cases, especially the ones who trace the cause of insanity in its outer manifestations and in the physical body. Every cause has an external effect, and yet it is a mistake to take the effect for the cause. Therefore, it is not generally a medicine or even surgical operations or any external application that can be of great use. It is more the work of a healer than of a physician to cure insanity.

As every disease of insanity could be cured in its earlier stage, it is the work of the healer to recognize the signs of insanity in their primary state, for such signs are not ordinarily noticed in a person, and they are passed over as something "funny" about a person or "queer." The first step in healing insanity is to get at the root of the complaint by association with the subject, and as soon as the root of the complaint is touched a great relief is brought, even before healing. Naturally, insanity being a mental disease, thought power alone is the remedy for it.

Loss of memory, confusion, puzzlement, instantaneous anger, and passion, all these are signs of the beginning of insanity. Insanity is inherited from the family, but it can also be traced to several weaknesses and vices. All of these—drink, and fondness for drugs, and unnatural habits, too much worry, anxiety, and allowing melancholy to develop in the nature—these are the things that cause insanity.

The work of the healer is first to catch the primary cause of insanity, and that is loss of memory. It is caused by weakness of the mind. The mind has not sufficient power to bring forward the thought entrusted to it at the command from within, and this is what may be called loss of memory, and it must be healed and cured in its very beginning. Another primary stage is the extreme activity of mind, which results in extreme thoughtlessness or passion. Then, when its spell is passed, repentance comes. This should be avoided at its beginning. A guilty conscience, fear of consequences, a doubting tendency, and all such things are as fuel to the fire of insanity. A pure, thankful, useful life, a constant thought of appreciating things and avoiding blaming things, people, and conditions—all these help to keep away the germ of insanity.

Spirit

There is a part of one's life which could only be called life. There is no other name appropriate for it, and the English phrase, "to pull oneself together," means to get that part of life to work. This part of life may be called spirit, and this part is both intelligence and power in itself. It is intelligence because any part of the body and mind, or every part of both that it dwells in, it makes sensitive; and it is powerful because whichever part of the body and mind it touches, it strengthens.

In games and sports, when people jump down from a great height, what is it that protects them from being hurt? It is this spirit, for they have made it their habit to call this spirit to their rescue. When people throw balls at each other, and even in boxing, the receiver of the blow awakens this spirit in the part that receives the blow. The sporting person does not know what this spirit is even though taking refuge in it. The mystic understands it by meditation, also by research into metaphysics. When a person awakes from a deep sleep, the first thing that rises through the mind to the body—when the tendency of stretching and contracting, and of twisting and turning, and of opening the eyes comes—is the rise of the spirit. It rises, so to speak, and expands.

By the mastery of this spirit diseases are cured, age is mastered, even death is conquered. When this spirit is lacking, energy is lacking, intelligence is lacking, joy is lacking, rest is lacking. And when this spirit is there, there is hope, there is joy, there is rest, because the nature of this spirit is to hold intact the body of atoms and vibrations. Comfort lies in its being held intact, and discomfort when this spirit is not sufficient to hold one's body intact. Therefore, it is the lack of this spirit in many cases which is the cause of a great many diseases. By the development of this spirit in oneself, the healer can give a part of this spirit to another, and that becomes the best source of healing.

The Origin of Disease

Almost every disease originates in the mind, even in cases of infectious diseases. It does not mean that it must be a wickedness of the mind. If it were so, good people would never have been ill; and yet it cannot be overlooked that it is the weakness of mind, in some way or other, which allows the disease to enter. Besides that, there is negligence, oversight, irregularity—mental and physical—which cause diseases. Life and death are two forces, constructive and destructive; and there is continual fighting between both these forces. And there are times when one power wins, and the success of that power is either better health or death. It is necessary that the body be ready and fit to fight this battle, but mind has a still greater part to perform. And when mind fails to perform its part, the body, with all its fitness, is incapable of retaining health. But if mind is capable of keeping health, the body, to a great extent, obeys it. Still, the harmony and power of both mind and body is needed to fight the battle of life.

The Effects of Food

It is the secret of nature that life lives upon life, and all carnivorous animals live upon the flesh of another animal and sometimes on their own kind. That shows that life sustains the body by the same element that it is made of. The human body is made of the food that one eats, and it is according to the life in the food one eats that one's life develops. Little insects which live on flowers create the beauty of the flower in their body. Insects that are fed on leaves sometimes become green and beautiful like a leaf, but insects living in the earth and in dirt have a similar body to the earth and dirt. This teaches that one's body depends upon the food one eats. Any decay in the vegetables one eats and any disease in the animal whose flesh one uses, all have an effect on one's health.

Brahmins, who have been the most scientific and philosophical people in the world, have always considered this subject; and one always finds in the Brahmins intelligent and superior minds. In the West, although there is continual scientific discovery and discussion on hygiene, there is great oversight in many things concerning food which, in a few words, can be explained as the lack of what may be called home life. Many have to take their food in public places where it is impossible to have a special consideration given to this subject. Among animals, there is a difference; there are some clean animals and others are unclean, and their flesh differs in that way and has a great influence on the health and the mind of a person.

The question as to what mind has to do with bodily food may be answered this way: just as an alcoholic drink has an effect on the mind, so every atom of food has a particular effect. There are three kinds of foods: *sattva*, which gives nourishment with calm and peace; *rajas*, which stimulates one to work and move about; and *tamas*, which gives sleep, laziness, and confusion.

A healer must become aware of all kinds of foods and their effects so as to prescribe for the patient, and to see whether the food is the cause of the illness, which is so in many cases, and to keep the healer in a condition to be able to heal successfully.

Examples of different kinds of food given in answer to a question:

Sattva foods: milk, butter, cereals, fruit.

Rajas foods: vegetables, spices, acids, curry; also tea and coffee.

Tamas foods: alcohol, flesh foods.

Self-Control

There are many people who may be said to be of nervous temperament, who have the tendency if they walk, to walk quickly; if they work, to work with a bustle; if they talk, to talk quickly, so quickly that they may drop words and make the hearer confused; and in a moment, they are up in a temper, inclined to laugh or cry easily. This condition gives a kind of joy in a way, but it weakens one and takes away one's self-control which, in the end, results in nervous disease. It begins as an indulgence in activity and ends in weakness. Many mental diseases are caused by this negative state of mind and body. From childhood there is an inclination to this, especially among children of nervous temperament; and if it can be checked from that time there is a sure result. No disease can be worse than an increasing weakness of nerves, which is the lack of self-control; and life is not worth living when control over the self is lost.

Human Being

One is not only constituted of matter in one's being but also of spirit. However well built a body one may have, with its mechanism in good working order, there is still something that is wanting. For the physical body is sustained by material food and drink, breath by the air, mind by thoughts, imaginations, and impressions; but that is not all. There is something besides mind and body that one possesses in one's being, and that is one's spirit, which is a divine light. It is therefore that sunshine makes one feel bright; but it is not only sunshine that is needed for the spirit. The soul is like a planet, and, as the planet is illuminated by the sun, so one's spirit is illuminated by the light of God. In the absence of this, however healthy and joyful one may look, one is not really healthy. One must have some spiritual touch, some opening in the heart, which will let the light come in, the light of God.

THE DEVELOPMENT OF POWER

The Breath

The breath is the principal power needed in healing. All the different manifestations of the magnetic current which come from the tips of the fingers, from the glance, and from the pores of the body are indirect manifestations of the breath. It is the strength of breath which is magnetic power in all its different aspects. Weakness of breath causes weakness of mind and body, and strength of breath is strength to both. One cannot lack energy and magnetism if one's breath is full of energy. Therefore, before developing any other means of healing, the power of the breath should first be developed.

There are two ways of developing the power of the breath. One way is to make it extensive, and the other way is to make it intensive. After that the breath should be mastered so that it can be directed to any desired part of one's own body; and second, it must be mastered so that it may be directed to any side: level, upward, downward, to the right or to the left. As one becomes master of aim when one is able to hit a target on any side, so one must master the breath.

There are Yogis in India who can put out a light at some distance by the power of the breath. And even the miracle of Tansen, who is said to have lighted candles by the power of his song when he sang the *dipak*, can be nothing else but the power of breath in its fullest development.

97

Purification

Science has always admitted—and values more highly every day—the importance of cleanliness around the patient and on the part of the physician; and things of different kinds have been used as disinfectants in many cases of disease. The healer who has to do more with the mind must, therefore, think how very important it is to consider purity of mind as well as of body for this purpose. No doubt it is difficult, after learning the nature of things, to say which is pure and which is impure. There is one way of understanding, and it is that everything in itself is pure, but when another element is mixed with it, then its purity is polluted. Deep thought in this direction would open a vast field of thought to a thinker.

Another way of understanding the pure and impure is that there is one thing alone that keeps things pure, and that is life; and when the life is gone out of them they are impure. There is a third way of looking at it: that death is impurity of things, but destruction is their purity. This also opens a vast scope of understanding to an observant student of life.

In short, it is necessary for a healer to observe the laws of hygienic life and to keep from partaking the germs of disease from the patients that are healed. Besides this, one should avoid all thoughts of bitterness, ill will, wrath, anger, jealousy, and purify one's mind from every spite or malice, and bathe, so to speak, in devotion to God, so that one's heart may become saturated with mercy and compassion. It is not only the power of mind that heals, but also the purity of mind. The mind free from all crookedness, deceit, treachery, is alone capable of emitting power, strong and pure in its nature, which can give to a patient a new life and relief from all pain.

Rhythm

The development of healing power depends upon the development of the breath. The breath can be developed by purification, by extension, by expansion, and by rhythm.

There are three different kinds of rhythm in the breath: first, the rhythm which cannot be distinguished in the continuation of inhalation and exhalation; second, the rhythm that can be distinguished by the two distinct swings of inhaling and exhaling; and third, evenness in breathing. Those who have not mastered their breath are under the influence of these three rhythms in their health, their mood, and their condition in life. But those who master the breath can put their breath in any of these rhythms; and when mastery is acquired then the healer has the key to wind any clock.

In reality, every disease means something is wrong with the rhythm. As a doctor says congestion is the root of diseases, so to a Sufi, congestion means lack of rhythm; it may be a lack in the circulation, in breathing, in activity, or in repose. A physician, in order to find a disease, examines the pulse, the beats of the heart, and the condition of the lungs. This itself is the proof that rhythm is the keeper of health. And when there is something wrong with the health, the rhythm, in some way or other, has gone wrong, as when the tick of the clock gets out of rhythm the clock goes too fast or too slow and it does not give the proper time.

The healer, therefore, must get the healer's own rhythm right, so that the healer may be able to work on the mechanism of another person's body. In India there is a custom of clapping the hands or snapping the fingers when somebody is yawning. The idea is that yawning is the sign of the falling of the rhythm. It is the rhythm of one's body that falls to a slower rate when one feels inclined to sleep, and the clapping of the hands and the snapping of the fingers set the pulsations of the other person in the same rhythm as before. It is just like shaking a person who is nodding, to bring the mechanism of that person's body to its proper working order.

The healer who is capable of regulating the healer's own rhythm, in turn becomes capable of making another person's rhythm regular also. This requires great knowledge and inspiration concerning the nature of the human mind and body. The healer who knows rhythm and knows how to work with it, is like the conductor in the orchestra. The health of everyone that is healed is kept regular, as the conductor keeps the rhythm of every musician who plays in the orchestra.

The Power of the Breath

It is the power of the breath that heals body and mind, since breath is life; and through the breath, life can be imparted to the mind and body of a patient. The breath is also a cord that runs through human beings, connecting them in one life. If it were not for the breath, the senses would never have perceived the external world. Therefore, all that one sees, smells, tastes, and hears is through the channel of the breath, and therefore no medicine can have such influence on a patient as the breath. Weak breath is susceptible to all contagious diseases, and a healer with weak breath could get the disease from a patient in one healing. Therefore, power of breath is the most essential thing before one should attempt to heal.

Power of breath can be developed in two forms: volume and length, which make it intensive and extensive. It is dangerous to try healing before one is fully sure of the power of the breath in both ways. The development of the power of the breath is felt, and one knows when one is ready to use it in healing.

One Common Cause of All Diseases

All pain, discomfort, disease, decay, and destruction of every sort are from a lack of life. The word *life* which we use in everyday language is the name of the result of two activities working harmoniously: one is the constant life of the spirit; the other the life that matter provides for it. There is a negative and a positive activity. It is the power of inner life which attracts outer life to it, and it is the strength of external life by which it clings to the inner life. In this way the reciprocal action of both keeps the flame of life burning, and the lack of either of these activities is the cause of disease.

There are five bodies through which the soul experiences life, the physical body being the poorest of all, for it is born of matter, fed with matter, attracted to matter, finds its life in matter, and has its return to matter. As it demands matter for its sustenance, so matter demands it in the end. This demand is called disease or death, when this body loses its strength by the loss of energy of the nerves, which, so to speak, pull together and keep the flesh, bone, blood, and skin not only intact but active and vigorous. It is the weakening of these nerves by exhaustion or by lack of sustenance or by lack of rest or by loss of energy, in whatever manner, which is the cause of all disease.

Therefore healing, in other words, may be called life-giving to that part that wants life, or to the body as a whole. The materialist believes that a person, however weak, could be saved and brought to life by injecting into that person's body the blood of another. If that be a successful remedy, how much more could the power of thought, of life, which has more power than matter, produce life in another! And even the fine essence of the [healer's] physical body may be passed through gases by the process of earth rising to water, water to fire, fire to air, air to ether—sending the finest atoms of physical energy and strengthening vibrations of mental energy to a person who needs it. The difference between medicine and healing is this: instead of sending a thing by railway train, it is sent through the sky by an airplane.

The question of whether it is worthwhile weakening oneself by giving part of one's life to another may be answered by saying that, of course, it would not do for a poor person to give a last penny to one who is starving, but it is the only thing for a rich person to do, to make use of riches for the comfort and happiness of those who are in need. A spiritual healer is rich with divine strength, and this healer's power will not be lessened if given out. Therefore material healing is a failure, however successful it may seem. It is powerless compared with spiritual healing, because on the side of the spiritual healer there is the power of God.

The Development of Power in the Fingertips

The human form may be called materialized light, the symbol of which in mysticism is the five-pointed star, which suggests the head, arms, and feet, which make five points. The nature of light is to spread its rays, and as the human form is made of light, the hands and the feet and the fingers and the toes and the organs of the senses and the hair all represent rays. It is the knowledge of this light that one sees in the Eastern custom of blessing with the tips of the fingers on the head, and of kissing the hand or touching the feet, for the fingers and toes are the source of the radiance.

The healer, therefore, develops the power of the fingertips. As by directing the breath in a certain direction through the body and mouth one can produce a certain pitch in a certain note, so by directing the energy through the fingertips and by developing the magnetic power of the fingertips one develops the power of healing. Moses is known to have possessed a light in his palm, which the poets call *yad-i baiza*. *Baiza* means "egg," "the form of an egg in the palm." And Zoroaster is always pictured with burning fire in his hand. Both suggest the radiance, the battery that can be developed in the human hand. When the power is developed in the palm, it pours out from the tips of the fingers and it shoots out when it is directed by the will. Then, by magnetic passes and by touch on the painful part, the healer is able to cure disease.

The Power of the Presence

It must be understood by the healer, that the healer's very presence must emit healing power. And in order to do this the healer must have overflowing life, power, and magnetism. In the first place, the body must be healthy, clean, and pure so that physical magnetism may be beneficial. Also purity of mind is necessary, together with sympathy for the patient and a desire to cure the patient instead of profiting by the cure. The soul speaks most in the form of the atmosphere; in other words, the atmosphere tells what the soul says. The development of the soul is brought about by a spiritual presence and a spiritual life. Therefore, the development of the mind, of the body, and of the soul is necessary in order to possess a healing power and presence.

The Power of the Mind

The power of concentration is the first thing necessary to develop healing power. The healer must be able to steadily hold the thought for the cure of a patient whenever this is required. Concentration is the most difficult thing, and if this is accomplished, there is nothing that one cannot accomplish. It is useless to try and cure the patient by any process, however successful and good it may be, if there is no power of concentration.

The work of the mind in healing is much greater than in anything else, for it is using the power of the mind on matter. And matter, which has been a disobedient slave of the spirit for ages through the mineral kingdom, through the vegetable kingdom, and even through the animal kingdom, always rebels against being controlled. No doubt mind can control matter and do with it whatever it likes, but when mind is enfeebled by serving matter it, so to speak, loses power over matter. If it were not so, everyone should cure oneself by controlling matter, and there would be no need of a healer. One's own power has a greater influence upon oneself than the power of another, and no one can feel so much sympathy as one can for oneself.

The nature of the mind is to slip from one's grip. Concentration is the practice which enables the mind and strengthens its fingers to hold fast to that which it may hold. Another secret of the mind is that, even with the power of concentration, the mind does not hold anything that is not interesting. And it is

sympathy in the mind which is a stimulus to the holding power
of the mind. Therefore no one can be a successful healer unless
one's sympathy comes forward with its hands extended to raise
the patient from pain.

The Power of Concentration

It is necessary that before one attempts to heal another, one
must develop in oneself the power of concentration. The concentration of a healer should be so developed that not only
when sitting in meditation and closing the eyes can the healer
visualize the desired object, but even with eyes open the healer
should hold fast to the picture that the mind has created in
spite of all things standing before the eyes.

In healing it is necessary to know what one should hold before one's mind. If the healer happens to hold the picture of a
wound, the healer would help the wound to continue instead
of being healed; and if the healer thought of pain, it might
perhaps be continued more intensely by the help of the healer's
thought. It is the cure that the healer should hold in mind. It
is the desired thing that the healer must think about, not the
condition.

In all things in life this rule must be considered: that even in
trouble one must not think about the trouble, and in illness
one must forget about the illness. A person often continues
life's miseries by giving thought to them. The healer must, from
beginning to end, hold the thought of cure and nothing else.

Sending Power to a Distance

The greater development in healing power is to be able to send
power over a distance. Neither land nor sea can prevent power
sent by the mind. Scientific discoveries such as wireless telegraphy prove that, by means of objects, thoughts can be sent over
a distance; but the mystic has always realized and practiced, to
a great extent, the sending of thought over a distance. As the
whole idea of a mystic is to serve humanity by love and good-

ness, the mystic naturally does not feel inclined either to prove to the world the greatness of the mystic's power or to utilize this power for any worldly thing except healing.

Hindu metaphysics says that *Nada Brahma*, meaning "sound-God," explains the secret of life: that sound is motion, and, therefore, nothing takes place unless it was moved by some force behind it. As for external action a physical movement is necessary, so for a mental action the motion must be caused by mind. As the voice of one person may reach to the other corner of the room, and the voice of another may reach to the other end of the street, so it is with the power of the mind. As it is necessary to develop the power of the voice by practice, so it is necessary to develop and practice the power of the mind. It must be remembered that a gift is necessary in all cases. A gifted person may progress much further and more quickly than a person without the gift.

There are three other things necessary in sending thought over a distance: first, faith in the theory; second, self-confidence, meaning confidence in one's own power; the third thing is the power of concentration. However great the power of concentration may be, without self-confidence it is of no use; and self-confidence without faith in the theory is powerless. Healing at a distance is the last stage at which a healer arrives after a long time's experience in healing; and for anyone to attempt this at the beginning it would naturally result in failure. Work gives experience, and experience gives confidence; and faith becomes firm when it is built by experience and strengthened by confidence.

THE APPLICATION OF HEALING POWER

Healing by Charms

There is a great power hidden in the mystery of the repetition of a sacred word. But there is a still greater power in writing a sacred word, because the time taken to write a sacred word carefully is perhaps five times or ten times as long as the time taken in speaking a sacred word. Besides that, action finishes thought power better than speech. In writing a sacred name it is the completing of a thought, which is even more powerful than uttering the word. But when a person thinks, feels, speaks, and writes, that person has developed the thought through four stages and made it powerful.

Sufis, therefore, give a charm to the faithful whom, they think, believe in the healing power of the charm. They call it *taviz*. The patients keep it close night and day, link their thought with the thought of the healer, and feel at every moment that they are being healed.

In India they put a charm in a silver or gold plate, or keep a charm engraved on stone or metal. And the very fact of realizing that they possess something in the form of a charm that has a healing influence upon them becomes such a help to the believers that they feel that every moment of the day and night they have the healer with them, and that they are being healed.

A gift is nothing without a giver, so a charm is nothing without a personality that gives confidence to the patient. Therefore, a charm written by any person has no effect; the personality of

106

the person who writes the charm should be impressive. That person's piety, spirituality, love, kindness, all should help the charm that is given, to make it valuable and effective.

Magnetized Water

Water is the most responsive substance, partaking of the color and effect of everything. The magnetism that runs through the fingertips enters into everything that a healer holds in the hands, and thus water can be charged with that electricity more than any other substance. Again, the breath that heals is powerful enough to produce an added life in all life-giving substances. Water especially, which is a most invigorating substance, partakes of that life from the breath.

Among the ancient Hindus there was a custom of giving water as a benediction to guests, which is observed even now. A Brahmin will, as a rule, first offer a guest water, which means not only to quench the thirst, but is like giving life to the guest. The Persians have called the water of life *ab-i hayat*, and in many verses one finds this word. The sacrament of the Catholic Church also has this secret behind it. It is the healing power or the life that the priest is supposed to have by his divine contemplation. He imparts it to the others by the substance, the bread or wine, that he holds. Among Sufis everywhere in the East, there is a custom that the sheikh gives a loaf of bread or a glass of water, milk, syrup, or buttermilk, or a fruit or some sweet, which is accepted as something that heals both mind and body. No doubt it is not only the effect of the breath or touch, but also it has the power of mind with it, which is hidden as a soul in the substance which is its body.

Healing by Breathing

A healer must know in the first place that breath is the very life, and breath is the giver of life, and breath is the bringer of life. One can live without food for some time, but one cannot live without breath even for a few minutes. This shows that the sustenance that breath brings to a person's life is much greater and much more important than any nourishment upon earth. Every atom of the body is radiant, but if the body is the flame, the breath is the fire. And as the flame belongs to fire, so the body belongs to breath; as long as breath dwells in it, it lives, and when breath leaves it, it is dead—for all its beauty, strength, and complicated mechanism. Therefore, the effect of the breath of a holy person can magnetize water, it can magnetize bread, it can magnetize milk or wine, fruit or flower.

The breath that is developed spiritually will have a healing effect upon any painful part that it falls upon. If one knows how to direct the breath, there is no better process than healing with breath; and in all the different methods of healing, breath is the main thing, since in breath is hidden the current of life.

Healing by Magnetic Passes

All scriptures have explained, in some way or other, that life is like light. In the Muslim scriptures the word *nur* is used; in the Vedanta it is called *chaitanya*. The nature of this light is to express itself in a particular direction, and that accounts for the face and back in our forms. At the same time the tendency of the light is to spread. This can be seen in the tendency of fire to spread and of water to spread; air shows the same tendency, and earth and all things on earth show the same tendency. A deep study of every form will show this nature of life to spread in four directions, which make north, south, east, and west, and from head to foot, right and left.

Life and light have a center in the center of every form, but they express themselves through the directions in which they spread. Therefore the power of the hand has been shown in the ancient symbology. Hindus have pictured divine incarnations with four hands. This means two hands of the mind and two hands of the body. When the four hands work, the work is fully accomplished; therefore, in healing the hands are most import-ant. The physical hands are needed to help the hands of the mind, and when thought is directed from the mind through the hands, its power becomes double and its expression becomes fuller.

Every atom of a human being, mental or physical, is radiant and throws its rays outward, which is life itself and gives life. All illness and every kind of illness is, so to speak, lack of life; and it needs life to be given to it. The power of electricity has been discovered by scientists, and they believe that it cures diseases when it is used for that purpose. But the mystic discovered ages ago the power of this hidden electricity, the life of the mind and the life of the body; and the mystic believes and knows that its application in healing is most beneficial. There are sores and wounds and painful parts which are too tender to touch. In such cases healing by magnetic passes, in other words, by waving the hands over the affected part and so allowing thought to heal, brings about a successful cure.

Healing by Touch

Every atom of a human body is in reality radiant, living, and powerful compared with other objects, herbs, or drugs. By the very fact of being a living body, besides being the finest and most perfect compared to other living bodies, it has a great power. Therefore, shaking hands, speaking to a person by touching that person have a certain effect. In India when a wrestler goes to a wrestling match, and when he comes back, his teacher pats him on the back, saying, "*Shabash!* Bravo!" In fact, this gives him added strength and courage and power, which otherwise he would not have had. People speaking in friendship, even in disputing and arguing, hold each other's hands, which brings about a better understanding. Discomfort and restlessness are taken away by the mother in one moment by patting the child. Therefore, massage is helpful when there is pain, and yet it is as a dead treatment when compared to the healing treatment; for the healer operates the power of the mind through the fingers, as a musician reproduces feelings on the violin. Is it everybody that can produce on the violin the same tone that an expert could? It is not the placing of the fingers on a certain place on the instrument, but it is the feeling of the musician's heart manifesting through the fingers that produces a living tone. So it is with the touch of a spiritual healer.

Healing by the Glance

The eye is the most wonderful and powerful factor in the body, conveying to another pleasure or displeasure, joy or sorrow, love or hatred, without a word being spoken. This shows that the eye is the most responsive instrument for the mind to express thought and feeling. Sometimes in an assembly two people can just look at each other and there is agreement between them. And then again two people may stare at each other, which may have a worse effect than shooting, and which again shows that fire and water, both, can manifest either to destroy or to inspire.

To a healer, therefore, there is no better means than the eyes to send the thought of healing; and there is no better means of receiving the healer's thought in the patient than the eyes. The healer can send the healing power through the glance to the painful part of the body, but it is more helpful when the healer sends power directly to the eyes of the patient. As there is a link between the mind and the eyes of the healer who sends the power, so there is a link between the eyes and the mind of the patient who receives it. Medicine can touch the physical body, but thought can touch the mind, which often is the root of every disease; and a suggestion that a powerful healer gives to a patient reaches the patient's heart and destroys the germ of disease.

The eyes of every person are not capable of healing. It is the penetrating glance and stillness of the eyes, and then the power of the glance and ability to aim that are necessary. These things are developed by certain exercises. Of course, some eyes have a natural ability for this purpose. Besides this, concentration of the mind, which gives power, is necessary in healing, for power of mind, directed by the glance, brings about a successful result.

Healing by Suggestion

There are five elements that constitute a human being: earth, water, fire, air, and ether. Air represents the voice and it reaches the ether, which means that the voice reaches farther than anything else in the world. It touches the depths of the human heart. Therefore, music is a living miracle; there is nothing that can thrill one's being through and through as sound can. This explains why suggestion is much greater and more beneficial in healing than any other remedy.

In India, where the daily life of the people is based upon psychic laws, they take great care in speaking to another person that it may not make a bad effect upon that person's physical, mental, or spiritual self. Healers who, by the power of zikr, develop healing power in the voice, impress their words with the power of their hearts on the heart of the patient.

Healers must be sincere in their suggestions, because all the power lies in their sincerity; they must also be self-confident; they must have psychic power developed in themselves; but beyond and above all they must be good human beings, so that at the time of healing no thought of humiliation or of any sort of discomfort should come to them. Their thoughts, feelings, and actions should be satisfactory to their consciences; if not, any discomfort, dissatisfaction, fear, or repentance weakens their power. Then they are no longer capable of healing, however learned and powerful they may be. When healers think they are healing, their power is as small as a drop. When they think God is healing, and when from this thought their own selves are forgotten and they are only conscious of the self of God, then their power becomes as large as the ocean.

Healing by Presence

There is warmth in fire, and there is a greater warmth in feeling. The presence of a person with warm feelings can create an atmosphere of warmth, and the presence of the cold-hearted can freeze one. No doubt warmth of heart is not the only quality the healer needs. The healer must have the power to heal, in addition to concentration and a desire to heal. But at the same time it is the name of Christ that is known as that of the Messiah. *Messiah*, in the East, means "healer," and for a messiah the power of love is the first quality, love in the form of sympathy. One sympathizes with another, thinking perhaps, "This person is my relation, friend, or acquaintance." But when sympathy develops to its fullest extent one begins to see in everybody "I," "myself," and the pain of everybody one begins to feel as one's own pain. This is a sign of a true messiah.

How can one heal the wounds of the hearts of the children of the earth and relieve them from pain and suffering, since life is full of them, when one's sympathy is not awakened to such a degree that one feels the pain of another even before feeling one's own pain? Every healer who has a spiritual aspiration must develop the spark of the fire of the heart of the Messiah; and then, even before trying to heal a person, one's very presence would heal. When a child is ill the mother goes near with the wish that it may be well, with a pain in her heart for the suffering of her child. For that moment she becomes a healer; her touch, her word, and her glance do more than medicine or any other remedy. When this mother quality is developed in the heart of the healer, when one heals not for any return except the happiness of seeing a soul released from pain, one becomes a healer who can heal merely by one's presence.

Healing by Prayer

Prayer is a wonderful means of healing oneself and another, for concentration only, without the thought of God, is powerless. It is the divine ideal which strengthens the healing power, which gives it a living spirit, and therefore, a spiritual healer has more hope of success than a material healer. For the material healer directs the material healer's own thought; however powerful it may be it is limited by the material healer's own personality. But the spiritual healer, who in the thought of God and God's divine power forgets the self, has much greater success than the former. It does not matter what form one has in one's prayer; sincere prayer in every form will bring a fruitful result.

Prayer, truly speaking, is the contemplation of God's presence—who is the power and origin of the whole creation—and considering oneself as nothing before God and placing the wish which stands before one's personality before the Almighty. Therefore, naturally, the result must be incomparably greater though it depends upon the contemplation of each individual.

In the first place, the one who prays for the cure of another must surely be blessed, because the goodwill and love from which one's prayer rises, of necessity, bring a blessing to one's own self. Also praying for one's own cure is not selfish; it is making oneself a fitting instrument to be more useful in the scheme of life. On the other hand, neglect of one's own health very often is a crime. Praying to God in thought is perhaps better than in speech, but it must be remembered that speech makes it concrete. Therefore, thought with speech makes prayer more effective than thought alone, and of course, words without thought are vain repetitions.

Absent Healing

When a healer has practiced healing for a certain time successfully, then the next step in the line of healing is to heal a patient from a distance. The method of absent healing is totally different from that of healing in someone's presence. In absent healing the power of thought alone is necessary, and those who are accustomed to use magnetism through the tips of the fingers, through the eyes, through the touch, find it difficult to direct their thought power without an external channel. Also when the patient is not present, in the first place the thought comes to a beginner whether one's thought power will reach the patient who is not present.

The mastery of *fikr* helps a healer to hold the thought of the patient before the healer's mind, and it is *fikr* that helps to heal a patient from a distance. Breath is, so to speak, an electric current that can be attached anywhere; distance makes no difference. A current of breath so established puts the ethereal waves in space into motion and, according to the healer's magnetic power, the space between the healer and the patient becomes occupied with a running current of healing power. No doubt spiritual evolution is the first thing necessary, for without this the mind power of a healer, however strong, is too feeble for the purpose.

By spiritual development is meant God-consciousness. There is a believer in God who may be called pious, but it is the God-conscious who become spiritual. It is the belief and realization that: "I do not exist, but God," which gives power to the healer to heal from a distance. Also it is this realization that gives a belief that one's thought can reach to any distance, because the knowledge of the all-pervading God gives the knowledge that the Absolute is life in itself, and even the space, which means nothing to the average person, is everything. In fact, it is the very life of all things.

VARIOUS METHODS OF HEALING

The Origin of Healing

Consciously or unconsciously, every being is capable of healing itself or others. This instinct is inborn in insects, birds, and beasts, as well as in humankind. All these find their own medicine and heal themselves and each other in various ways. In the ancient days the doctors and healers learned much from the animals in the treatment of disease. This shows that natural instinct has manifested in the lower creation as well as in the higher. The scientists of today may not, therefore, claim with pride that they are the inventors of chemical remedies, but may humbly bow the head in prayer, seeing that each atom of this universe, conscious of its sickness, procures for itself from within or without a means for its restoration. In other words, medicines were not discovered by physicians, but only instinctively found in creation as the necessity for them appeared.

The excess of humanity's artificial remedies has had the effect of increasing disease. This is also mainly due to the modern artificial way of life, so different from the natural living of the ancients which is today ridiculed by so-called civilization. Thus, the luxuries and needs of life are obtained at the sacrifice of true health and comfort.

Healing without drugs and medicines is the most natural thing, although the absolute neglect of them is inadvisable. There are cases in which the tools of surgery are also permissible, but only when absolutely necessary. If the engine can move the wagons, why should horses be used? In the same way, if a disease can be cured by a simple remedy, mental power should not be wasted, for it may be used in a more serious case. If every malady were to be healed mentally, why then were all drugs and herbs created? On the other hand, diseases which will yield more easily to mental treatment should not be left entirely to material remedies, for their root must first be healed. So many patients temporarily recover by the help of medicines and again become sick, and in such cases healing is especially needed. It is much to be deplored that such important work as healing has in the present age been undertaken by people who are in many cases most materially minded and do not understand its psychology, making a profession of it and thus bringing discredit upon it.

Self-healing is more desirable than healing by others; the former strengthens the will, the latter weakens it. Many people think that hypnotic and psychic power alone can heal, but they do not realize how the healers must first heal themselves by the practice of the strictest morality, from the lowest to the highest phase of their existence. They must purify themselves by *iman*, or confidence. Then alone can they claim to be healers.

There are five kinds of diseases caused by various disorders in different planes of existence. Some diseases in the physical plane are contracted from without, while others spring from within. There are several supposed causes, but in reality the true cause of disease is weakness, while the cause of health is strength. Thereby is not meant physical weakness or strength only, but strength and weakness on all planes of existence. Activity causes what is called life, while the reverse brings about death. The former causes circulation and the latter congestion. Circulation gives health, while congestion causes disease.

The scientists of today are giving electrical treatment as a comparatively new discovery, and it is proved to be the most beneficial of all remedies. Healing is also electrical treatment and has been given throughout the different planes of life for ages. Every being has a natural gift of healing in a greater or less degree, but it may be developed. The physical and mental faculties should be opened out in such a way that the electric vibrations in the various planes of existence may be enabled to operate.

Physical vibrations depend upon the purity and energy of the body, and they can be projected through the finer organs, such as the palms of the hands, the tips of the fingers, the soles of the feet, the tongue, the cheek, the forehead, the ear, the lips, nose, and eyes. The finest of all these is the eye; it is much more useful than all the other organs, for it is through the eyes that the electric rays can be emitted. The nose has also an important part to perform, it being the very channel of breath. The ears can work when the healer is spiritually advanced; and the vibrations can also pass through the tips of the fingers.

The Oriental custom of placing the eyes upon the holy hands or feet of the sage is not only expressive of humility, but it has a still greater meaning. It signifies the healing by the holy hands or feet which illuminate the devout.

The sages who bless those aspiring souls by placing their hands upon the head inspire them by sending forth the rays of their power through the fingertips. In kissing the hands or feet of the holy ones, the Orientals have the same object in view. In the same way the caress of the mother heals the child of all its pain and soothes it to sleep. Courage and consolation is given to another by placing the hands on that person's shoulders; the vibrations in this action give a new life and courage.

Physical Healing

Patients can be healed only if they have sufficient faith in the power of healing and confidence in the healer. In the case of self-healing, self-confidence, the power of breath, and concentration are most necessary. There is a well-known story told among Sufis that Shams-i Tabriz, the Shiva of Persia, was once most respectfully entreated by the priests of the day to awaken the crown prince from his last long sleep. The shah, his father, issued a decree that if there was any truth at all in religion his only son must be restored to life by prayer, otherwise all the mosques should be destroyed and the mullahs be put to the sword.

In order to save many lives Shams-i Tabriz complied with their request and sought the dead body of the prince. He first said to the dead body of the prince, "*Kun bismillah*," "Awake at the call of God." The dead body did not move. He then, under the spell of ecstasy, exclaimed, "*Kun bismi*," "Arise at my command." At this suggestion the prince immediately arose. The story goes on to relate that this abrupt command, although it restored the prince to life, brought the charge of the claim of Godhead upon Shams-i Tabriz, and according to the religious law, he was condemned to be flayed alive. He gladly submitted to this punishment in order to keep religion intact, as it is the only means of governing the masses.

By this we understand that Shams-i Tabriz in his first suggestion to the dead spoke conventionally, entreating God as a third person, which had not the slightest effect on the dead body. But in his next command, he lost his individual self from his consciousness and felt himself to be the whole Being of God. This story makes it clear that healers must be confident of their at-one-ment with God, and during the time of healing they should most assuredly feel the power of the Almighty working through them, thus absolutely losing the thought of an individual self.

The electric battery which heals is recharged in three ways:
1. By controlling the breath
2. By strengthening the will
3. By absorbing the electricity of the sphere

In order to make use of the healing battery, it is most essential that the eyes should be made to work as projecting electricity. They must be first cured of their nervousness, that ever-moving condition to which they are addicted from birth. The eyes are naturally weakened and tired by being allowed to respond from morning to night to every attraction which invites their attention. The healer, in order to make use of them for healing, first trains them to be steady. The electricity can be absorbed by striking, with the fingers, the finer vibrations in space, and it can be discharged in the same way, by slowly passing the tips of the fingers in the space above the affected part of the patient's body.

Sometimes passing the fingers closer to the body and sometimes slightly touching the affected part is helpful. It depends upon the intensity of pain suffered by the patient and the amount of electricity required. It is very necessary that each time the fingers have passed over the affected part, they should be shaken in order to disperse the poisons collected there—in other words, that the poisonous germs collected on the fingers may be thrown away. It is advisable to shake the fingers over a fire so that the germs may not be left on the floor, and also to have incense burning in the room. Some healers, in order to protect the fingers, make use of peacock feathers, which sweep away all such germs.

Healers can test their healing power by feeling the electric current running through their fingers as they shake them. Healers, even when playing an instrument, can heal their listeners with their music. If their fingers touch either food or drink it becomes a sacrament, powerful to heal. If the healer gives a gift with a good wish it brings good luck, and if the healer writes a word it becomes a charm, a healing in itself, which heals the possessor and keeps that person free from death and disaster.

Mental Healing

Mental healing is performed by suggestion. Mostly parents are the first healers, for they convey their thought to the child by the knitting of the brow or the looking at the child fixedly. Even the animals can be trained in the same way.

There are many diseases of the human mind produced by self-consciousness. They develop unconsciously, and are such as love of praise and flattery, intolerance of insult, irritability, infatuation, jealousy, anger, passion, and greed, besides the craving for alcohol and drugs. In order to cure such diseases healers must first have a great control over themselves, for their own shortcomings may keep the patient back.

The Holy Prophet was once requested by an aged woman to speak to her son, who spent all his daily wage on dates, leaving her penniless. The Prophet promised to do so after five weeks' interval. On the appointed day the boy was brought before the Prophet, who spoke to him very kindly, saying, "You are such a sensible lad that you ought to remember that your mother has endured much suffering for your sake, sacrificing all her wages in order to bring you up. And now she is so old and you are in a position to support her, you are squandering your money on dates. Is this just or right? I hope, by the grace and mercy of Allah, you will give up this habit."

The boy listened very attentively and profited by what he heard. The disciples of the Prophet wondered and asked why the reproof was delayed for thirty-five days. The Holy Prophet explained saying, "I myself am fond of dates, and I felt as if I had no right to advise the lad to abstain from them until I had myself refrained from eating them for five weeks." Healers of character should never for a single moment try to heal others of weaknesses to which they themselves are addicted.

Spiritual Healing

Spiritual healing is still higher in its nature than either of the former. It can be performed by a single being just as well as by a group of people. In this case the heart of the healer can send forth its feelings as vibrations, and in accordance with their intensity the subject is healed. In absent spiritual healing the desire spreads forth its rays and reaches the patient wherever the patient may be, curing the patient without the presence of the healer. The concentration of several people united together works still more wonderfully.

The power of the healer depends upon the warmth of the heart. Devotees by their power of concentration and by their purity of life and by their divine love become wonderful healers. Their every tear and sigh becomes a source of healing for themselves and those around them. Devotion is the fire in which all infirmities are consumed, and devotees become illuminated within themselves. And the joy of devotees and their pain cannot possibly be compared with any other joy of life.

Spiritual healing does not require the fixed gaze; the touch of the fingers, or the power of breath, and *tawajjeh* (a kind glance) or *du'a* (a good thought) of the healer serves the purpose.

Abstract Healing

In abstract healing, the soul, heart, and body are healed of all diseases and weaknesses therein. This healing is only possible during the ecstasy of the healer. The strong psychical vibrations which run through the pores of the healer's body from the healer's inner self naturally pierce through the bodies, hearts, and souls of all around the healer, who receive them in accordance with their power of receptivity. Murshids have frequently inspired their murids without reading or discussing, and such murids have reached perfection. It is a wonderful phenomenon which an exceptional murid once in a while experiences under the guidance of a murshid.

There is a story told of Hafiz Shirazi, who, together with ten other *huffaz*, was being trained under the same murshid. A certain time was set apart for their meditation and other practices, and a certain time for food and sleep. Hafiz Shirazi kept awake during the night in rapt contemplation of Allah. After years of patient waiting, one evening the murshid, in ecstasy, called for Hafiz.

The wakeful Hafiz was the only one who heard, and he answered the call and was blessed by the murshid, who chose this ideal time to inspire all his murids. Each time he called for Hafiz, the same Hafiz answered the call, all the others being

121

asleep. So the wakeful one received an elevenfold blessing—his own and that of the ten others who lost this precious opportunity by their sleep. And Hafiz became the greatest spiritual healer of his time, whose every word from that day to this has been powerful to heal.

MENTAL PURIFICATION

MENTAL PURIFICATION

While speaking on mental purification, I should say that as much as it is necessary that the body is cleansed and purified, so is it necessary— or perhaps more necessary— that the mind is cleansed and purified.[1] All impurities cause disease as well as irregularity in the working of the physical system. It is the same thing with the mind. There are impurities which belong to the mind which also cause different diseases, and by cleansing the mind one helps to create health in both body and mind. By health I mean the natural condition. And what is spirituality? To be spiritual means to be natural, yet very few think so. So many think to be spiritual means to be able to work wonders, to be able to see strange things, wonderful phenomena. And very few know how simple it is, that to be spiritual means to be natural.

Mental purification, therefore, can be done in three different ways. The first way is the stilling of the mind, because it is the action of mind which very often produces impurities. The stilling of the mind displaces impurities in it. It is like tuning the mind to its natural pitch. Mind is likened to a pool of water. If the water in the pool is undisturbed, the reflection is clear. And so it is with the mind. If the mind is disturbed, you do not get intuition and inspiration clear in it. Once the mind is still, it takes a clear reflection as a pool of water does when the water in the pool is still.

1 Lecture, Sufi Center, San Francisco, February 19, 1926.

This condition is brought about by the practice of physical repose. By sitting in a certain posture, a certain effect is created. Mystics had, in their science, different ways of sitting in silence; and each way has a certain significance. And it is not only an imaginary significance: it produces a certain result. I had, personally and through other persons, many experiences of this question of how a certain way of sitting changes the attitude of mind. And the ancient people knew this, and they found different ways for different persons to sit. There was the warrior's way, the student's way, the way of the meditative person, the way of the businessperson, of the laborer, of the lawyer, of the judge, of the inventor. Imagine the mystic knowing this for ages and having the experience of this for thousands of years—the fact that sitting in a certain posture has a great effect on a person, especially on the person's mind. We experience it in our everyday life, but we do not think about it. We happen to sit in a certain way and feel restless. And we happen to sit in a certain way, and we feel peaceful. A certain position makes us feel inspired, another way gives enthusiasm, and still another way of sitting makes us feel unenergetic, with no enthusiasm. By stilling the mind with the help of a certain posture, one is able to purify it.

The second way of purifying the mind is the way of breathing. It is very interesting for an Eastern person to see how sometimes those in the West, in their inventions, apply those principles unknown to them in mystical realms. They have got a machine which sweeps carpets, which sucks up the dust. It is the same system inside out. The proper way of breathing sucks up the dust from the mind and pushes it out. The scientist goes so far saying that a person exhales [carbon dioxide]; the bad gasses are thrown out by exhaling. The mystic goes further, saying not only from the body but also from the mind. If one knows how to do it, one can throw out more than one can imagine. Impurities of mind can be thrown out by the right way of breathing; therefore, mystics combine breathing with posture. Posture helps the stilling of mind, breathing helps the cleansing of mind. Therefore, these two things go together.)

And the third way of purifying the mind is by attitude, by right attitude toward life. That is the moral way and the royal road to purification. A person may breathe and sit in silence with a thousand postures, but if one does not have the right attitude toward life, one will never develop. That is the principal thing. And one might ask, "What is the right attitude?" The right attitude is this: it depends on how favorably one regards one's own shortcomings, for most often one is ready to defend oneself in one's faults and errors. And very often, even knowing that something is a shortcoming, a fault, one is ready to defend oneself and is willing to make one's wrong right. But one does not take that attitude toward others. One takes them to task when it comes to judging them. It is so easy to disapprove of others. It is so easy to take a step further and to dislike others, and not at all difficult to go a step further and to hate others. And while one is acting in this manner, one does not think one is doing any wrong. It is a condition that develops within, but one only sees it without. All the bad that accumulates within, one sees in another person. Therefore, one is always in an illusion, always pleased with oneself and always blaming another. And the most wonderful thing is this: that it is the one who is most blameworthy who blames the most. But it can be said in the other way: that the one who blames most becomes most blameworthy.

There is beauty in form, in color, in line, in manner, in character; and in some persons it is lacking, in other persons it is more. And it is only the comparison that makes us think that this person is better than the other. If we did not compare, then every person would be good. It is the comparison that makes us think one thing more beautiful than the other, but if we looked better, we would see the beauty that is in that thing. Very often our comparison is not right for the very fact that what we determine today in our mind as good and beautiful, we are liable to change that conception within a month's or a year's time. That shows us when we look at something, we are capable of appreciating it if that beauty manifests to our view.

There is nothing to be surprised at when one arrives at a stage that one says, "All that I see in this world, it is all worthwhile. I love it all in spite of all the pains and struggles and difficulties; it is all worthwhile." Another says, "It is all miserable. Life is ugly; there is no speck of beauty in this world." Both of these are right from their point of view. They are sincere, but they are different because they look at it differently. These two have their reasons to approve of life and to disapprove of it. But one benefits by the vision of beauty, and the other loses by not appreciating it, by not seeing the beauty in it. By a wrong attitude, therefore, a person accumulates in the mind undesirable impressions coming out of people, since no one in this world is perfect. Everyone has a side that can be criticized and wants repairing. When one looks at that side, one accumulates impressions which only make us more and more imperfect, because we collect imperfections, and then that becomes our world, those accumulated shortcomings and errors. And when the mind has become a sponge full of undesirable impressions, then what it emits is also undesirable. No one can speak ill of another person without making it one's own, because the one speaking ill of others is the one who is ill.

The purification of mind, therefore, from a moral point of view, must be learned in one's everyday life: to try and look at things sympathetically, favorably, by looking at others as one looks at oneself, putting oneself in their position instead of accusing them at the sight of their infirmities. Souls on earth are born imperfect and show imperfection, and from this they develop naturally, coming to perfection. If all were born perfect, then this creation would not have any purpose. And manifestation has taken place so that every being here may rise from imperfection toward perfection. That is the object and joy of life, and for that this world was created. And if we expect every person to be perfect and conditions to be perfect and all things to be perfect, then there would be no joy in living and no purpose in coming here.

Purification of mind, therefore, means purifying it from all undesirable impressions, not only of the shortcomings of others but also arriving at that stage where one forgets one's own shortcomings. I have seen some righteous ones accusing themselves of their errors until they became error themselves. Concentrating on error all the time means engraving the error upon the mind. The best principle, therefore, is to forget others and to forget ourselves, and to put our mind to accumulating all that is good and beautiful.

There is a very significant occupation of the street boys in India. They take the earth from a certain place, and they have a certain way of finding in that earth some metal such as gold or silver. And all day long their hands are in the dust. But looking for what? Looking for gold and silver. In this world of imperfection, when we seek for all that is good and beautiful, there are many chances for us to be disappointed. But at the same time, if we keep on looking for it, not looking at the dust but looking for the gold, we shall find it. And once we begin to find it, we shall find more and more. There comes a time in the life of a human being where one can see some good in the worst person in the world. And when one has reached that point, if the good was covered with a thousand covers, one will put one's hand on what is good, because one looks for good and attracts what is good.

And now we come to the phenomenon of a pure mind. The pure mind does not only create phenomena, but is a phenomenon itself. Someone who thinks of having a good fish, a nice fried fish, in the office, finds that the cook did the same thing: made a nice fried fish. Why is it? Reflection of the pure mind. It was just a thought; this person was not concentrating. A thought just passed through the mind, but it took the right direction. In other words, it struck the mind which was respon-sible for preparing the fish. Someone who wanted to look for a certain bracket for a room did not know where to go in the city and where to find it, but had an idea it should be like this. And as soon as the person went out, the first shop that this person'ss fall upon had that bracket there, and that is the only thing nec-essary. Perhaps throughout the whole city one could not have found it, but the mind brought the person to the object that was desired. Where does all this come from? It all comes from purity of mind.

Besides that, mind is likened to water. Even just looking at a stream of pure water, running in all its purity, is one of the great-est joys one can have. Drinking pure water is the greatest joy. And so it is with the mind. The contact with the pure-minded, association with the pure-minded, is the greatest joy, whether that pure-minded one speaks with you or not. There is a purity that comes out of such a person, a natural purity which is not human-made but which belongs to the soul and gives you the greatest pleasure and joy. There are others who have learned to speak and entertain, and their manner is all polish and fineness, and their wit exaggeration in artistic speech. What is it all? If there is no purity of mind, nothing can give that exquisite joy for which every soul yearns.

And now, coming to the question, they say that the pure-minded one very often seems to be too good to live and very often seems to be void of common sense. Very often the pure-minded one seems not to belong to this world. Yes, it is true. But it is not the fault of the pure-minded, it is the fault of the wicked world. That world has gone from bad to worse. Those that show purity of mind begin to be outcasts and to be incapable of doing whatever they can do. But what does it mat-ter? One can just as well be pure-minded and wise at the same time. The difference between wise and clever is this: the clever cannot be wise, but the wise can be clever. The pure-minded one can also work in worldly matters as thoroughly and as capably, as a worldly person. But even though the one without a pure mind may be able to make a success in the world, it will not be an everlasting success.

When we come to the question of success and failure, there is no principle upon which this is based. It is not true to say you must be honest and good and pure-minded in order to make a success; very often it's the opposite in order to be successful. But very often the dishonesty and lack of purity of mind is what brings one to a great failure. And if there can be said to be any rule pertaining to this, that rule is that the one who makes a success through honesty and through goodness has that success depend upon honesty and goodness. The day that person lacks these, that success will go down. And the one who makes a success without honesty and goodness, the day that person is honest and good, that person will have a failure, because their paths are different. The whole attitude of mind works upon one's life's affairs. It is most wonderful to watch. The more you think about it, the more it will prove to you that success and failure absolutely depend upon one's attitude of mind.

I was very interested in hearing from a friend who was a seller, a salesman in a big firm of jewelers. He used to come to me to talk philosophy. He said, "It is very strange. I have seen so often on arriving in a house where I thought they are able to pay more than the actual price of things, that when I was tempted to ask a much greater price than what I knew the price to be, every time I gave in to this temptation, I did not succeed. And again I was encouraged to do the same when I saw my fellow salesmen, who sold a stone to someone who took a liking to it, at a price perhaps four times more than its worth. Why did they succeed, and why do I not succeed?" I told him, "Your way is different. Their way is different. They can succeed by dishonesty; you can succeed by honesty. If you take their path, you will not succeed."

Therefore, sometimes the one who is busy developing mentally, by mental purification, may have to go through little sacrifices, little failures. But they are only a process toward something really substantial, really worthwhile. If they are not discouraged by a little failure, they will certainly come to a stage when success will be theirs. Purity of mind sets forth springs of inspiration which otherwise are kept closed. And it is through inspiration that one enjoys and appreciates all that is beautiful and creates all that is good for the joy and pleasure of others.

Once I visited the studio of a painter. After I sat there for fifteen minutes, such a depression came upon me that I asked the widow of the painter, "What was the condition of your husband, who made these pictures?" And she said, "A terrible condition, his spirit was torn to pieces." I said, "That is what his pictures show," and the effect is that whoever sees those pictures gets the same influence.

If we have the purity of mind we create purity. In all we do—art, politics, business, music, industry—we pour out the purity of mind even to such an extent that those around us, when we see strangers, friends, they all have part in our joy. They say diseases are infectious. But I say purity of mind is infectious. Also its effect creates purity in others. Some keep it for a long time, others keep it for a short time. It depends upon the mind.

And now we come to the question of what are the ways that Sufis prescribe for the purification of mind? Repetitions of the sacred names of God, prayers, sitting in a certain posture, breathing in a certain rhythm, focusing one's mind on a certain object of concentration in order to become single-minded, and the changing of one's attitude toward life. All these things are practiced to bring about desired results.

* * *

Question: *Murshid, would you please repeat what you said about the searchlight?*

Answer: I said the mind is a storehouse, a storehouse of all the knowledge that one has accumulated by studies, by experiences, by impressions, through any of the five senses. In other words, every sound, even once you have heard it, is registered there. Every form that you have seen, if only a glimpse of it, is registered there. And when our heart is pure, it projects the light of the soul, just like the light is projected from the search-light. And the most wonderful phenomenon is that this light is thrown by the power of will on that particular spot in the storehouse I call mind, on the spot which you want to find. For instance, you have seen a person once ten years ago, and this person comes before you, and you look at this person and you say, "I have seen this person, but where?" In that moment your will throws the light of your soul on that picture that was once made on your mind ten years ago. It still is there. You had forgotten it all, but the picture is there. The moment you desired to see it, the light of your soul projected its light on that particular spot. And the most wonderful thing is that there are perhaps a million pictures—why must your light be put on that particular image? That is the phenomenon. It is that the inner light will have a great power; it is a power which is cre-ative by nature. And therefore, when it throws light, it throws it on that particular spot.

Question: *Murshid, would you kindly help me? What is the sub-conscious mind?*

Answer: I very seldom use the words *subconscious mind*. But by the word *mind* I mean subconscious mind. What I have said just now is there is a storehouse. That storehouse is the subconscious mind. In that storehouse there are things, and they live, are living things. And so all thoughts and impressions are living also. There is nothing in the mind that dies. It lives and lives long. But when we are not conscious of it, it is in our subconscious mind. For instance, a person was told to go and see a friend on such a day at such a time. He had written it in his notebook, but then forgot it. In his daily occupation there came a moment when he thought, "I ought to be in that place! I have not gone there. I have quite forgotten. I should have been there. Why am I not there? Why did I forget it?" Now, this idea that came to his memory was in the subconscious mind. And as his will wanted to know, it came up. He knew without doubt that he had an engagement, that he was meant to be there, only for the time being it had been forgotten. Where was it? In that part of the mind which some call the subconscious mind. The more words, the more complications. Higher mind, lower mind—I would just say mind.

Question: *What becomes of this storehouse after death?*

Answer: It comes to greater life, a life more real than here. For instance, a pupil who was very interested in spiritual exercises and metaphysical questions once went away from me and then became a businessman. All his time was taken in business. He forgot me altogether. For ten years he never did his practices. One day I happened to go in the city where he lived. And then he remembered his old teacher who had come again. After he heard the lecture, all things which he was taught ten years before, it all became living for him; but it all became alive in one moment's time. He said, "It is all living to me. Please tell me what to do." He was so eager to do things now. And so it is. All that is in the mind, all one has never thought about, all one never troubles about is there; and when one has leisure from worldly occupations—at death comes leisure—it all becomes living. Therefore comes the realization they say about heaven and hell: we have made in ourselves what we have accumulated in our mind, and in the hereafter it will be our own. Today our mind is in us. In the hereafter we shall be in our minds. And therefore that mind which is mind just now, in the hereafter will be the world. If it is in heaven, it will be heaven; if it is in the other place, it will be the other place. It is what we have made it. No one is attracted and put there. We have made it for ourselves, for our own convenience. What we have sought after we have collected. A valuable dress, if it was really important, it is there. If you find out that it is not important, that it is foolish, it is there just the same.

Question: *Do useless things take a form in the mind?*

Answer: Well, everything has a form. But it has a form akin to the source of impression. Now, for instance, a painting, a picture, is a form. Not only that, but music also is a language that the eyes do not see, but the ears see it. So mind accumulates all such forms as sour, sweet, bitter, pungent—all different tastes. We do not see them, but they are in a form distinguished by us, registered in the mind. The eyes do not see that form, but the mind sees them, actually in the same way as one had once tasted in the mind. They are all intelligible to the mind in exactly the same way, as intelligible to the mind as when it came through different senses.

Question: *Do various impressions remain?*

Answer: Yes, they do. Because, what is an individual? An individual is a unit. When different physical organs cannot any longer hold the spirit, then they fail and the spirit is finished with them. The body departs, the spirit remains. The spirit is as much of an individual as the person was an individual in the physical body. After the physical body has gone on, the contrary impressions are more distinct because the limitation of the physical body has fallen away. The physical body is a great limitation. When it has fallen away, individuality becomes more distinct, more capable of working than on the physical plane.

UNLEARNING

It is the most difficult thing to forget what one has once learned.[1] There is one thing, learning, and another thing, unlearning. The process of spiritual attainment is in unlearning. People consider their belief their religion. Really speaking, belief is a stepping-stone to religion. Besides, if I were to picture belief, it is just like a staircase that leads to a higher realization. But instead of going up the staircase, people stop on it. It is just like flowing water that does not run anymore. People have made their belief rigid, crude; and therefore, instead of being benefited by their belief, they are going backward. If not, I would have thought that all those believers in God, in truth, and the hereafter would be better off than the unbelievers. But what happens is that they are worse, because they have nailed their own feet with their belief.

And very often I am in a position where I can say very little, especially when people come to me with their preconceived ideas and want to take my direction, my guidance on the spiritual path. And at the same time their first intention is to see if their thoughts fit in with mine and if my thoughts fit in with theirs. They cannot make themselves empty to the direction given, they want to see if it fits in—my thoughts with theirs. They have not come to follow my thoughts, but want to confirm to themselves that their idea is all right. Among a hundred persons who come for spiritual guidance, ninety come out of

1 Lecture, Sufi Center, San Francisco, February 22, 1926.

that tap. What it shows is that they do not want to give up their idea, but rather they want to be confirmed that the idea they have is all right.

Spiritual attainment from beginning to end is unlearning what one has learned. But how to unlearn? What one has learned is in oneself. Yes, one can do it by becoming wiser. The more wise you become, the more you are able to contradict your own ideas. The less wisdom you have, the more you hold on with a fast grip to your own ideas. In the wisest person there is willingness to cede to others. And the most foolish are always ready to stand in support of their own ideas. The reason is that the wise person can easily give up a thought; the foolish person holds on to it. That is why the foolish do not become wise, because they stick to their own ideas. That is why they do not progress.

Mental purification, therefore, is the only condition by which one can reach the spiritual goal. In order to accomplish this, one has to look at another person's point of view. Whether that person has evolved less or more does not matter. One can easily let oneself go for a moment and try to see from another's point of view. And that is what a person does not do. A person always rejects that one thing, and that is looking at something from another person's point of view. For in reality, every point of view is our point of view. The vaster we become, the greater the realization which comes to us, the more we see that every point of view is all right. And the more we see from the point of view of others, the more we are able to expand ourselves to the consciousness of another. It does not mean that we limit ourselves to our own point of view, but that we are able to expand to others. Our consciousness becomes as large as two persons. And so it can be as large as a thousand persons when we accustom ourselves to seeing from another point of view, always trying to see what another thinks about it. And by that we do not necessarily have to lose our own point of view. I do not mean to say that we must lose it, but only that we try to see from the point of view of another. By that we do not lose ourselves. And this comes by making a habit every day of trying to see how another person looks at the same thing, when we look at it from certain point of view.

And the next step in mental purification is to be able to see the right of the wrong and the wrong of the right, and the evil of the good and the good of the evil. It is a difficult task, but once one has accomplished this, one rises above good and evil. You must be able to see the pain in pleasure and the pleasure in pain, and the gain in the loss and the loss in the gain. And what generally happens is that one is blunted to one thing and that one's eyes are open to another thing, and that one does not see the loss or that one does not see the gain of it. If one recognizes the right, one does not recognize the wrong, if the good, one does not know the bad. That is mental purification: that impressions such as good and bad, and wrong and right, and gain and loss, and pleasure and pain, these opposites which block the mind must be cleared by seeing the opposite of these things. Then you can see the enemy in the friend and the friend in the enemy. When you can recognize the poison in nectar and the nectar in poison; that is the time when death and life become one too. Opposites no more remain opposites before you. That is called mental purification. And those who come to this stage, those are the living sages.

And now the third field of mental purification, and that is to identify yourself with what you are not. By this you purify your mind from impressions of your own false identity. I will give you an example. There is a very interesting story of a sage in India. The story begins by saying that a young man in his youth asked his mother, who was a peasant woman living in a village, "What is the best occupation, mother?" And the mother said, "I do not know, son, except that those who searched after the highest in life, went in search of God." "Then where must I go, mother? In anything in the world, I would rather pursue God," he said. He intuitively felt what Christ has said,

"Seek ye first the kingdom of God and all other things shall be added unto you."[2] "Yes, son," she said, "I do not know whether it is practical or not, but so they say: the best pursuit is the pursuit of God." He said, "Well, mother, give me leave, I will go somewhere in the pursuit of God. Where must I go, mother?" "I have heard in solitude, in the forest." So he went there for a long time and lived a life of patience and solitude. And once or twice in between he came to see his mother. Sometimes his patience was exhausted, his heart broken. Sometimes he was disappointed in not finding God. And each time the mother sent him back with stronger advice. When at the third visit he said, "Now it is a long time since I am there." "Yes," said his mother, "now I think that you are ready to go to a teacher."

So he went to see a teacher. And there were many pupils learning under that teacher. Every pupil had a little room to meditate in. And this pupil also was told to go in a certain room to meditate. The teacher asked, "Is there anything you love in the world?" This young man, being away from home since childhood, having not seen anything from the world, could know no one except the little cow that was in the house. He said, "I love the cow in our house." The teacher said, "Yes, then think of the cow in your meditation."

All the other pupils came and went, and sat in their room for fifteen minutes for a little meditation; then they got tired and went away. But this young man sat there from the time the teacher told him to. The teacher said, "Where is he?" They said, "We don't know. He must be in his room." They went to see him; the door was closed and there was no answer. The teacher went himself and opened the door and there he saw the pupil sitting in meditation, fully absorbed in it. And when the teacher called him by his name, he answered in the sound of the cow. The teacher said, "Come out." He said, "My horns are too large to pass through the door." The teacher said to his pupils, "Look here, this is the living example of meditation. You

2 Matthew 6:33.

are meditating on God and you do not know where God is. He is meditating on the cow and he has become the cow. He has lost his identity. He identifies himself with the object before him, the object on which he meditates." That is our difficulty, friends, that we cannot come out of a false conception. All the difficulty in our life is from that.

I will give you another example. Once I was interested in helping a person who was ill, who had had gout for twenty years. And for twenty years this woman was in bed; she could not move her joints. I came to her and said, "Now, you will do this, and I will come back after two weeks." And when I came back after two weeks, she was already beginning to move her joints. And I said, "Now, I will come back after six weeks." And in six weeks she began to move her joints much better; she got down from the bed and had a still greater hope of being cured. Nevertheless, her patience was not as great as it ought to be. One day she was lying in bed and thought, "Can I ever be cured?" The moment she had that thought she went back to the same condition, because her soul had identified itself with a sick person. For her to see her own well-being, that she could be quite well, was something she could not imagine. She could not believe her eyes that her joints could be moving; she could not believe it. People can be well in their bodies but not in their minds. Very often, therefore, they hold on to an illness which they could get rid of. And the same thing with misery. Very often a person who is conscious of misery attracts miseries. They are their own misery. It is not that misfortune is interested in them, but they are interested in misfortune. Misfortune does not choose people; people choose misfortune. They hold that thought, and that thought becomes their own. When one is impressed that one goes downward, one goes downward; weight is helping one to sink.

Therefore, the third aspect of mental purification we have just now explained is to be able to identify oneself with something else. Of course the Sufis have their own way of teaching it. Very often one has the idea of one's spiritual teacher, and with that idea one gains the knowledge and inspiration and power that the spiritual teacher has. It is just like a heritage.

There is a story of a pupil and a teacher, that a candidate came to a great teacher and said, "Will you accept me as your pupil?" The teacher said, "Yes, why not?" He said, "Perhaps you do not know, I have great many faults." The teacher said, "I do not mind. What faults have you?" "I am a great gambler." "That does not matter at all; that does not matter." Then he said, "But I get drunk, teacher!" The teacher said, "Oh, that is all right. Just two, three faults." He said, "That does not matter." The teacher then said, "Will you accept my condition now? I have accepted all your faults, you must accept my condition." "Yes." The teacher said, "You may not do any of your faults in my presence. In my absence, you may do it." "Quite easy, I can manage it," and so the pupil went. And after some time he once wanted to go to the tavern, and as soon as he came near the tavern, he saw the face of his teacher. Then he went one day, thinking, "Well, I have not gambled for a long time." At the gambling house, he saw the face of the teacher and could not go there. He came back to the teacher who said, "Have you done any faults anymore?" "I could not do it, could not get rid of you. Wherever I went, you were also." That is the idea. The one who cannot concentrate so much as to forget oneself and go deep into the object on which one concentrates, will not succeed in mastering concentration.

The fourth mental purification is to free oneself from a form and have a sense of the abstract. Everything suggests a form to the eyes; everything does this even so much that, for a person whom one has not seen, if the name is mentioned, one makes a form. Even such things as fairies and spirits and angels, as soon as they are mentioned, they are always pictured in a certain form. It is this that hinders you from attaining to the presence of the formless. And therefore this mental purification is of a very great importance, and that is being able to think of an idea without form. This, of course, is attained by great concentration and meditation, but once it is attained, it is most satisfactory.

And the fifth way is to be able to repose your mind; in other words, to relax your mind. Imagine, after having toiled for the whole day, how much the body stands in need of rest and how much more the mind must stand in need of rest, for the brain has worked too, the mind has worked too. The mind works much faster than the body; naturally, the mind is much more tired than the body. And not every person knows how to rest the mind. When you are asleep, the mind goes on just the same. What you call dreaming is nothing but the action of mind. The mind is busy, and, therefore, the mind never has a rest. And then what happens after a little time is that the mind becomes feeble. Having no rest, it loses memory, the power of action; it loses reason. And the worst effects are mostly brought about by not giving the mind proper repose. If such infirmities as doubt and fear happen to enter the mind, then a person becomes restless and never has a rest, for at night the mind runs on the track of the same impressions.

Very few know, as simple as it seems to be, about the resting of the mind and how wonderful it is in itself. And what power, what inspiration comes as a reaction from it, and what peace one experiences by it. And how it helps, for the body and the mind, that the spirit is picked up once the mind has had its rest. And the first step in answering the question of how to rest the mind is the relaxation of the body. If one is able to relax one's muscular and nervous system at will, then the mind is automatically refreshed with the body. Besides that, the power of will to throw away anxiety, worries, doubts, fears, and to put oneself in a restful state is accomplished with the help of breathing properly.

There is a great magnetism produced by having stilled and purified the mind. And the lack of it produces the lack of magnetism. Those whose mind is not purified and stilled, their presence becomes a source of unrest for others and for themselves. And they attract little because the power of attraction is lost. A person is tired in their presence, and their atmosphere causes uneasiness, discomfort. They are a burden for themselves and for others.

Once the mind is purified, the next step is the cultivation of the heart quality, which culminates in spiritual attainment.

* * *

Question: *What should one do if one has the desire to go into these things, but if one's life is too busy?*

Answer: I have heard from many persons who say they have the greatest desire to give their time and thought to spiritual things, but because they have not attained the manner of living so that their mind will be free to keep these things, they think they cannot take up anything spiritual. And I saw the reason for their argument: that it is quite true that in this world, as life is today, it is difficult to move without money.

Material things apart, even spiritual things one cannot do without money. If I were to give you the same lecture, and if I would not be sitting in a room, not a person would come. And so it is that, if the newspaper had not had the advertisement, if a notice was not printed, you would not have known; perhaps two or three persons would oblige me to be kind enough to listen to me. It is therefore natural that a person thinks like this, and one is not to be blamed. But at the same time, when we look at it from a different point of view, we shall see that every moment lost in waiting for spiritual attainment is the greatest loss conceivable. And besides, one may go on thinking that, "The day will come when I shall change my life and give in to something higher, spiritual," and that day will never come. I should say that today is what one has, just now, instead of saying, "Tomorrow I will do it." If not, one repents. Life is assimilating; time passes. Hours, months, years slip by before one realizes that they have slipped. And to the one who understands the value of time, spiritual attainment is first. As Christ has said, "Seek ye first the kingdom of God and all these things shall be added unto you."[3] He did not say, "Let all things go in order to pursue spiritual things." But at the same time, that spiritual attainment does not deprive one of material gains. One only has to fix the spiritual things before one first; the other comes along. And in order to become spiritual it is not necessary that you must give up worldly things or all that is good and beautiful and valuable from the point of view of the material world. Solomon, with all his wealth, was not less wise. You need not give up all you have in order to become spiritual. If you think that, it is a great pity. But to wait, saying, "Till my ship comes I shall wait, then I shall become spiritual"—who knows when the ship will come? It is never too late to go into the spiritual path, and it is never too early. The best thing, therefore, is the moment you think that, "It is already too late, I must begin." One must begin and go through all the tests and trials of this path, confident that there is nothing that cannot be accomplished once the spiritual path is taken.

Question: [*not given*]

Answer: Mental purification is to be able to see the two opposite things: good in evil and evil in good. Why is evil a greater reality than good? Both are the same. It is we who have made it evil and made it good; it is our conception, our way of looking at it. We can look at good and make it evil following our conception. Therefore, to say there is no such thing as evil and call it all good, one and the same thing we turn into two things. Besides, as I have said, everything in its wrong place is evil, everything in its wrong time is evil. It is time and place that turns things from good to evil and from evil to good.

Question: *Is it the right thing to do to see the ideal in a picture?*

Answer: It is natural to see the ideal in a picture. But to get above it is to try and get to the essence. In other words, there

---
3 Matthew 6:33.

is one way of hearing the music, which is to think of the form, the technicality, the form of it. And the other way is to grasp the feeling, the sense that it suggests. So it is with life: that we can look at life in one way and see it in different forms and make a rigid conception of it, or to see that it could suggest the essence of it.

Now, for an instance, a person comes to you and speaks a thousand false things. And then you go over it and think, "This was false because it was composed like this. It cannot be true, it cannot be reasonable." That is one way. The other way of seeing it is when one says, "It is false from top to bottom," and not to see it in detail. This is quite enough, and it has saved your mind great trouble because you have just seen it. Sometimes a person says, "You are my friend, my acquaintance. All right, I am going to find out how you work." That is one way of realizing. The other way is to see the person and, in one glance, to know what the person is. And then it is finished. That is the idea.

Very often murids come to me for spiritual training. And those who are not sure of their mind come to me and say, "I was very interested in what you said, but I want to read more of your books, of your teachings, before I put myself under your guidance." It amuses me very much. This person has seen me and had an impression, whether wrong or right, whatever impression. And now that impression is not enough, and this person wants to read my books. What is a book? After all, it is a dead thing. This person has seen the living book, and that has not given confidence to that person. But perhaps in six months' time, when I have gone to Europe, this person will fit in with the idea, "It is that" or "It is not that." This is called not being sure of oneself. It is looking at something in form instead of looking in spirit. Once one sees, one knows, "This is my friend." If one waits for six months' time, the one who is not sure of oneself will not find a friend, will not find a friend in all of life. If in one glance one says, "This is my friend, I can trust this person," it makes one brave, venturous; and that makes one come nearer to the essence. It will give generosity, liberality. If not, one is small and narrow and confused. One does not know oneself. So thousands and millions of souls are buffeted along in the sea of life, not knowing where they are going, not sure of themselves. The moment a person says, "I don't know you, perhaps I will know you someday," that person will never know you, or all through life that person is not sure.

THE DISTINCTION BETWEEN
THE SUBTLE AND THE GROSS

There is a verse in the Bible, "It is the spirit that quickeneth, the flesh profiteth nothing."[1] So what we call living is subtle, and what is dead is gross; in other words, what is dense is gross, and what is fine is subtle. It is true as it is said among Hindus that there was a golden age, then a silver age, a copper age, and an iron age. Certainly we are in the iron age. So much grossness we find now that never before in any period of history was there such grossness and denseness as humanity shows today. And how it has come is by the law of gravitation. When consciousness is absorbed in gross matter, then a person gravitates toward the earth. When consciousness is released from gross matter, then it gravitates toward heaven.

I do not mean to say that people were not gross before, two thousand or three thousand years ago. But when you study traditions, you will find that they were very fine and subtle in perception, more than we are today. Our contact with earth and earthly things has made us more rigid. They were more placid. And if you want to find it out, you have only to study an ancient language, such as Sanskrit, [Avestan], Persian, or Hebrew, and see the manuscripts of the ancient times and the way they explain things. It may be that they are quite strange to our mentality and perception, yet their fineness is beyond words.

And I am afraid we are going from bad to worse, and that we are becoming grosser every day. If we only realized how far

1 John 6:63; lecture, Sufi Center, San Francisco, February 23, 1926.

147

we are removed from what may be called fine perception. No sooner has a person come to understand subtle things only by mathematical calculations, then that person has come in the dense sphere and does not want to become fine. And the spirit, which is the finest thing, that person wants to make it gross to make it intelligible.

Friends, it is therefore of the greatest importance, in order to attain to spiritual attainment, to develop fine perception. I have seen some people going into a trance or diving into a deep meditation, and yet, if lacking fine perception, then it is of no value. They are not really spiritual. A really spiritual person must have a mentality like liquid, not like a rock—something that is moving, not crude and dense.

And now I come to the metaphysical side of it. There are two experiences of life. One realm of experience is sensation; the other realm is exaltation. And by these two things, what is experienced? By these two experiences one tries to experience happiness. But by sensation, or in the form of sensation, what is experienced is not necessarily happiness; it is pleasure. It might for a moment give the appearance of happiness, but it is only a suggestion of happiness. Now, exaltation is something that the mystic experiences. And those who have not been mystics, they experience it also, but they do not know what it is and they cannot distinguish between sensation and exaltation. Furthermore, sometimes exaltation is the outcome of sensation. It is possible. But at the same time, exaltation that depends upon sensation is not an independent exaltation.

As much as we need sensation in life to make our experience of life concrete, so much or even more do we need exaltation in order to live life fully. The lower creation, such as birds and beasts, also have glimpses of exaltation. They do not only rejoice in grazing and in picking grains, in making nests or in flying in the air, in singing, and in running about in the forest, but there are moments when even birds and beasts feel exaltation. And if we go into this subject deeper, we shall say the same as the Prophet Muhammad has said in the Qur'an. There is a most wonderful couplet, a *sura*, which says that there are moments when even rocks become exalted and trees fall in ecstasy.[2] If that is true, a human being, who is made to complete the experience that any living being can have, must experience exaltation as much as sensation.

And now, coming to the idea, what do I mean by sensation? The admiration one has for line and color, the preference one has for softness in structure, the appreciation one has for fragrance and perfume, the enjoyment one gains by tasting sweet and sour and pungent, the joy one experiences in hearing poetry, chanting, and music—all these experiences are manifest in the realm of sensation. Therefore, the world of sensation is one world; the world of exaltation is another world. And these two worlds are made for humanity to experience and live life on earth fully. And imagine, with this possibility and this opportunity in life, human beings continue to live the life of sensation, forgetting that there is a life besides it, a life that can be experienced here on earth, and something that completes life's experience.

And now I shall explain to you what I mean by exaltation. There is a physical aspect of exaltation which comes as a reaction or result of having seen the immensity of space, having looked at the wide horizon, or having seen the clear sky, the moonlit night, and nature seen at dawn. Looking at the rising sun, watching the setting sun, looking at the horizon from the sea, being in the midst of nature, looking at the world from the top of the mountain, all these experiences, even such an experience as watching the little smiles of an innocent infant, these experiences lift you up and give you a feeling which you cannot call sensation. It is exaltation.

And a still higher aspect of exaltation is a moral exaltation: when you are sorry for having said or done something you did

2 See Qur'an 55:6.

149

not like to do; when you have asked forgiveness, and humbled yourself before someone before whom you were inconsiderate. You have humbled your pride then. Or if you felt a deep gratitude for someone who has done something for you; you have felt love, sympathy, devotion which seems endless and which seems so great that your heart cannot accommodate it; when you have felt pity for someone so much that you have forgotten yourself; when you have found a profound happiness in rendering a humble service to someone in need; when you have said a prayer which has come from the bottom of your heart; when you have realized your own limitedness and smallness in comparison to the greatness of God—all these experiences give you a lift up. And the moment when one feels these experiences, one is not living on earth, one is living in another world. The joy of such experiences is so great, and yet these experiences can be gained without paying anything, and sensations cost something. We have to go to the theater, pay in order to go to entertainments. They all cost something; they cost more than they are worth. And exaltation, which is beyond price, comes by itself no sooner than you have shown a leaning toward it. That is all. It is a matter of changing your attitude.

Once I visited a great sage in Bengal in India. I said to him, "What a blessed life is yours, that gives pleasure and happiness to so many souls." But he said that, "How privileged I am myself that a thousand times more pleasure and happiness comes to me."

Exaltation is a purifying process. A moment's exaltation can purify the evil of many years, because it is like bathing in the Ganges, as Hindus say. It is symbolical. Exaltation is the Ganges; if one bathes in it, one is purified from all sins. It does not take much to feel exalted: a kind attitude, a sympathetic trend of mind, and it is already there. If you took notice of it, the moment your eyes shed tears in sympathy with another, you are already exalted, your soul has bathed in the spiritual Ganges.

It comes by forgetting self and by destroying selfishness. But remember, we can never claim to be unselfish. However much we may be unselfish, we are selfish just the same, only it is wisely selfish. If we show ourselves to be selfish, it is just as well to be wisely selfish and profit by it. This is the same as what we call unselfish, and it is profitable to be that instead of being foolishly selfish, because the former gains and the latter loses.

And now we come to the third aspect of exaltation. The third aspect of exaltation comes by touching the reason of reasons and by realizing the essence of wisdom, by feeling the depth, the profound depth of one's heart, by widening one's outlook on life, by broadening one's conception, by deepening one's sympathies, and by soaring upwards to those spheres where the spiritual exaltation manifests.

Today a person of common sense or a person who is called practical has the habit of laughing at the idea that a certain person has dreams, that a certain person has the experience of ecstasy, that a certain person experiences what they call trance. But there is nothing to be surprised at, nothing to laugh at. And yet all these things are laughable when done by those undeserving, and mostly those who claim such things by saying they have gone into a trance or had a wonderful vision, and so show themselves extraordinary and look for approbation from others, and exaggerate their experiences. Those who really experience these things do not need to tell people, "I had this or that experience." Their own joy is their reward. No one should be recognized for it; the less others know, the better it is. Why must we show ourselves to be different from others? It is only vanity. And the more vanity, the less progress in the spiritual path, because the worst thing in the spiritual path is to try and show oneself to be different from others. Those who are really evolved are glad to act as everyone else acts.

To novelists, it is always a beautiful thing to write about masters who are in the caves of the Himalayas or who are moving about in the forest, somewhere where one cannot go and find them, who are always keeping aloof and remote so that no one having curiosity about them can reach them. But, friends, every soul has a divine spark. And therefore, if there is any higher stage of human evolution, it is for the human being, not for those outside of the human world. And if they are outside the human world, there is no relation between us and them. The great spiritual souls have lived in the world, in the midst of the world, and proved to be the greatest masters. Imagine the life of Abraham, of Moses, the life of Jesus Christ, and again the life of Muhammad in wars and battles and yet as exclusive and remote, as spiritual as anyone could be. And Krishna, picture him in Vrindavan, and fighting in the battle, giving a scripture to the world. If they had all lived in the caves in the mountains, we would not have been benefited by them. What is the use of those holy ones who never see, never experience, from morning till evening, the tests and trials of the dense world, where at every move there are a thousand temptations and difficulties, a thousand problems. What can those who are outside the world do for us, we who are exposed to a thousand difficulties at every moment of our life? And they are increasing. With the evolution of the world, life is becoming heavier, more difficult. No, the mastery, the holiness, the evolution must be shown here on earth. It is very easy to be exalted in the seventh heaven. But exaltation experienced and imparted to others here on the earth is exaltation which is worthwhile.

And now we come to the grossness and subtleness of human nature. The heroes, kings, masters, prophets, those who won the heart of humanity, they have been fine in perception and fine in character. They have not been gross. And at the same time, their fineness was simple. There is a side to it that is always so simple, and at the same time it is so subtle; that is the beauty of it. A person who can say without saying and who can do without doing is a subtle person, and that subtlety is worth appreciating. One who sees and does not see, knows and does not know, the one who experiences and does not experience at the same time, the one who is living and yet dead, that is the soul who experiences life fully.

* * *

Question: *Is the horoscope a science?*

Answer: Yes, the horoscope is a science, there is no doubt about it. And there is a science of numbers and their mystical significance. But at the same time, I consider it as one of the fine sciences.

Question: *It has become so popular that one can hardly imagine that it is really a science.*

Answer: There is always something false standing by the side of the real. And there can be nothing existing in this world that has not a false side to it. Both are existing at the same time. And so there is a possibility of astrology being real science, and also of astrology not knowing that science. That is the case with all things.

Question: *Is the knowledge of astrology intuition or knowledge?*

Answer: Well, now coming to this subject, not only astrology, but even with a concrete science such as medicine, its beginning is always intuition. I can show a thousand proofs that the medicine we have today as a science, promoted and improved by scientists who perhaps never think about intuition, had its origin in intuition. If such a science as medicine can come from intuition, it must have been a very fine perception with which the science of astrology was learned. It is a science which has come, as many other sciences, from intuition. Now the other idea is that every soul has its relation with the cosmic mechanism which is working, and in relation with that cosmic mechanism a soul continues to live. Therefore, the soul is always under the influence of this whole cosmic influence. And those who have gathered some experience, no doubt they have perhaps one thousandth of the real science, or even less than that. But still it is a science, if really studied.

The third point is that I would rather not ask anybody what would happen to me next year. Perhaps the less known, the better it is. To know that something evil will come means it is an impression which grows and works. Maybe that brings a worse result than if one had not known it. I would be very interested if someone said, "Last year this happened because the planets were in this condition," but I would not like to hear about it a year before, unless the astrologer had a very good news. But an astrologer does not always have good news. On the contrary, if there are fifteen bad remarks, there are perhaps five remarks that make one hopeful, because life is such. There are more pains than pleasures.

Now for the fourth idea about the same question, I want to tell you that one need not be a seer in order to make astrological predictions. If it were so, every astrologer would be a seer. But if one is a seer and astrologer at the same time [. . .], intuition helps in every science. But if a person were a real seer, one need not have the help of astrology. One knows it. One need not be dependent upon the calculation of numbers to throw one's own light on the present or future. The seer knows more than the astrologer knows and does not only know, but can change it too. Therefore, a seer is one thing, and an astrologer is another thing.

Question: *Is it better to have desire, or is indifference preferable?*
Answer: It depends upon what we desire. If we cherish a desire, we must keep away from indifference. Desire is fulfilled by motive power. Motive power is at the back of it. Indifference is the weakening of motive power. If a person wants to have money, and if that person says, "What does it matter?" indifference will ruin motive power. And whether indifference is right or wrong depends. If you wish something and you are indifferent to it, then you are your own enemy. But if you are indifferent to something that wants you, then indifference is the best thing to help.

Question: *But as a general rule is it better to have desire or interest?*

Answer: It all depends. That is why I say a living person is better than a book. One may perhaps show in my books a thousand contradictions in my own words. That's the large view. If you pin yourself to the words, it is small. Indifference is as good as interest, only it must be used when it is required. Sometimes interest is required, sometimes indifference is profitable. For instance, you are in a situation where people laugh at you. There is something that you want to accomplish, and people mock you. Or perhaps people antagonize you, don't like you, or are apt to criticize you. If you put your interest in all these things, you will lose your work, lose your way. You should have no interest in it. Be indifferent in that situation. But then you have a business; you have to see someone to promote your business, to get more customers, to advertise it, to get connections. It will all come about according to your interest. The more interest you have, the more profitable it will be. If you are indifferent about it, then you defeat your own cause.

I was very amused visiting a certain province in India. I went in a shop to buy something, and the man in the shop was smoking his pipe, sitting with cushions in his shop, cross-legged. I said, "Have you got this thing?" He thought for a minute or two and said, "I don't think I have it." He did not take the trouble to make himself sure, yes or no. I should have thought he would have some enthusiasm about having a chance of selling. I asked, "Where can one get such a thing?" He said, "I don't know." I said, "I would like so much to get this." He says, "I don't know." He would not budge. He remained quite comfortable in the place where he was sitting. I greeted him and thanked him for this kind silence and indifference, and I went to the shop next to his. And there I found what I wanted. Imagine, the shopkeeper easily knew the shop of the other man who was eager to sell, but that lethargy, that indifference! It is all right, indifference, if you sit in thought in a forest, and not care about a shop. But if one has a shop, or if one has business to do, then no amount of interest is foolish. Indifference and interest must be studied, used properly. Both are useful.

Question: *Do Orientals not promote desirelessness?*

Answer: Well, I should think, whether Orient or Occident, the moment you come to desirelessness, you must go in the forest, you must not live in the world. At the same time, desirelessness is a sign of evolution. But at the same time, for a person who has to live in the world, if one has no desire, one must act as if one had desire. A seer, a sage, acts like an actor on the stage: one must play the role, whatever role one is put into. That is what makes the seer or sage superior to others. The others who are also playing a role, if they are in a wretched condition, in an inferior condition, they think, "I am inferior." But this blessed soul does not think so. In all conditions, the seer or sage keeps the spirit high and knows, "I am playing a role. It is all right."

Question: *How could one cultivate intuition?*

Answer: By having self-confidence and trust in intuition. Very often people who are fine and are capable of intuition lose that faculty by not having confidence in intuition. Sometimes they are doubting, fearing, thinking, "My intuition will not come right, I shall be put to a loss." And in order to escape that position of having the loss, they lose their intuition, and their loss is greater. If they sacrificed their gain once or twice or thrice, if they would hold on to intuition, they would have success in life, whatever they will do. . . . In other words, in order to follow intuition, be brave, be courageous. One who says, "Is it true? I don't know," confuses one's own self, makes the intuitive faculty blunted. It is not everyone who is ready to lose. They would rather lose intuition than lose anything in the world. I have heard from many people, "It is too dangerous to follow intuition." I say, "Yes, it is true, when you do not distinguish between imagination and intuition. But it is the only way to come to that stage where you can trust intuition." A person learns to ride on a bicycle by falling once or twice or thrice. The same thing with intuition. If you fear, then you lose that faculty. Besides, it is fineness, a sympathetic nature, good action, right thinking, fineness of perception, all these things that help a person to be intuitive.

MASTERY

Life is purposed to attain to mastery, and this is the motive of the spirit; and it is by this motive at the back of it that the whole universe is created.[1] Through the different stages—from mineral to vegetable, from vegetable to the animal kingdom, and from animal to humanity—the continuing waking of the spirit is toward mastery. Human beings are in first place by using the mineral kingdom, utilizing the vegetable kingdom, and controlling the animal kingdom for their service. This shows that spirit by which the whole universe was created is wakened in them. Their power of knowing, of understanding, of utilizing to the best advantage, is the sign of mastery. In the whole creation human beings show that mastery in life. But at the same time, it must be known that there is one enemy that humanity has, and that enemy is limitation. And in realizing the spirit of mastery and in practicing it, this spirit of limitation is always a hindrance.

Those who have realized, at some time or the other in their lives, this principal object with which the human being is born, have then tried to develop that spirit of mastery in order to perfect themselves. And the process of going from limitation to perfection is the process which is called mysticism. Repeating it again, I will say that mysticism means developing from limitation to perfection.

---

1 Lecture, Sufi Center, San Francisco, February 26, 1926.

158

All pain and failure belongs to limitation; all pleasure and success belongs to perfection. Among those whom you know in your own surroundings, you will find those who are unhappy, dissatisfied with their lives, who make others unhappy, are those who are more limited. And those who can help themselves and help others and those who are happy and bring pleasure to the life of others, are the ones who are nearer to perfection.

And by knowing this, we must now find out what I mean by limitation and what I mean by perfection. These are only conditions of the consciousness. When one is conscious of limitation, one is limited; when one is conscious of perfection, one is perfect, because it is the same one who is limited in the limited consciousness who is perfect in the perfect consciousness. In other words, there was a son of a rich man who had plenty of money put in his name in the bank. But he did not know it, and when he had the desire to spend some, he found very little money in his purse. This made him limited. In reality, his father had put a very large sum in the bank, but he was not conscious of it. It is exactly the same case with every soul. Every soul is conscious of what it possesses and is unconscious of what is put in its name. In other words, what is within one's reach, one is conscious of being one's own. But what does not seem to be within one's reach, one considers to be outside. It is also natural. But wisdom opens a door to look out, to see, "If it is not meant, or if it is also meant that I knew it." Sometimes the mystery of life is known to a person; one may not be a mystic, but if one's time comes, one knows it.

One day I was very interested that a man who did nothing but business all through life and made himself rich—he was perhaps one of the richest men of the country—wanted to show me his park. He had a beautiful park around his house. While I was his guest we were taking a walk. He said, "This is a park I have; it is wonderful to come here in the morning and evening." I asked him, "How far does your park extend?" And he said to me, "Do you want to know it? Do you see the horizon from here?" I said, "Yes." He said, "All this ground is mine, and the sea besides. All that you see." It was a wonderful answer. This answer was an example of the theory I have spoken about: he was not only conscious of what he possessed, but of all that was there. He did not make a dividing line between what was his own and what was beside it. It is a mystery, and for every person it is difficult to look at life in this way. But I wish to tell you that even this man, who was in business, this man who never thought of mysticism, also could arrive at that conception which the mystic finds out after the meditation of years. It was purely a mystical conception.

When dervishes address to one another—sometimes dressed in their patched coats, and sometimes they are scantily clad, sometimes they have food and sometimes not—they address one another saying, "O King of kings, Emperor of emperors." It is the consciousness of what is king or emperor which is before them, as the boundary of their kingdom is not limited. All the universe is their kingdom. It is in this way that a soul proceeds toward perfection by waking the consciousness, raising it higher. It is exactly the same as when you are standing at the foot of a mountain: what you see is a narrow horizon compared with the horizon you look at from the top of the mountain. When the soul evolves spiritually, it rises to a height where it sees a wider horizon. Therefore, its possession becomes greater. But you might say, "By looking at the horizon, it does not become our possession; what we possess is what we call our own." First Columbus saw America. He did not possess it first, the possession came afterward. The first thing is to see; afterward one possesses. But if we do not see, how can we possess? And without seeing your possessions, it is not your possession.

There are two different ways, or two different angles from which you must look at perfection. One way is likened to a perpendicular line, and the other way is likened to a horizontal line. The way which is likened to a perpendicular line is the raising of the consciousness within. And one might say, "How does one raise this consciousness?" First of all, by concentration one raises consciousness within, which means one is able to see concretely and to be conscious of something which is apart from one's physical body. A person may be conscious of a poem, a word, a picture, an idea, or something. A person being conscious of it—if one can be so conscious of it that one can lose one's limited body out of one's consciousness for a moment—that is the first step. Although it seems very easy, it is not so easy. When one begins to do it, no sooner one closes one's eyes in order to concentrate than a thousand things come before one. Besides, this physical body becomes restive. It says, "This person is not conscious of me." And then a person gets nervous and twists and turns in order to be conscious of the body. The body does not like a person to be unconscious of it. Like a dog or a cat, it likes that one is conscious of it. Then a kind of nervous action comes in the body. It feels like moving, turning, scratching, or something. As soon as one wants to discipline the body, the body does not want to take discipline.

The second stage is that instead of being conscious of a thought, one is conscious of a feeling, which is wider still, because thought is a form and even mind sees the form, but feeling has no form. Therefore, to fix your mind on a feeling, and to keep it with the intention of keeping it, is not an easy thing. If once a person has done it, and one has not given oneself to the restiveness of mind, then no doubt one feels uplifted and has gone further.

This is the boundary of human progress, and further than that is divine progress. And you may ask me, "What is divine progress?" When you go further still, then instead of being active, you become passive. Being passive is a state. There you do not need concentration; what you need there is meditation. There you get in touch with that power which is audible and visible within you, and yet one is ignorant of that power which is busy moving toward materializing its intended object. And once you come in contact with this experience, you no longer can say even once that there is such a thing as an accident in your life. Then you will see all that happens is destined and prepared when you catch it in its preparatory condition, before it has manifested on the earthly plane.

And if you go further, there is consciousness in its aspect of being pure intelligence. It is knowing and yet knowing nothing. And knowing nothing means knowing all things, because it is the knowing of things that blunts the faculty of knowledge. In other words, when a person is looking in a mirror, that person's reflection covers the mirror, and in that mirror nothing else can be reflected. Therefore, when the consciousness is conscious of anything, it is blunted: at that moment it is blunted or, in other words, it is covered by something that it is conscious of. The moment that cover is taken away, it is its own self, it is pure intelligence, it is pure spirit. And in that condition its power, life, magnetism, force, its capacity is much greater, incomparably greater than one can imagine it to be except that one, by the help of meditation, reaches that condition. And if you go higher still, it is not even consciousness. It is a kind of omniscient condition which is the sign of inner perfection.

This is one direction of progress. There is another direction of progress, and that is to see oneself reflected in another. When you are friends with another person, naturally your sympathy, love, friendship, makes you see yourself in another, and this gives a person the inclination to sacrifice. No one will sacrifice for another except when the other is oneself. If this feeling develops, it extends further, not only with friend, with neighbor, but with a stranger, with anyone, with the little beast and bird and insect, as Buddha has said that harmlessness is the essence of religion—being in at-one-ment with all living beings. And it gives you insight into others as much as the others know about themselves. You know about them as much as they know, or even more. This is the simplest phenomenon of this consciousness, not to work wonders. It brings you a quick proof that one knows as much about others as they know themselves.

But there is another, moral proof: that you become friends with the wise and foolish, with the virtuous and wicked more and more, as you attract them to you. You cannot help it. Sympathy is so powerful that even enemies sooner or later are melted. It is not only a story when they say that Daniel was sent to the cave of the lions and the lions were calmed. But in order to see this phenomenon, one need not go to the mountains. In this world there are worse than lions: good natures and bad natures, possible and impossible people. And if you can tame them, you have accomplished something, for it requires a greater power than calming lions. One can think of the different ideas, agitated ones, antagonized ones, blunted ones, ignorant ones, drunken with falsehood or with jealousy, all sorts of poisons—there are many in this world. And it is only one power, the power of your sympathy, that assimilates all poisonous influences. It assimilates them; it takes away their poison, and it does not hurt you. You sooner or later purify them, revivify them, melt them, mold them, and direct them toward their purpose in life.

The world seeks for complexity. If I were to give a lecture on how to get this magnetism in order how to make people listen to you, and in order to draw them to you, if I were to give twenty exercises for doing these things, there might be a great success for me. But if I told you simple things like the deepening of your sympathy, the wakening of that sympathetic spirit in you, is every power and magnetism there is, and the expansion of which means spiritual unfoldment, then there will be few to understand. For human beings do not want simple teaching; they want complexity.

And then there is another stage of expansion, and that is trying to look at everything from another's point of view, trying to think as the other person thinks. This is not an easy thing, because from one's childhood one learns to think so that one stands upon one's own thought. One does not move whether it is right or wrong to another's thought; for the very fact that one has thought it oneself, one must keep on it. Therefore, know that it is a sign of expansion to be able to see from the child's point of view, or from the point of view of the foolish person, how another looks at things. And the most interesting thing is one needs only to be tolerant in order to see from the point of view of another and to be patient. In that way one extends one's knowledge to such a degree that no reading can give that knowledge. Then you begin to get from all sources; from every plane you will attract knowledge as soon as the mind becomes so pliable that it does not only stick to its own point of view.

In my books I have called it unlearning. If you say, "This is a very nice person," and another person comes and says, "That is not a nice person. You are quite wrong," the general tendency is to stick to that idea. But the greater evolution is to see from the other's point of view also. That person has a reason for it, maybe that person is too unevolved to see or more evolved or less interested in the other person or something. But by seeing from another person's point of view you do not lose your own. Your own point of view is there, but the other point of view is added to yours. Therefore, your knowledge becomes greater. It takes a greater tolerance and a greater stretching of the heart, and sometimes it pains when you stretch it. But by stretching the heart and by making it larger and larger, you turn your heart into the sacred book.

And the third aspect is to feel another, because when it comes to their feelings, people are very often different from what they appear and from what they think. Sometimes others act quite differently from their feelings and talk quite differently about their feelings. And if your feelings can sense the feeling of another, this is a high aspect. You become a very high personality when the feelings of another can tell you much more than that person's words and actions can. And sometimes they can give you quite a different opinion of a person than if you had only seen that person and heard that person speak.

And if one has arrived here, human evolution finishes and divine evolution begins. Then, no doubt, a person gets insight into what happens in the spirit of others—if they are going to succeed or going to be happy, or what they are going to accomplish. Because there is something going on within a person preparing that person's plan for tomorrow, and you begin to touch it and begin to get the impression of it. And that impression is as clear, sometimes, as anything visible and audible could be.

And if you go further, then you unite with everything. In this consciousness distance remains no distance; if you can extend your consciousness so that your consciousness touches the consciousness of another, then not only the thoughts of that person but the whole spirit of that person is reflected in your spirit. Space does not matter; your consciousness can touch every part of the world and every person, at whatever distance that person may be.

And if you go still further, then you can even realize that you are connected with all beings, that there is nothing or no one who is divided or separate from you. And you are not only connected by chains with those you love, but all those you have known and do not know are connected by a consciousness which binds you faster than any chains. Naturally, one begins to see then the law working in nature; one begins to see that the whole universe is a mechanism working toward a certain purpose. Therefore, the right and wrong one, the good and bad, they are all bringing about one desired result, by wrong power and by right power—a result meant to be, which is the purpose of life.

Then, naturally, one holds oneself back from that priestly spirit of "You are wrong," and "You are right." But one gets the sagely spirit: saying nothing, knowing all, doing all, suffering all things. This makes one the friend of all and servant of all. And with all the realization of mystical truth and spiritual attainment, what one realizes is one thing, the only thing worthwhile, and that is to be of some little use to one's fellow human beings.

CONTROL OF THE BODY

Many think that the physical has little to do with the spiritual.[1] Why not, they ask, cast aside the idea of the physical in order to be entirely spiritual? If without the physical aspect of our being the purpose of life could be accomplished, the soul would not have taken the physical body, and the spirit would not have produced the physical world. A Hindustani poet says, "If the purpose of creation could have been sufficient, could have been fulfilled by the angels, who are entirely spiritual, God would not have created humanity." And that shows that there is a great purpose that is to be accomplished by what is called the physical body. If the light of God could have directly shone, there would not have been a manifestation such as that of Christ. It was necessary, in other words, that God should walk on the earth in the physical body. And that conception that the physical body is made of sin, and that this is the lowest aspect of being, very often will prove to be mistaken, for it is through this physical body that the highest and the greatest purpose of life is to be achieved. It is when a person is ignorant of it that a person calls it a physical body. And once the knowledge has come, that person begins to look upon it as the sacred temple of God.

And now we come to the five aspects of our experience of life through the physical body. The first aspect is health, the presence of which is heaven, and the absence of which is hell.

1 Lecture, Fine Arts Building, Chicago, April 30, 1926.

No matter what we have in life—wealth, name or fame, power or position, comfort or convenience—without health it is all nothing. When one is healthy one does not think about it, one does not value it. One cares about things one has not got. One tries to sacrifice health for pleasures, health for the material wealth; one is ready to sacrifice health for intellectual fancies, for gaiety, for merriment, for a cheerful time, for an ambition one wants to accomplish. Very often, before the ambition and the desire is accomplished, the collapse comes. Then one begins to realize what health means. Nothing can buy it; nothing can be compared with it. If you gather together all the blessings that can be received in life and weigh them on the scale, you will find health will weigh heavier. No other blessing can be compared to it. It is health which enables us to be material as well as to be spiritual. The lack of it robs us of materiality as well as of spirituality. It robs us of materiality because our condition is not in order; it robs us of spirituality because it is the completeness of health that enables us to experience spiritual life fully. I do not mean that it is a sin to be ill and it is a virtue to be well, but I mean health is a virtue and illness is a sin.

The other aspect of the physical existence is balance. It is balance which gives control of the body. It is by balance that a human being is able to stand, and that a human being is able to walk, and a human being is able to move. Every action, every physical movement is sustained by balance. And the lack of balance always will show some lack in the human character, and, at the same time, some lack in the condition of one's life. In whatever form the lack of balance manifests, it always means lacking something in the personality. You can study the walking of a person, the moving of a person, the way of looking of a person. In everything one does, whenever balance is lacking, something is lacking which you have not known, which you will find out in time. For instance, with a wobbling person, do not think for one moment that it is only an outside defect. It has something to do with that person's character. As a person is

wobbling in walking, so that person is wobbling in determination, wobbling in belief. Just like the physician sees the internal
condition in the eyes and on the tongue of the patient, so the
wise sees all that is pertaining to a person in that person's every
movement, especially by watching the balance.

Many Western readers of Oriental philosophy have talked
with me on this question. They asked me, "Why is it that your
adepts in the East practice acrobatics, sitting in a certain posture, standing on one or the other leg, standing on their heads,
sitting cross-legged in one posture and one pose for a long time,
and many other strange things that one could not think of a
spiritual person doing? What spirituality is there to be attained
by it, for what we know about these things is of acrobatics
and athletics?" And I have answered that, "In all such things
as sports and athletic practices and acrobatics, which others do
for a pastime, they abuse energy, time, and work. They do not
get the full benefit out of it. The adepts use it toward the higher
purpose." And, in addition, I have told them that, "There is
not one thing in this world, if properly practiced, which will
not prove to be beneficial in spiritual attainment." Therefore,
do not think that going to the church or temple, and making
offering of prayer, and sitting in silence with closed eyes only is
the means to spiritual attainment. But all things we can do and
we do in our everyday life, if we turn them to a spiritual goal,
will help us in our spiritual attainment. Besides, it is doing very
little spiritual work if we went once in a week to church. It is
even very little spiritual work done if we said our prayer every
day before going to bed, because every moment of the day we
live in the illusion. Everything we do has an effect of covering
our spiritual vision. Do you think that going to church once
a week, or saying a prayer once at night is sufficient? Never.
Every moment of the day we must have a concentration. And
how can we do it if we have business, industry, profession, if
we have a thousand things to do in everyday life? And the answer is that we must turn all things that we do into a prayer.

Then, whatever be our profession, work, occupation in daily life, it all will help us to spiritual attainment. Then our every action will become a prayer. Every move we make toward south, north, west, or east will point to the spiritual goal. Not everyone thinks about to what extent one is lacking a balance in one's life. And among a hundred persons you can hardly find one really balanced. There is a spiritual balance also, but this spiritual balance is attained by first balancing the physical body and its movements.

And now I come to the third aspect of our physical existence. The third aspect of our physical existence is the fullness of our body. In other words, the fineness, the sensitiveness of the body. There is a spiritual temperament, and you can see that temperament from a person's body. There is a sensitive person, maybe a little bit nervous. And then there is a dense person, which is quite a different aspect. A sensitive person who can appreciate music, who can respond to the beauty of line and color, who can fully enjoy salt and sweet and sour and bitter tastes, who can feel cold and heat, who can perceive fragrances, distinguish them, it is that person who is born with a spiritual temperament. The person who has no love for music, who cannot appreciate fragrance, who cannot understand the beauty of line and color, that person is a dense person. It takes time for that person to develop. Therefore, the experience of all the joy and pleasure that life offers is not in materiality, it is in spirituality. It is not that the material person experiences life fully; it is the spiritual person who does it.

And one might ask, "Then what about these ascetics who have lived the life of a hermit in solitude, who did not eat proper food, and who kept themselves away from all the comfort and beauty of life?" I say, "They are not for everyone to follow," and at the same time, it is a mistake if we criticize them. Such people are the ones who make experiments of life by the sacrifice of all the joy and pleasure that the earth can give. They make an experiment by their solitude. Just like scientists who close themselves up in a laboratory for years and years, so these ascetics, who left everything in the world, also attained a certain knowledge that they give us. But at the same time, it is not a principle to follow for everyone, for spirituality does not depend upon such things. Why are the eyes given if not to appreciate all that is beautiful? Why are the ears given if one cannot enjoy music? Why have we been sent on the earth if we do not look on the earth because we shall be material? Those who make of spirituality something like this, they make of God a bogey, something that frightens. Really speaking, spirituality is the fullness of life.

And now, I come to the fourth aspect of our physical existence. Human beings wrongly identify themselves with their physical body, calling it "myself." And when the physical body is in pain, they say, "I am ill," because they identify themselves with something which belongs to them but which is not themselves. The first thing to learn in the spiritual path is to recognize the physical body not as one's self, but as an instrument, a vehicle, to experience life by it. This instrument is equipped so that one may be able to experience all that is worth experiencing outside oneself, and all that is worth experiencing within oneself.

When a child is born and brought up, its first tendency is to enjoy and experience all that is outside itself. And so it never had a chance in its life to experience what is within. But at the same time, the body is equipped with the instrument, with the means by which to experience the life outside and the life within. If one did not use one's hand for many years, or one's leg for many years, the outcome will be that it will lose the vitality, the life, the energy; and it will no longer be of any use, because it was not used. We know the use of our hands and feet, which are outer particles of the external physical mechanism. But then there are inner and finer parts of the physical mechanism, which mystics have called centers, each center having its particular object, intuition, inspiration, impression, revelation. All these are achieved through the mediumship of these centers. As our organs of senses can experience life that is before us, so the nervous centers can experience life that is within us. And when these centers are not used for many years, they become blunted—not destroyed but blunted—and are no longer of that use for which they exist.

Many who begin to do spiritual work, guided by a proper teacher, begin to feel a sensation here in the midst of the forehead, as if something is awakening. After some time they begin to notice more and more a sphere of which they have been quite ignorant. There are some who begin to notice a feeling in the solar plexus which they did not have before. If that feeling is wakened they naturally become more intuitive. Some feel a sensitiveness on the top of their head, some in the midst of the throat. With their growth they feel more and more. And remember that among these people there are to be found those who are intuitive. The difference between such people whose nervous centers respond, and those whose nervous centers don't respond, is the difference between rock and plant. The rock does not respond to sympathy, but the plant responds to it. If you take care of a plant with love and sympathy, if you rear it wholeheartedly, that plant begins to respond to your sympathy. In other words, the plant begins to waken to your sympathy, whereas the rock does not. And so the ones whose intuitive centers are wakened to some extent, they begin to feel intuition; and after this, inspiration and revelation follow.

But remember that there is so much talk about these things, things that may not be talked about. Those who know little, they talk more. And then the ones who are not yet ready to know the secret of this, if they get hold of some little theory of this kind, they speak about it before everybody. And then they write a book about it, their own wrong conception. Perhaps they never have patience, perseverance, and right guidance to help them. Perhaps they go astray. And many of them and many people have damaged their health and gotten out of balance trying to waken centers; and they make a fuss about it and discuss it and tell everybody about it. They make a play of something which is most serious, most sanctified, and something which leads to spiritual attainment. And there are others who make fun of it, those of the wrong quality who cannot perceive as a plant perceives sympathy. They do not see those qualities in themselves and mock those who perceive them. And in this way a science, which is the highest, has been abused and laughed at by not studying it thoroughly. In the East a teacher does not give guidance until the teacher has full confidence in the pupil, that the pupil will not get the most sacred theory mocked and laughed at by others. They give an initiation. The pupil takes an oath not to speak about these things before those unaware of their value, importance, and sacredness. Then the pupil is guided. And every individual is guided by the teacher separately. Nevertheless, by this we learn that the body is not only an instrument for experiencing the physical sphere, but an instrument at the same time to experience the inner spheres. And it is the experience of the outside life and the life within that makes one live a fuller life.

And now I come to the fifth aspect of our physical existence. There are two things: sensation and exaltation. By sensation one experiences pleasure; by exaltation one experiences joy. There is a difference between joy and pleasure. What one is accustomed to experience by the mediumship of the physical body is pleasure, the pleasure of eating, the pleasure of drinking, the pleasure of looking at beautiful things. And therefore, everything comforting that one knows is that which is experienced by the physical senses. But besides that, there is a joy which does not depend upon the senses, which only depends upon exaltation; and that exaltation is achieved by the mediumship of the body. And now you might ask, "How is this to be achieved?" There is action and its result, and there is repose and its result. It is the result of action which is called sensation; it is the result of repose which is called exaltation. In the book of Rumi, the most wonderful poet of Persia, we read about the blessing of sleep where he says, "O sleep, there is no greater bliss to be compared with you, that in sleep the prisoners are free from their prison and the kings do not possess throne and crown. The suffering and patients lose their pain or worries, and sorrows are forgotten."[2] This shows that sleep is a form of repose automatically brought about, which lifts us up from anxieties, worries, discomforts, from sorrows and troubles. If this condition of repose can be brought about at will, that could give one an experience of mastery, because then one is not dependent upon an automatic condition. For sleep is an automatic condition. If this condition can be produced within ourselves, which raises us above our worries, troubles, sorrows, anxieties, pains, and suffering, it is accomplishing a great thing. And the way of accomplishing this is by the practice of repose.

The first thing an adept does in life is to attain these five different things of which I have spoken and to master them first before taking the next step in the path of spiritual attainment.

---

2 *Masnavi* 1:3.

CONTROL OF THE MIND 1

The tendency to be worried over nothing and the tendency to become anxious about little things—to be fidgety and restless, to be afraid, to be confused—and the tendency to move about without any reason, the tendency to speak without purpose, the tendency to be sad without any motive at the back of it, all these things come owing to the lack of control of the mind.[1] And now you will ask, "Is there any other effect besides the effect that is made upon one's own personality?" Yes, all weaknesses, errors, and mistakes that one makes against one's own wish, all these come from the lack of control over one's own mind. And if there is a secret of success, the key to it is the control of mind. Intuition, inspiration, revelation, all come when mind is controlled. And all worries, anxieties, fears, and doubts come from the lack of control.

One might ask, what is mind? Today the idea of mind is divided into two different parts. There is one part of humanity which considers mind as something still inexplicable, and another part of humanity who considers mind as an action of the brain: all that is registered in the brain is impressed on the atoms of the brain, and it is the composing and decomposing of these little pictures in the brain that brings about a thought. It is a very limited conception of mind. If the voice is such a great thing that it reaches through the wireless miles beyond, the mind is finer than the voice. It cannot be limited and restricted to the

1 Lecture, Twentieth Century Club, Detroit, February 7, 1926.

174

brain, although the brain is the medium by which thoughts are made clear.

Mind, according to the mystic, is the real person; the body is a garb which a person wears. This word *mind* comes from the Sanskrit *mana*. And from that comes *man*. In other words, *man* means "mind." It is true too. When a person says someone is sad, seems downhearted, someone seems courageous, seems enthusiastic, well balanced, all these attributes belong to that person's mind. What a person is, is not that person's body, but it is that person's mind. There is a saying that what you are speaks louder than what you say. That means the voice of mind reaches further than the spoken word and has greater effect than a spoken word, as it is mind which creates atmosphere. One often wonders why it is that one feels uncomfortable in the presence of someone without that person having done any harm, or that one feels excited in the presence of someone, and that one gets out of tune or tired or confused in the presence of someone else. Why is it? It is the effect of that person's mind. The mind that is going into a fire creates a fire in the atmosphere. Everyone in that atmosphere is burning also in the same fire. The mind that is restful and peaceful emits its effect, giving rest and peace to those coming into the atmosphere of that mind.

Once I asked my spiritual teacher how we can recognize the godly. And my teacher replied, "It is not what the godly one says and it is not what the godly one seems to be, but it is the atmosphere that the godly one's presence creates. That is the proof. For no one can create an atmosphere which does not belong to one's spirit."

The first thing about the mind we can learn is to know that mind is independent of the body as far as its existence is concerned. But the mind is enriched by the experience one gets through one's senses. No doubt, mind is within the body but also without the body, just like the light is within the lantern and also without the lantern. The body is the lantern in which there is the light, but the light is not covered by the lantern. The light is independent of the lantern. It shines out, and so does the mind. Neither is the brain the mind, nor is the piece of flesh in the left breast the heart. It's only that feeling is felt more deeply in the breast, and thought is made more clear in the brain. In other words, spectacles are not necessarily eyes; spectacles only enable one to see things more clearly. The sight is independent of the spectacles, but the spectacles are dependent upon the sight. So the body is dependent upon the mind, but the mind is independent of the body. The body cannot exist without mind, but mind can exist without the body. The mind is the invisible being of the body. It has its seat in the physical being, and it is that seat which is called brain, as the seat of feeling is the heart. Neither, therefore, is the mind visible nor is the heart. Mind is the surface of the heart, and heart is the depth of the mind. It is two aspects of one and the same thing. Very often we confuse these two words, the heart and the mind, not knowing that they are one and the same; only they are distinct in this way: that thinking belongs to mind, and feeling belongs to heart.

Mind can be explained in five different aspects. The first aspect is the power of thinking. And thinking can be divided into two parts: automatic thinking and intentional thinking. Automatic thinking is imagination, and when we think with intention that is called thought. Both thought and imagination have their place in life. A person who does not allow imagination to work is as much mistaken as a person who does not allow a thought to act. Many laugh at an imaginative person. They say the imaginative person is in the sky, in the clouds, floating in the air, flying in space, in dreams. But all works of art and music and poetry, they all come from imagination, because imagination is a free flow of mind. Mind is allowed to work by itself and brings out the beauty and harmony it has. And when it is restricted by a certain principle or rule, then it does not work freely. No doubt, among artists and musicians you will find many who are dreamers and impractical people, but that does not mean they are backward in their gift. Perhaps their impracticality, in a way, is a great help so that they accomplish something that practical people cannot accomplish. One need not follow their example, but one can appreciate it just the same. Besides, no one has believed in God, no one has loved God, and no one has reached the presence of God who has not been helped by imagination. Those who come with arguments before the believer and say, "But where is God? Can you show me? How can you conceive of God? How do you explain God?" they are the ones without imagination. And no one can give them one's own imagination. And can anyone believe in the belief of another? If one believes in anything one must do it oneself. And that belief is formed of what? Of imagination. A philosopher says that if you have no God, make one. And no one has ever reached God who has not been able to make God. Those who trouble about the abstract God, they have no God. They only use the word *God*. They have the truth, but they have not God. But truth without God is not satisfying. You ought to reach truth through God. It is that which gives satisfaction. All the strength that one derives from food, if it is given in one pill, perhaps it would keep a person alive, but it would not give the joy of eating. If one took the pill of truth, it may be that a part of one's being would be satisfied, but that is no satisfaction. The idea of God feeds a person. That idea one must first make in oneself, one must make it with one's imagination. If one is not willing to imagine, if one is only waiting for God to come before one, one ought to wait a long time. And if one wants to find the truth of life without the idea of God, it is a pill which will keep one alive; but it is not food.

The next aspect of mind is memory. Memory is likened to a photographic plate: it takes impressions, and the impressions are there. And when a person wishes to recollect something, this faculty helps. It is within one's reach. As soon as one wants to recall an experience, one, so to speak, puts a hand on that particular plate which had taken the impression of a certain experience. There is no experience taken from sight or smell or hearing or touch or taste which is lost. But every little experience once gained, be it for a moment, is impressed upon the memory, and the plate of that picture is there. But some say, "My memory is not good. I cannot remember things, I am absentminded." The reason is that they have lost the control over this faculty. But the impression is there. Very often a person says. "I know it, but I cannot recall it to my memory." In other words, in the mind one knows it, but in the brain it is not yet clear. For instance, if a person has lost the memory of the name of a person, the face of a person, then that person says, "I think I know it and yet I cannot make it clear." That means that my mind knows it. It is there, but I cannot make it clear in my brain.

The third aspect of the mind is the retaining quality, the ability to retain a thought. Those who concentrate practice retaining a thought, an impression. But those who do not practice concentration automatically retain things of great interest, things that impressed their mind most. It is therefore that some carry with them a fear which perhaps is there from childhood. It is carried along through life. Some have a sad impression of disappointment. They carry it throughout life, they retain it in their mind. Mind is keeping it alive by revivifying it, by keeping that impression, whether an impression of revenge, of gratefulness, of success, of failure, of love, of admiration. It is kept there, and the cells of the mind give it food and a means to be kept alive. Sometimes this is helpful, and sometimes this is against oneself. Now, the psychologist calls it a fixed idea, and is always ready to call it insanity and to put it on the list of the insane. But it is not insanity, everyone has got it. It is one of the attributes of mind. It is a faculty, a quality, to retain what one likes to retain or happens to retain. No doubt, sometimes it is a fact that it may seem to be insanity, but insanity only comes from the abuse of that faculty. But it is not only that. Any faculty can be abused, and a person can become unbalanced by it.

The fourth faculty of mind is reasoning. This is a department of mind which is always balancing and which is always enlightening, enlightening in the way that mind asks "Why has that person done it?" Mind says, "That person is senseless, that is why that person has done wrong." That is what mind says is reason. What mind knows it says immediately. But what mind says may not always be right; it may also be a wrong reason. But at the same time, there is always some answer. And it is very wonderful to watch the trick of the reasoning faculty, that when another person has done something wrong, reason says because that person is wicked, that person has done ten wicked things, and now has done another wicked thing. And when one's own self has done a wicked thing, reason says it was "Because I could not have done otherwise. I could not help it."

Reason takes the side of the ego. Reason is a slave and a servant of mind. It is ready at the call. Mind only has to turn its face to reason, and reason stands there as an obedient servant. It may not be right at all, but it is always there. No doubt, there is always a reason behind a reason, and if we penetrate the thousand veils of reason we can touch the reason of all reasons, and we can come to an understanding that the outer reasons cannot give. And by that we understand all beings, those who are in the right and those who are in the wrong. They say the apostles, in one moment's time, were inspired to speak in many languages.[2] It was not the English language, the Hindustani, or Chinese language, it was the language of every soul. When a person has reached that state of mind where it touches the essence of reason, then it communicates with every soul. It is not a great thing to know thirty languages. If a person knows a hundred languages and does not know the human heart, that person knows nothing. But there is a language of the heart. Heart speaks to heart. That communication makes life interesting. Two persons may not speak, but their sitting together is an exchange of lofty ideal and harmony.

2 See Acts 2:2–4.

And it will interest you to know that when first I became initiated at the hands of my spiritual teacher in India, I was as eager as any could be to assimilate, to grasp as much as I could. Day after day I was in the presence of my teacher, but he did not once talk on spiritual matters. Sometimes he spoke about herbs and plants, about milk and butter. I went there for six months continually, every day, to see if I could hear anything about spiritual things. After six months, one day the teacher spoke to me about the two parts of a personality, the outer and the inner. And I was overly enthusiastic. The moment I heard I took out a notebook and pencil. As soon as I did it, my teacher changed the subject, going on to other things. I understood what that meant. It meant in the first place that the teaching of the heart should be assimilated in the heart. The heart is the notebook for it. When it is written in the outer notebook, it will remain in the pocket. When it is written in the heart, it will remain in the soul. Besides this, one has to learn that lesson of patience, to wait, for all knowledge comes in its own time. I asked myself further, after six months' time of making a long journey to get to the place, if it was worthwhile going there every day to hear of nothing but trees and butter. And my deepest self answered, "Yes, more than worthwhile, for there is nothing in the whole world that is worth more than the presence of a holy person. If the teaching is not said in theories, it is in the atmosphere." That is a living teaching, which is real upliftment.

And now we come to the fifth aspect of mind, the heart, which is the feeling. But thought, reasoning, maintaining of thought, and memory, all these faculties are nourished by this one faculty of feeling. People today divide intellectuality and sentimentality, but in reality intellectuality cannot be perfect without sentimentality. Neither the thinking power can be nurtured, nor the faculty of reasoning can be sustained without a continual outflow of feeling. In this age of materialism we seem to have lost the value of feeling. We know the name *heart*, but we have never seen such a thing. We don't know of its existence. We don't use it. We don't see its importance. But really speaking, that is the principal bank, that is the root of the plant of life. The heart quality is something that sustains the whole life. All virtues such as sincerity, respect, thoughtfulness, consideration, appreciation—all those qualities come through the heart quality. If one has no heart, one is not capable of appreciating, nor of being grateful, nor capable of expressing one's own soul, nor of receiving favor, goodness, or help from another. A person without heart quality remains selfish, even foolishly selfish. If that person was wisely selfish it would be worthwhile. People say very often, "But we have no time to show our heart quality, we have no time to allow the heart to develop. We are so busy." But we can be busy every day, every moment of life, every minute from morning till evening, but everything we do, we can do it with our whole heart, express it from the depth of our heart. When the heart quality is shut out, then all one does is lifeless.

Mind is likened to a pool of water. When the water in the pool is troubled, it cannot take reflection. So is mind. When mind is troubled, it is confused, it cannot take reflection. It is the stillness of mind that makes one capable of receiving impressions and of reflecting them. In the Persian language the mind is called a mirror. Everything that stands before the mirror appears reflected in it. But when it is taken away, the mirror is pure. It does not remain. It is only in the mirror as long as the mirror is focused to it. So it is with the mind.

It develops by concentration, contemplation, meditation, that quality in mind which makes it still at times and active at other times, which makes it reflect what it sees at one time, and makes it avoid every reflection, so that no outer influence can touch it. The mind is trained by the master trainer by diving deep, by soaring high, by expanding widely, and by centering the mind on one idea. And once the mind is mastered, a person becomes a master of life. Every soul born, from the time it is born, is like a machine, subject to all influences, influences of weather, of all that works through one's five senses. For instance, no one can pass through a street without seeing the placards and advertisements. One's eyes are commanded by what is before one. A person has no intention of looking, but everything outside commands the eyes. So one is constantly under the influence of all things of the outside world, which govern without one knowing. A person says, "I am a free human being, I do what I like." But one never does it. One always does what one does not like, many times. The ears are always subject to hearing anything that falls on them, whether it is harmonious or disharmonious. And what one sees, one cannot resist. And so a human being is always under the influence of life, then planetary influences, then living influences of those around. And yet a person says, "I have free will, and I am a free human being." If one knew to what extent one is free, one would be frightened for one's life.

But then there is one consolation, that in a human being there is a spark somewhere hidden in the heart which alone can be called a source of free will. If this spark is greater, a person has a greater vitality, a greater energy, a greater power. All that person thinks comes true, all that person says gives impression, all that person does will make an effect. What does a mystic do? The mystic blows this spark in order to bring this spark to a flame, till it comes to a blaze. This gives that inspiration, that power which enables the mystic to live the life of free will in this world. It is this spark which may be called the divine heritage of humanity, in which the mystic sees the divine power of God, the human soul.

Spiritual quality, therefore, is the developing of this spark. To become spiritual means by blowing this spark you produce light from it, and see the whole life in this light. And one is more able to think, to feel, and to do by bringing the inner light to a blaze.

CONTROL OF THE MIND 2

In Sanskrit language mind is called *mana*, and from that word comes *manu*, which means "man."[1] The [English] word "man" is also is much the same as *manu* in Sanskrit. And from that we gather that the human being is the human mind, not the body or the soul; for the soul is divine, it has no distinction, and the body is a cover. Therefore, the human being is the human mind. Once you begin to look into the minds of human beings, you begin to see such a phenomenon that no wonder in the world can be compared to it. To look in the eyes when they are afraid, when they doubt, when they are sad and they want to hide it, when they are glad. When they have a guilty conscience you can see lions turn into rabbits. As flowers emit fragrance, so minds produce the atmosphere. To see it in the aura apart, even in the expression of a person you can clearly see the record of the mind. Nothing can express one's mind better than one's own expression. Mind, therefore, is the principal thing. We distinguish a person as an individuality. It is the culture of mind which develops individuality into a personality.

One thing is the mind, and the other thing is the heart. Both of these are the two different aspects of one object. The mind is the surface, the heart is the bottom. The mind thinks, the heart feels. What the heart feels, the mind wants to interpret in a thought. What the mind thinks, the heart assimilates, expressing it in a feeling.

1 Lecture, Sufi Center, San Francisco, April 17, 1926.

183

The mind can be seen in five different faculties working together: thinking, remembering, reasoning, identifying, and feeling.

Thinking is of two kinds: imagination and thought. When the mind is working under the direction of the will, it is thought. When the mind is working automatically, without the power of the will, it is imagination. The thoughtful person is the one who reigns over the activity of the mind. The imaginative person is the one who indulges in the automatic action of the mind. Both thought and imagination have their place in life. The automatic working of the mind works out a picture, a plan, which is sometimes more beautiful than a plan or an idea thought out carefully under the control of the will. Therefore, artists, poets, musicians are very often imaginative; and the beauty they produce in their art is the outcome of their imagination.

Now, the secret about imagination that needs to be understood is this: everything that works automatically must first be prepared to work automatically, just like a watch must be prepared to work automatically. We must wind it up, then it can go on automatically; we need not trouble about it. That shows that the mind needs preparing to work automatically for the best advantage in life. If those who do not prepare their mind for imagination then become imaginative, that lack of preparation can lead to insanity, or at least an unbalanced condition. It is the imaginative person who afterwards becomes unbalanced, which leads to insanity, because that person has no control of the mind.

Now the question is how to prepare it? The mind is just like a moving-picture film: all the single photographs make the film, and it produces what was put into it. The one who is critical, who looks at the ugly side of human nature, who has love of evil, love of gossip, who has the desire to see the bad side of things, who wishes to find the bad points of people, prepares a film in the mind. And that film, projected on the curtain, produces undesirable impressions in the form of imagination.

The great poets who have given us beautiful teachings in
morals, in truth—where did they get it? Here. This life is the
school from which they have learned; this life is the stage from
which they have seen and gathered. They are the worshippers
of beauty in nature and in art. In all conditions of life they are
meditating upon it and finding the good points of all those
they see. They gather together all that is beautiful from the
good and the wicked both. Just like the bee takes the best from
every flower and makes honey from it, so they gather together
all that is beautiful and express it through their imagination in
the form of music, poetry, art, and also in their thoughts and
deeds in everyday life.

In my early life I began a pilgrimage in India, not a pilgrimage to the holy shrines, but a pilgrimage to holy people, going
from one place to another and seeing sages with different natures and characters. What I gathered from all was their great
love-nature, their outgoing tendency, their deep sympathy, and
their inclination to find some good in every person they see.
They are looking for some good, and therefore, they find it in
the most wicked person; and by that they become themselves
goodness, because they have gathered it. We become what we
gather. In their presence there is nothing but love and compassion and understanding, which is so little to be found in
this world. In our domestic life, in our life in the world, in our
social life, political life, in business, commerce, national activities, if we had that one tendency it would make life different
for us, more worth living than it is today for so many souls.
The condition today is that people are rich, they have all convenience and comfort, and what is lacking is the understanding.
The home is full of comfort, but there is no understanding,
there is no happiness. It is such a little thing and yet so difficult
to obtain. No intellectuality can give understanding. That is
where a person makes a mistake and wants to understand with
the head. Understanding comes from the heart. The heart must
be glowing, living. When the heart becomes feeling, then there

is understanding. Then you are ready to see from the point of view of another as much as you can see from your own point of view.

And now we come to the other aspect of thinking, and that is the thought which is heavier, more solid, more vital than the imagination because it has a backbone, and that is willpower. Therefore, when we say, "That is a thoughtful person," that makes a distinction between the imaginative and the thoughtful. Those who are thoughtful have a weight about them, something substantial about them; you can rely upon them. The imaginative person one day comes and says, "I love you so much, you are so good, so high, so true, so great." It is just like a cloud of imagination that rises. Then it is scattered away next day, and the same imaginative person who had yesterday followed this cloud of imagination would try to find some fault. And nothing is left in that person's hands. How very often it happens. They are angelic people perhaps, but they ride on the clouds, and they are of no use for this earth. You cannot rely upon them; they are as changeable as weather. The thoughtful person, on the contrary, takes time to express both praise or blame. The mind of the thoughtful is anchored and under control. And the one who learns how to make the best of imagination and how to control thought shows great balance in life.

How is it to be achieved? By concentration. In India there is a Hindu sacred legend that two sons of God were in a country. And the younger son saw a horse which was set free by the government, and the one who could catch this horse would be brought to become the king of that country. And this youth was so attracted to the horse and the idea that was behind it, that he ran after this horse, but he could not catch it. For this horse would sometimes become slow, but as soon as he got nearer, the horse would run away. The mother was worried and asked the elder brother to go and find him. Then the elder brother comes and he sees that, "My brother is in pursuit of the horse." So he said to his brother, "It is a wrong method by which you will never be able to catch it. The best way of catching it is not to follow it, but to meet it." Instead of following the horse, he met the horse and then caught it. The mother was very pleased and proud that, "My son was able to catch it." So he became entitled to the throne and crown of the father. The horse here is the mind. When the mind is controlled, then mastery is gained, God's kingdom is attained. The younger brother is the pupil, the elder brother is the guru, the teacher. And the way of controlling the mind is not to follow it, but to concentrate. By concentrating you meet it.

There is a story of a Sufi and a pupil. The pupil said, "Teacher, I cannot concentrate on one thing. If I try to concentrate on one object, other objects come in. Then they become so muddled that I do not know on which object [to concentrate], and it is difficult to hold the mind on one object." The teacher said that, "Your difficulty is your anxiety. The moment you begin, you are anxious your mind would wander away. If you were not anxious about it, your mind would have poise. Your anxiety makes it more active. If you just took what it gives you instead of looking from behind where it goes, if you meet it before it comes, with what it comes to you—if you change this tendency—you will be able to concentrate better."

In this story there is a great lesson to learn. For it is always the case: the moment one sits to concentrate, the mind changes its rhythm from the very fact that the person is anxious to keep it under control. The mind does not wish it. It wants its freedom. As you stand for your right, the mind stands for its right. And the best way is to greet the mind as it comes to meet you, to let it bring what it brings; and then you stand face-to-face with your mind and do not become annoyed with what it brings. Just take it. Then you have the mind under control. Because the mind comes to you, it will not go further. Let it bring what it brings. In this way you make a connection with your mind, and as soon as you begin to look at your mind, you have your mind in hand. The photographer has the subject in hand when the photographer has focused the camera on the subject. The same thing with a person and the mind: as soon as one has focused oneself on one's mind, one has got the mind in one's control.

The concentrations can be considered as different stages of evolution. The first concentration is the concentration on a certain designed object. And this is divided into two sections. One is the making of the object and then holding it in the mind. It is just like a child takes the little bricks and pillars and different things, and makes out of them a little house. The first action is the making of the house. The second action is looking at it. That is one kind. And the other kind is that there is an object already, and our mind must reflect that object by focusing on that object.

The next stage of concentration is improving on the object. For instance, you imagine a tiger. But then you also imagine the background of the tiger: the mountain, the rocks behind it, the trees, the forest, the river. That is improvement: holding at the same time the background, changing it according to the activity of our mind. Even if the tiger is changing, it does not matter as long as we have that particular kind of concentration.

And the third concentration is concentration on an idea. An idea has an inexpressible form, but the mind makes it.

And now coming to the realm of the feeling. Feeling is such an important thing in our lives that our whole life depends upon our feeling. A person once disheartened, sometimes for a whole life, loses enthusiasm. A person once disappointed, for a whole life loses trust. A person heartbroken, for all of that person's life, loses self-confidence. A person once afraid sustains, in the heart, fear forever. A person who has once failed, keeps all through life the impression of failure.

There is a love of bird fighting in the East, and two men bring their birds to fight. And the man sees that the other bird will win in the end. And as soon as he sees it, he takes his bird away while it is in the action of fighting, before it has accepted defeat. And this man admits defeat while the two birds were fighting, but he does not allow his bird to go so far as to be impressed by defeat. Once so impressed it will never fight. That is the secret of our mind. And just as with the bird, once you learn to take care of your mind so that you can make any sacrifice but do not let your mind be badly impressed, you would make the best of your life.

Besides, you will read in the lives of great heroes and great personalities, how they went through all difficulties and sorrows and troubles, and yet always tried to keep their heart from being humbled. That gave them all the strength. They always escaped humiliation. They were prepared for death, wars, suffering, poverty, but not for humiliation. That is something.

I will tell you an amusing story. I was in Nepal once, near the Himalayas, and I wanted a servant, so I sent for one, and he was of the warrior's caste, Kshatriyas, from a fighters' tribe in the mountains. But what amused me the most was when I asked what work he wanted to do. He said, "Any work you like, anything you like." I said, "And pay?" "Anything you will give." I was amused. He wants to do any work I give him, accepts any pay I give him. "Well," I said, "then there is no condition to be made." He said, "One." I said, "What?" He said, "You will not speak a cross word to me." Imagine, ready to accept any amount of money, willing to do any work, but not humiliation. I appreciated that spirit of the warrior beyond words. That is what makes him a warrior.

Friends, our failure and success, all depends upon the condition of our mind. If mind failed, the failure is sure; if mind is successful, it does not matter what the condition; in the end we shall succeed.

* * *

Question: *Is it possible, when humiliated, for us to be able to see that the person who is humiliating us is beneath us, in that way and spare our mind the injury of humiliation?*

189

Answer: That is not the way, because as soon as we accept humiliation we are humiliated, whether we think it or not. It does not depend upon the other person, it depends upon ourselves. No sooner we admit humiliation, there is humiliation. If the whole world does not take it, it does not matter if our mind is humiliated. If our mind does not accept it, it does not matter if the whole world took it as such. If a thousand persons came and said that, "You are wicked," you do not believe it as long as your heart says, "I am not wicked." But when your heart says, "I am wicked," if a thousand persons said, "You are good," your heart will continue to say, "No, no, I am wicked." The heart keeps you down just the same. If we ourselves give it up, then nobody can sustain us.

Question: *Then is it possible to develop a state of mind that lifted us out of humiliation?*

Answer: Yes. Well, the best thing would be to avoid a humiliation. But if one cannot avoid it, then one must be like a patient who must be treated by a physician. Then one wants a person powerful enough, a master mind, a spiritual person who can help. And then one can be doctored, attended to, and can get over that condition. But when one is a patient one cannot help oneself very well. One can do much, but then there is the necessity of a doctor.

Question: *Can that condition be treated by counter-irritation?*

Answer: Yes, it can be met with that.

Question: *What to do when the feeling of humiliation has entered into the mind?*

Answer: To take it as a lesson. To take poison as something which must be. But poison is a poison. What is put in the mind will grow just the same. It must be taken out. If it remains it will grow—every impression, humiliation, fear, doubt. What is there is there. There will come a time that the person will be conscious of it, then it will grow. Because it is growing in the subconscious mind, it will bear fruits and flowers.

Question: *Would the study of mathematics be good for the imaginative poet?*

Answer: Yes, it can bring about a balance. I have seen it in the case of one of my pupils, very extremely imaginative. He could not stay on the earth. But later on, by getting into a business where he was obliged to count figures, after some time he obtained a great deal of balance.

THE POWER OF THOUGHT

There are some who, by life's experience, have learned that thought has some power; and there are others who wonder sometimes if thought really has some power.[1] But there are many who listen to this subject with the preconceived idea that even if every thought has a power, it also has its limits. But if I were to give my candid opinion on the subject, I would say that it is no exaggeration that thought has a power which is unimaginable. And in order to find proof of this idea we do not have to go very far. All that we see in this world is but a phenomenon of thought. We live in it, and we see it morning till evening, and yet we doubt if it is so. This doubt gives us a pride and shows that we understand things better. The less one believes in the power of thought, the more positively one thinks one stands on the earth. Nevertheless, consciously or unconsciously, one feels one's limitation and is searching for something that will strengthen one's belief in thought.

Thought can be divided into five different aspects: imagination, thought, dream, vision, and materialization. Imagination is that action of mind which is automatic. From morning till evening, either a person is working or is resting; and if resting, that person's mind is working just the same through imagination. It is automatic thinking; what it produces is called imagination. And then we come to the word *thought*. Thought is thinking which has willpower behind it. And in this way we

1 Lecture, Sorbonne, Paris, March 24, 1925.

192

distinguish between the imaginative and the thoughtful. And therefore, these two kinds of people cannot be confused, for one is imaginative, whose thinking is powerless, automatic; and the other is thoughtful, whose thinking is powerful.

And when this automatic action takes place in the state of sleep, it is called a dream. No doubt, this is distinct and different from imagination, because while a person is imagining, the senses are open to the objective world, and therefore, the imagination does not take a concrete form. But the same automatic action of mind goes on in the dream, and there is no objective world to compare it with. Therefore, the dream brings more imagination than a wakeful state. Therefore, the mystic can always see the person's condition of mind by hearing the dream of the person, by knowing about how a person dreams; because in the dream the automatic working of the person's mind is much more concrete than in the imagination.

There are some who can perhaps read the character of a person, some who can read what they call the future by knowing what a person imagines. They always ask a person, "Give me a name of a flower, of a fruit, of something you love, you like," so that they can find the stream of imagination, where it goes. And from that stream of imagination they find out something about the character of that person and about that person's life. And it is not necessary for a person to be a character-reader, or a fortune-teller in order to know what any wise and thoughtful person can understand by the way someone dresses or by someone's environment. A thoughtful person can understand what way someone's thoughts go, what someone's imaginations are. Since the state of dream gives the mind the possibility to express itself more concretely, the dream is the best way to understand in what state of mind a person is. And once that is understood, there is little reason left to doubt whether the dream has any effect upon a person's life and future. For I would repeat the same thing again which I have said at the commencement of my lecture, that a human being does not know, and cannot imagine, to what extent thought works upon life.

And now, coming to the question of what we call vision. In order to make it simple, I would explain vision as that state of dream which one experiences in the wakeful state. A person who is imaginative or a person who is capable of imagining is capable of making a thought. And when this thought which one has created becomes one's own, an object upon which one's mind is focused, then all else becomes hidden; there is only that particular imagination that stands before one as a picture. No doubt, the effect of this vision is greater than the effect of a dream. The reason is that this imagination, which can stand before one's mind in one's wakeful state, is naturally stronger than the imagination which was working in one's state of sleep.

But then the fifth aspect is materialization of thought, and it is in the study of this subject that we find the greatest secret of life. No doubt, a person if asked will accept that it is by the architect's imagination that the beautiful building is built, that it is by the gardener's imagination that a beautiful garden is made. But when it comes to nature and all things that spring from nature, then one begins to wonder how far imagination or thought has any power upon it. Nowadays, as psychology is beginning to spread throughout the Western world, people would at least patiently listen to what it is. But otherwise there are many who would take a medicine and have a great belief in it, but if they are told that a thought can cure you, they will smile at it. And this shows that, with all the progress that humanity seems to have made, it has gone backward in one direction; and that direction is in regard to the higher thought, the elevated thought. For a person today generally disbelieves in thought and still less believes in what one calls emotion. And in the point of fact, if there is a soul to be found in thought, that soul is the feeling which is at the back of it. The reason is that souls become confused when there are only words and there is no feeling behind them. What convinces in a thought is the power behind it, and that power consists of feeling. The general tendency is to wave off what is called imagination. "Those ones imagine" means that "those ones amuse themselves." When a person says, "Oh, you think it, but it does not exist in reality. You just think it." But in reality when one has imagined, that imagination is created, and what is once created exists. And what is thought exists, and that lives longer, because thought is more powerful than imagination. And what a person today calls sentimentality, which means nothing, in this way ignores that power which is the only power and the greatest power that exists. It is with this power that the heroes have conquered battles. And it is with this power that, if anyone has accomplished a great thing in the world, it is with the power of heart that one has accomplished it and not with the power of brain. The music of the most wonderful composers and the poetry of the great poets of the world—it has come from the bottom of their heart; it has not come from their brain. And if we close the door to sentimentality, to imagination, and to thought, that only means that we close the door to life.

And now, coming to fancies and fantasies. Perhaps some, if not all of you, have read the stories of fakirs and dervishes in the East. Perhaps you have read about them in a novel, and perhaps they have been exaggerated in some way in order to make the book more beautiful. Nevertheless, I ask you to study the matter a little more and to understand something of a race, a nation, that has for so many thousands of years devoted itself, at the sacrifice of the whole life, to thought.

There exists perhaps in every little district, in every little village, a person who is called the healer of the scorpion sting. And in the heat, as it is in India, scorpions can be found in the house, especially in summertime. And it is not seldom that a child or a grown-up person is stung by a scorpion, and the sting is very poisonous and very painful. But, in spite of all that, there are healers, and several of them. And sometimes there is a healer who says, "You are cured. It is gone." And immediately the person is well. And then we come to the sting of the snake-bites. The poison of the serpent is such that hardly a person lives after a serpent bite. There are some who by the passing of their hands have cured it. There are some who have cured it by saying, "It is cured."

And then I will tell you my own experience, that once there was a dervish to whom a person came and said, "There is a case going to be in the court next week." And he said, "I am so poor that I cannot even have a lawyer to speak for me. And the other person, being rich, he will use every influence, and I am without it." And that dervish said, "Tell me what is the condition." And after hearing it all he said, "As you are not found guilty in this, I dismiss this case." He told him simply to go, "All will be well." When the man went to the court, he was asked everything by the judge; at the end, the judge wrote exactly the same words that the dervish had said. If I were to give any explanation, words fail to explain it. Only this can be said, that the heart of the judge, for this dervish, was just like the receptive machine of wireless telegraphy.

The great seer and mystic of Persia Jalal ad-Din Rumi says that, "Fire, water, earth, and air are dead things to those who see in them no person. But before the Creator they are all live beings; they are the Creator's obedient servants." And the great thinker of the Hindus says in the Sanskrit language that this whole creation is the dream of Brahma, which means the Creator.

And now I come to Sufism and what the Sufi thinks of the idea of the Creator and the creation. The Sufi sees both, the Creator and the creation, in humanity. The limited part of the human being is the creation, and the innermost part of the human being is the Creator. And if that is true, then the human being is both limited and unlimited. If one wishes to be limited, one can be more and more limited. If one wishes to be unlimited, one can be more and more unlimited. If one cultivates in oneself the illusion of being a creation, one can be more and more that. But if one cultivates in oneself the knowledge of the Creator, one can also be more and more that.

With every kind of weakness, every kind of illness, every kind of misery, the more one gives in to it, the more it falls upon one's back. And one can even give into it to such an extent sometimes that the whole world falls on one's back and one is buried under it. And then there is another person who gets out of it. It may be difficult, but at the same time it is possible. Little by little, gradually, but with courage and patience, one can get out of it and stand upon the same world which would have otherwise crushed one under it.

The former thing is going down, the latter thing is coming up. Both things depend upon the attitude of our mind, and it is changing this attitude that is the principal thing in life, whether from a material point of view or from a spiritual point of view. All that is taught in the Sufi esoteric studies and practices is to gain that mastery in order to arrive little by little, gradually, at that fulfillment which is called mastery. But, you will say, it is a great struggle. But, I will answer, the struggle is in both ways; in coming down and in going up; in both ways there is a struggle. It is just as well to struggle and come up instead of struggling and going down. And whenever a person goes down, it only means that person is feeble in thought. And why that person is feeble in thought is because that person is weak in feeling. If feeling protects thought, and if thought stands firm, whatever be the difficulty in the life of a human being, it will be surmounted.

CONCENTRATION

Concentration is a subject which is interesting to every thoughtful person.[1] But to have knowledge of concentration requires not only study, but also balance. Before touching this subject, I would like first to explain what motive we have behind concentration. There are two aspects of life: the audible life and the silent life. By audible life I mean all experiences, all sensations we experience through our five senses, namely sight, hearing, smell, taste, and touch. All that we experience through these senses is sensation. This is separate from the life which I call the silent life.

Now, the question is: What benefit does one derives from getting in touch with the silent life? In answer to this one can say that the benefit is as abstract as the silent life. The life of sensation is clear; its benefit is clear. And yet as limited as is the life of sensation, so limited is its benefit. Therefore, at the end of the examination we find all our experiences of little value. Their importance is for as long as we experience them, but after the experience the importance of the life of sensation is finished. But the value of the silent life is independent. Naturally, we consider of value that which our outer life considers so. By touching the silent life, we do not touch a certain benefit, but a general benefit. In other words, if there is a certain hurt on the skin, a little wound on the body, an external application of medicine can cure it. But there are medications which can cure

1 Lecture, Kunstgewerbehaus, Munich, March 20, 1925.

198

the general condition, and this is better than the outer cure. This latter cure is not noticed as much as the former. Naturally, one cannot exactly say what profit is gained by concentration, but in reality, every kind of profit is to be attained through concentration, in all directions.

Concentration can be divided into two parts: first, automatic concentration; and second, intentional concentration.

Automatic concentration is found in many people who do not know that they concentrate, and yet they do. They concentrate automatically, some to their disadvantage, some to their advantage. Those who concentrate to their advantage are the ones whose mind is fixed on business, on any occupation they do. And they are the ones who can be most concentrated and can work more successfully. Be it a composer, a writer, a musician, according to one's power of concentration, one will have success. One may not know it, but one's power of concentration may be great. For instance, I had the pleasure of hearing Paderewski[2] in his house. He began gently on his piano. Every note took him to a deeper and deeper ocean of music. Any meditative person could see clearly that he was so concentrated on what he did that he knew not where he was. Great composers who left such works which will always live, which win the hearts of others, from where do they come? From concentration. So it is with a poet, so it is with an artist, that it is concentration which brings color and line, which makes the picture. Naturally, be it an artist or a writer, a musician or a poet, somebody who is in business or industry, in the absence of concentration a person can never succeed.

Now, we come to the kind of concentration that works to one's disadvantage. There are some who get to think that, "I am unlucky, everything I do goes wrong," some who think that everybody dislikes them, that everybody hates them. Then some begin to think that, "I am unable to do anything, I am incapable,

---

2 Ignacy Jan Paderewski (1860–1941), Polish composer, pianist, and statesman.

useless." Some, out of self-pity, think that they are ill. In that way, if they are not ill, they create illness. Some, by concentration, cherish illness, always think of it. No physician could be successful with them. As an old physician has said, "There are many diseases, but there are many more patients." Once a person has become a patient through concentration, that person is difficult to cure. Never think for a moment that there are few such cases. There are many cases of automatic concentration to the disadvantage of human beings.

And now we come to intentional concentration. This, no doubt, is taught by thinkers, philosophers, meditative people. The whole of mysticism, esotericism, is based upon the idea of concentration. This mystical concentration can be divided into four different grades. The first is concentration, the next contemplation, the next meditation, the fourth realization.

The definition of the first grade is to fix one's thought upon one object. No doubt the question arises, "Which object?" A person need not concentrate upon any object that comes along, because what you concentrate upon has an effect upon you. When you concentrate on a dead object, it has the effect of deadening the soul. If you concentrate on a living object, it naturally has a living effect. In this the secret is to be found of the teachings of all prophets and mystics. This concentration is made in three different ways. The first way is by action. One does a certain movement or action which helps the mind to concentrate on a certain object. The other way is with the help of words. By the repetition of certain words one learns to think automatically on a certain object. The third way is made with the help of memory. Memory is like the storehouse of an architect. From it the architect takes everything the architect likes—tiles, pillars, bricks—whatever the architect wants. To give an illustration, it is much like the play of children using toy bricks to build toy houses. It is the same thing for the one who does this concentration: that person gets things [from memory] and composes objects in order to concentrate on the wished-for end.

Now, coming to the subject of contemplation. Only when a person is advanced enough can that person contemplate, because contemplation is not on an object, it is on an idea. No doubt, one can think one is ready to do anything, that after concentration one can contemplate. The nature of the mind is such that it slips out of your hands the moment you try to hold it. Therefore, before one has thought, the mind has thrown off the object of concentration like a restive horse. Mind is not always so unruly. It proves to be unruly when it wants to rule. It is like the body. You may feel restful sitting naturally, but as soon as you keep it still for five minutes, it begins to feel restless. It is still more difficult to make the mind obey. Yes, automatically it will, but when one wishes, it will not. Mystics, therefore, find a rope to tie the mind to a certain place where it cannot move. What is that rope? That rope is breath. It is by that rope that they bind it and make the mind stand where they wish it to stand. It is like the bird which puts out its saliva to make its nest. So it is with the mystic who out of the breath creates atmosphere, creates light and magnetism in which to live.

Before speaking on the third subject, the third grade, I should first like to say what qualities the mind has. There are two characteristics of the mind that must be understood. First, it is like a gramophone record: whatever is impressed upon it, it is able to produce. So it is with our mind: all it takes upon itself it repeats. If it is a pleasing impression, a happy impression, it gives happiness. If it is an ugly, depressing impression, it produces unhappiness. How few there are who think about this. How more ready one is to see the bad side than the good side of things. The other characteristic of the mind is that not only is it a gramophone record, but it creates what is impressed upon it. If ugliness is recorded, it will produce disagreement, disharmony. Learning concentration clears the record, making it produce what we like, not what comes automatically. In this world one is so open to impressions; one goes about with eyes and ears open. But it is not only the eyes, not only the ears which are open; the lips are open to give out what the eyes and ears take in. That is the dangerous part. Suppose one goes on in life like that? Where does it end? It would end in nothing.

The third part of concentration is meditation. In this grade one becomes communicative. One communicates with the silent life, and naturally, communication also becomes open with the outer life. It is then that we begin to realize that all of the outer and inner life—all of it—is communicative. Then we begin to learn what can never be learned by study or from books: that the silent life is the greatest teacher and knows all things. It does not only teach, but gives that peace, that joy, that power and harmony which make life beautiful. No one can claim to be meditative, for a meditative person need not say it with the lips. One's atmosphere says it. One can say that it is true or that it is false, but atmosphere alone can say if it is true or false. Once I asked my spiritual teacher what was the sign of knowing God. He said, "Not those who call out the name of God, but those whose silence says it." Many go about looking, searching for something worthwhile, something wonderful. But there is nothing more wonderful than the human soul.

Realization is the result of the three other grades. In the third kind of experience, a person pursued meditation; but in this, meditation pursues that person. If I may say it in other words, no longer is it the singer who sings the song, but the song that sings the singer. This fourth grade is a kind of expansion of consciousness. It is the unfoldment of the soul; it is diving deep within oneself. It is communicating with each atom of life existing in the whole world. It is realizing the real "I" in which is the fulfillment of life's purpose.

THE WILL

No doubt words such as *wish, desire, love,* and their like mean more or less the same thing, but the word *will* has a greater importance than all other words. And the reason is that will is life itself.[1]

The Bible calls God love. Love in what sense? Love in the sense of will. The Creator created the universe by what? By love? It is by will—love came afterward. Love is the will; when it is recognized by its manifestation, then it is called love, but in the beginning it is will. For instance, the Taj Mahal, the great building located in Agra, is said to be the token of the love that the emperor had for his beloved. And at the same time, if you look at it only with reason, you cannot call it an expression of love; but you can, with good reason, call it a phenomenon of will. For the beginning of the building at least, you may call that spirit, that impulse which brought it about, the phenomenon of the emperor's will. After it was made, then you can say it was the expression of his love. When a person says, "I desire it," "I wish it," it is an incomplete will, a will which is not conscious of its strength, a will which is not sure of what it wills. In that case it is called a desire, a wish. But when a person says: "I will it," that means it is definite. A person who can never say "I will it"—that person has no will.

We come to the conclusion that will, therefore, is the source and the origin of all phenomena. Hindus have called creation

1 Lecture, Paris, October 17, 1925.

the dream of Brahma, which means the dream of the Creator. But may I add that dream is a phenomenon of an unconscious will, when the will works automatically.

And now we come to the question of the difference between the imaginative and the thoughtful person. The difference is that one thinks with will, the other thinks without will. When a person once knows the value of will, that person then recognizes that there is nothing in the world which is more precious than will. Naturally, therefore, a question arises in the mind of the thoughtful: Have I will in me? Have I a strong will, or have I a weak will? And the answer is that no one can exist without a will. And therefore, everyone has will.

And now the question arises: How can we maintain our will? The nature of the life that we live is such to rob us of our will. Not only is it the struggle through which we must go in life, but also our own self, our thoughts, our desires, our wishes, our motives—they all weaken our will. And the person who knows how our inner being is connected with that perfection of will will find that all that makes will smaller, narrower, limited, is our experience throughout life. Our joys rob us of our will, as do our sorrows, our pleasures, and our pains.

And the only way of maintaining the power of will is by studying the existence of will and by analyzing, among all the things we have in ourselves, what will is.

The other thing is that—as in the saying in English, "Man proposes, God disposes"—one is always faced with a power greater than oneself which does not always support one's desire. And naturally a person with will, faced with a greater power, must sooner or later give in and be impressed with the loss of will. This is only one example, but there can be a hundred examples given to show how one is robbed of one's will without one's knowing. Very often one thinks that by being active, by being determined, one maintain one's will. Very often a person thinks that by being passive one loses one's will. But it is not true. Where there is a battle, there is an advance and there is a retreat. By a retreat one is not defeated, and by an advance one has not always succeeded. A person who exerts will all the time strains it, and very soon it is exhausted. It is like being too sure of a string that one has in one's hand while rubbing it on the edge of a sharp stone. Very often one sees people who profess great willpower fail much sooner than those who do not profess it.

There is also always a battle between willpower and wisdom, and the first thing and wisest to be done is to bring about a harmony between wisdom and willpower. When one says, "I wish to do this, I will do this," and at the same time that one's sense says, "No, you cannot do this, you must not do this," with all one's willpower, one either cannot do it or does something without sense. But this also shows us life in another light: that those who are wise but without will are as helpless as those with willpower but without wisdom. There is no use in keeping wisdom at the front and willpower at the back, nor is there any use in keeping willpower at the front and wisdom at the back. What is necessary is making the two as one.

There is another enemy of willpower and that is the power of desire. This very often robs willpower of its strength; but very often willpower becomes stronger by a conflict with desire. The self-denial taught in the Bible often meant the crushing of desires. It should not be taken as a principle; it must be taken as a process. Those who have taken it as a principle have lost; those who have taken it as a process have gained.

And the enemy of sense, of wisdom, is the lack of tranquility of mind. When the mind is tranquil it produces the right thought, and wisdom naturally springs forth as a fountain. The Sufis, therefore, have taught different exercises in physical and in meditative form for making the mind tranquil, so that the wisdom which is there may spring up as fountain. It is not in disturbed water that one can see one's image reflected; it is in still water that one can see one's image clearly. Our heart is likened to water, and when it is still, wisdom springs up by itself. It is wisdom and willpower together that work toward a successful issue.

* * *

Question: *What value do you give imagination in comparison with will?*

Answer: As I have said, an automatic working of mind produces an imagination, and the value of imagination depends upon the cultivation of mind. If the mind is pitched to a higher pitch, then the imagination will naturally be at a higher pitch; but if the mind is not pitched to a high pitch, then naturally the imagination will not be at a high pitch. Imagination has its place, and imagination has its value. But when? At the time when the heart is tuned to such a pitch that the imagination cannot go anywhere else but to paradise; the heart which is so tuned by love and harmony and beauty that, without willing, it begins to float automatically. And in this automatic movement, whatever it touches it reacts to or it expresses in some form, such as in the form of line or color or musical notes. It is then that imagination has value. But when it comes to business and science and all things which are connected with our everyday life and world, it is better to leave imagination inside and work with thought. As both night and day are useful, as both resting and acting are necessary, so thinking and imagination both have their place in our life. For instance, if a poet used will to direct imagination, it will become a thought and it will become rigid. The natural thing for a poet is to let the mind float into space, and whatever it happens to touch, let the heart express it. And then what is expressed is an inspiration. But when one has to attend to a business affair, one must not let one's heart float in the air; one must think of the things of the earth and think about figures very carefully.

Question: *There again imagination is superior; one's thoughts still rule above the will, and mind is the factor.*

Answer: There is one thing which is done by control, and the power or will is controlling. The other thing is done without control, for if one controls it, one spoils it. Nothing can move in the world, either in the sphere of mind or in the physical plane, without the power of will. But at the same time, in one thing the power of will is absolutely controlling it, in the other it is working automatically.

Question: *What is the way of strengthening the will? Is it by practices?*

Answer: Practice is the most important thing to strengthen the will.

Question: *It must be guided by wisdom, no?*

Answer: One must always think of these two things in doing everything; one must not be carried away by willpower without listening to what wisdom says.

Question: *How to bring the two together?*

Answer: By becoming conscious of the action of both in all one does. But at the same time, one can practice in one's everyday life by depriving oneself of things one likes. If one always has what one likes to have, no doubt one spoils one's will, because the will has no reaction.

Question: *One can always will what one wants?*

Answer: Yes, but that does not give a stimulus to the will. A stimulus to the will is given by depriving oneself of what one desires. Then the will becomes conscious of itself as living. It says, "Why am I not to have this?" For instance, a person wishes to have a peach, a flower from the plant. One is very much attracted to it, the flower is beautiful. But at the same time the idea comes: why not let it remain on the plant? Then a person says, "Well, I will not pick it." This gives will a stimulus, because first desire wanted to take hold of it, then sense wanted

207

to work with it, and as light comes from friction, so will comes as a flame from friction.

Question: *Then next time it is more powerful?*

Answer: Yes.

Question: *But exercises made?*

Answer: Of course, exercises help; meditative exercises are most useful.

Question: *There are instances when you find people with very powerful imaginations succeed, and for those having little willpower, the contrary.*

Answer: Only the thing is this: that they both have their domain. For instance, if a poet wants to use poetical imagination in business, the poet may by chance make a success; but at the same time, a poetic inspiration will not help in counting figures.

Question: *In both cases imagination is supreme?*

Answer: In my words I have distinguished these two as imagination and thought: imagination when the will is acting automatically, and thought when the will exerts a direct control.

MYSTIC RELAXATION 1

I am going to speak on the subject of mystic relaxation, a subject of the greatest importance, because the whole spiritual culture is based and built upon this one subject, and yet there is so little spoken and written about it. It is a subject which is experienced and studied by all sages, and it is by the full understanding of this subject that they attained to greater power and inspiration.[1]

To begin, I would like to explain that life is rhythm. This rhythm can be divided into three stages, and in every stage this rhythm changes the nature and character of life. The one rhythm is mobile, the other is active, and the third is chaotic. The mobile rhythm is creative, is productive and constructive; and through that rhythm all power and inspiration is gained, peace is experienced. Then the further stage of that rhythm which I have called active, that rhythm is the source of success and accomplishment, of progress and advancement, the source of joy and fulfilment. And the third stage of this rhythm, which I have called chaotic, is the source of failure, of death, of disease and destruction, the source of all pain and sorrow. The first kind of rhythm is slow, the second kind is faster, and the third kind is most quick. The direction of the first is direct, of the second is even, and of the third is zigzag.

When they say, "That person is wise and thoughtful," that person is in the first rhythm; and when they say, "That person is

1 Lecture, Sufi Center, Steinway Hall, New York, May 27, 1926.

209

persevering and successful," that person is in the second rhythm. And when they say, "These people have lost their heads, and have gone astray," those ones are in the third rhythm. They are either digging their own grave or the grave of their affairs. They are their own enemy. Everything they want to accomplish, if they wanted to advance or to progress, it all goes down to destruction because they have taken this third rhythm, the chaotic and destructive rhythm. Therefore, it is up to us to tune ourselves either to the first, to the second, or to the third rhythm, and accordingly will become our condition in life.

But then you might say, "Have not planetary influences to do with our life?" Yes, but even planetary influences—how do they work on you? If you have put yourself in a particular rhythm, these influences have no power to bring about success or failure; if you only put yourself in that rhythm, there will be a similar result, and the environment follows in the same way. If you are in favorable or in unfavorable or in congenial surroundings, it all means that you have put yourself in that particular rhythm. When you experience success, good luck or bad luck, good or bad fortune, it is according to the rhythm you have brought about.

Now, you might ask, "Where is this power to be found? How is it to be realized?" If a person thinks about it, that person can very easily realize it physically, mentally, and spiritually. And how? There is a time when the body is in a perfect calm condition, and there is a time when the body is excited; the breath has lost its rhythm and it is not regular, not even, but uneven. That is a chaotic condition. And when the body has a regular circulation and proper rhythm and even breath, then a person is capable of doing things, accomplishing things. And when the body is restful, comfortable, relaxed, at that time one is able to think about things, inspirations come, revelations come, one feels quiet, one has enthusiasm and power. In Sanskrit the first rhythm is called *sattva*, the second *rajas*, and the third *tamas*. It is from the middle rhythm that the word *raja* comes, which means "the one who has persevered with the sword and made a kingdom." That rhythm is the middle rhythm. The first rhythm, now and then, is called *sant*, which comes to the same meaning as *saint* in English. From the first rhythm comes goodness, which brings about greater rhythm. And *tamas* is which leads one astray and brings about all destruction. Now, since I have explained these three rhythms, we also have in our life a certain time in one rhythm, a certain time in another rhythm, and a certain time in the third rhythm. And yet in our life one rhythm is predominating with all changes, whether a person has the third, or the second, or the first rhythm.

One who has the first rhythm always has a power to accomplish things. And as it is in the body, so it is in the mind. Body and mind are so much connected together that whatever rhythm the mind has, the body has; and then the rhythm which is predominating in body and mind, that same rhythm is the rhythm of your soul.

I have known of a king who, when there was a certain problem brought by his ministers, used to say, "Read it again," and the minister would read it again. Maybe after four lines he would stop him and say, "Read it again," and the minister would read it again. And after he had heard it three times, his answer would be perfect. But what do we do sometimes when we converse with people? Before the conversation has stopped, we have answered it. We are so impatient and eager to answer and excited about it, that one among a hundred persons stops to hear what another person says. It is the wrong rhythm, the chaotic rhythm, which brings about chaotic results. Where does war come from? Do you think any nation wanted a war? No nation does. War comes from chaotic action. When there is chaotic action, nations can become involved in the war. Whenever there is chaotic action, the whole world may be involved in war. When people doubt that word, that religious belief of Christ having saved the whole world, they cannot understand it. They say, "Human beings save themselves." But

211

they do not know that one person can ruin the whole world, and one person can save the whole world. By that rhythm one can save the whole world. When there is a chaotic influence, it goes just like a liquor into thousands of people. It is just like a germ of disease, of plague, going from one person through the whole country, from just one person. If that is true mechanically, then psychologically it can be true that one person's chaotic influence can put the whole world in despair, though it is very difficult for people of common sense to understand and digest it. But at the same time it is logical just the same. Very often it is one person in the nation who brings about disaster. It is according to that person's rhythm.

The Turkish nation was so depressed on every side, and wars had made the country so poor; with nothing but disappointment all the time, it had gone down to the depths. And there came only one man, Kemal Pasha, and his rhythm put action in thousands and thousands of dead souls who were waiting for some result, hungry from lack of food, disappointed with every effort. And one man cheered them all up and picked up the whole country. We can see the condition in Italy, where every action was powerless because of so many different thoughts and parties, with thoughts going everywhere, depressed. There was no united effort, no concentration. After the tiredness of the war, there comes one man, Mussolini, who lifted up the thoughts of the whole country.

And this is the outer plane. In the spiritual plane it is still more powerful, only those who work on the spiritual plane do not manifest to view. What happens in the political world is known, but in the spiritual world great things happen and they are not known. And why is their influence greater and more powerful? This comes from their rhythm.

Now, there is an interesting story about a *majzub*, who is a highly evolved soul who acts before people like someone who is insane, who is not in a normal mind. But in the East some people recognize the *majzubs* and give them due respect. The *majzubs* do not care for it; on the contrary, they do not like to be recognized. Their every action is like the action of an insane person because they want to shield themselves from the eyes of others, to be in the midst of the crowd in the world and yet out of the world. A *majzub* was allowed in Kashmir to wander about in the garden of the palace of the maharaja, who lived not long ago. And there was a little miniature cannon at the gate of the garden. And this *majzub* used to get in a condition and would make a sound like gunfire and would feel very excited. People used to go and tell the maharaja about it, knowing that now war was anticipated. When the *majzub* came into that rhythm there was a war, there was an enemy waiting somewhere, and they had to prepare because there was going to be war. Now how did this mystic feel it? By the rhythm. His consciousness was all around the world. When there was war coming, this rhythm then came in his being, and he acted in the same way as the world in order to give warning of what was coming.

And now we come to the life of Napoleon. Some appreciate his life and some not, but at the same time, during the war he was the inspiration and power and backbone of the whole movement, he was the spirit of the movement. The army has another strength now; it does not have that patriotism—it has no idea of it! It was all Napoleon's spirit. And at the same time, during his anxiety about war, his activity of war, he used to have some moments of silence, even sometimes on horseback. And while he was sitting on horseback and going into this silence, he would recuperate all the strength lost in his responsibilities and in the continual calls of war. It must be remembered that war at that time was not such as it is now, with so many people being responsible. At that time he had all the responsibility. After five minutes on horseback, he would feel fresh after having closed his eyes. What was it? He had the key to relaxation. What is relaxation? It is tuning oneself to a desired rhythm.

One should not be surprised or laugh at pupils of sages who keep one hand raised up or who stand on their heads with their feet up or who remain sitting in one posture. There is some reason for it. There are the different ways used by those who know the art of relaxation. They know how to bring about a relaxed condition in the body and in the mind. If I could tell you of my own experience, that continually for about twelve years I had three hours sleep at night and sometimes not even that—perhaps a little rest in the day, a little nap, but that does not provide all the sleep necessary. And in all those twelve years I never felt sick. I was never ill. I had all the strength necessary and was perfectly well because of the practice of relaxation.

And now we come to the idea: How do we relax? It is not by sitting silent with closed eyes, because when the mind is giving attention to the body of thought, of feeling, then the body is not relaxed because the mind is torturing the body. And when the feeling is giving attention to the mind, then the mind is tortured. And in this torture, even if the eyes are closed, even if we are sitting in a certain posture, it does no good.

Where relaxation comes is in considering three points of view: the point of view of the physical body, the point of view of the mind, and the point of view of the feeling. The point of view of the physical body is this: that one must accustom one-self to get power over or to have influence on one's circulation and pulsation, and one can do that together with breath, with the power of thought, and by the power of will. By willpower you can bring about a condition in your body so that your circulation takes a certain rhythm. It can be decreased according to will. You can do the same thing with regulating your pulsation by the power of will. No sooner has the will taken in hand the circulation and the pulsation of the body, then the will has in hand a meditation of hours. It is for this reason that sages can meditate for hours and hours, because they have mastered their circulation in body and blood, and they can breathe slower or quicker at their will. And when there is no tension in your nervous system, in your muscular system, then you get such repose as the sleep of ten days cannot bring about. Therefore, to have relaxation does not mean to sit quiet; it is to be able to remove tension from your system, from your circulation and your pulsation, from your nervous and muscular system.

And now we come to the subject of mind: How do we relax the mind? Relaxation of the mind is first making the mind tired. The one who does not know the exercise of how to make the mind tired, that person can never relax the mind. Concentration is the greatest action you can give to your mind, because the mind is held in position on a certain thing. Naturally, after that it will relax; and when it relaxes it will gain all power.

And now coming to the question of how to relax feeling. It is by feeling deeply. The Sufis in the East, in their meditation, have music played that stirs up the emotions to such a degree that the poem they hear becomes a reality. Then comes the reaction, which is relaxation. All that was blocked up, all congestion is broken; and inspiration, power, and a feeling of joy and exaltation come to a person.

It is by these three kinds of relaxation that one becomes prepared for the highest relaxation, which is to relax the whole being: body in repose, mind at rest, heart at peace. It is that experience which may be called nirvana, that ideal of the thinkers and meditative souls. It is that they want to reach, because in it there is everything, because it is by that condition that each person becomes as a drop that is assimilated or submerged in its origin for that time. And being for one moment submerged means that all that belongs to the origin is extracted by this drop, because the origin is the essence of all. The drop has taken from its origin everything it has in life. It is newly charged and has become again illumined.

* * *

Question: *The question is if accidents are meant to be, or if they are preordained by God?*

Answer: In this the questioner wants me to commit myself. If I say they are preordained by God, it would be a great blame to God, because very often a person becomes unhappy by an accident. And one might think there is a great cruelty there. And at the same time, there is not one action that takes place without the command of God. Not one tittle can move; there is no movement without the command of the Supreme Spirit, because every motion is under the control and command and directed by the wisdom of the Supreme Being, only it cannot be said. As soon as we say that it is so, we have to give the reason why a person broke a leg in the street, why this cruelty was done. Therefore, one cannot answer that question, because a person only sees, "Poor person, that person must suffer so much." That is all one sees, all one can say. One does not know the greater justice, the adjustment of the whole action of the universe, because one has no insight in the scheme of the whole universe. Therefore, our knowledge is so limited. When from our knowledge we judge the action of God, we judge wrongly, we go astray. Therefore, the prophets always taught, "Remember God, the most merciful, the father and mother and most beloved. Do not go astray in judging God wrongly. You cannot see the justice of the justice of God." The best thing to do, the best we can do is to judge ourselves, not even to judge another person. In this way we can advance.

Question: *How can we have success in concentration on business and in our private affairs at home?*

Answer: As I have said, there are three rhythms. If one keeps tuned to the third rhythm, one is sure to have failure in everything. If one keeps tuned to the second rhythm there will certainly be success. But we cannot tune ourselves to the second rhythm in order to come to the first rhythm, because if you will force yourself into the first, the world will bring you to the second rhythm. Therefore, always seek the first rhythm. That is said, "Take the first rhythm." "Seek ye first the kingdom of God and all things shall be added unto you."[2] Then all will come.

2 Matthew 6:33.

Question: *Is it God who plans and rules human destiny, or one's own mind? And if so, what part does intuition play in it?*

Answer: It is true that God plans human destiny. It is also true that one's own mind plans and rules one's own destiny. How is it done? It is true that one wants to put on one's coat. One wishes to put it on, but one's hand has to do the work also. In that way one has a part in doing the will of God, and one calls it one's own free will. And now comes the question, Where does intuition come from, from God, or from a human being? My answer is that intuition is from within, in other words, from God. A human being only knows it according to one's evolution.

Question: *How can we change the rhythm of another?*

Answer: It is very difficult. First of all one must be able to change one's own rhythm, then to change the rhythm of others too. But as I say, one who cannot stand on one's own feet cannot save others from falling. But the one who is strong enough to stand on one's own feet, can take hold of another and keep that person from falling. Naturally, if we gain strength in ourselves, we can give it to another. When a person is in a slippery place, if that person holds the hand of another, that person will be safe. Very often people are foolishly enthusiastic. They want to help others when they have not yet strength to help themselves. And that is the wrong thing. If one gets strength in oneself, one does not need to do much. One's presence, one's atmosphere, one's thought will act and turn things into shape.

MYSTIC RELAXATION 2

Call it mystic relaxation or meditation, it is one and the same.[1] I have called it mystic relaxation in order to make it less complicated, easier to explain. Very often people are puzzled about the word *meditation* because it is used so often and by so many people who have different ideas about it. By mystic relaxation the meaning becomes simple and clear. From a physical point of view there is one condition, the condition of contracting and stretching, which enables us to bring the inner vitality outside. Relaxation is a contrary condition. Either the energy is brought to the outer plane or the energy is put to repose in its natural, normal condition. When a person lifts something heavy or does something with determination, that person brings that energy which is within into the physical body. It expresses itself through the muscles and nerves. When a person is asleep, that energy is put to repose. This energy is valuable, most precious; when used outwardly it brings outer gains; when used inwardly, it brings about inner attainments.

Meditation is reached by two stages. The first stage is concentration, and the next stage is contemplation. After having reached these two stages, the third stage is meditation. What comes after is realization.

Nothing in this world can be thoroughly accomplished without concentration, whether it is in business or a profession, or whether it is spiritual work. Those who cannot make a suc-

1 Lecture, Twentieth Centry Club, Detroit, February 8, 1926.

218

cess in life, in business, or in a profession, are the ones whose concentration is not right. And with many of those who have succeeded in their lives, the mystery is that their concentration is great. They may not know it. There have been so many great inventors in the United States who have produced wonderful works. Perhaps they themselves do not know that it is from their concentration that they have been able to produce wonderful things. Some are naturally born with that gift, and it is because of that gift that whatever they have undertaken, they make a success of it. If one is an artist, by the help of concentration one can produce wonderful works. If one is a scientist, one can accomplish wonderful things in science. If one is a poet, poetry will be easy to write. If one is a mystic, mystical inspiration will flow. But without concentration, however qualified a person may be—in the first place, one cannot be qualified, but if one were—one cannot make the best use of the qualification one has. It is by the power of concentration that one can express oneself fully.

Concentration can be regarded from a metaphysical point of view in three aspects: reflecting, constructing, and improvising. The first kind of concentration is reflecting any object that one has placed before oneself. This is the mirror quality of mind that enables one to concentrate in this way. A person who is impressed by a certain thing that person has seen, without trying to concentrate upon it, holds it in mind. In other words, that person has focused the mind on that object with which that person is impressed, and the mind is doing nothing but reflecting it.

The other kind of concentration is constructing, or in other words, composing. For instance, if an artist was told to make a most fanciful picture, the artist creates the face of a person with the horns of a buffalo and with two wings of a bird in the mind. The material is there in the artist's mind. The artist has only to put it together in order to produce a certain form. This is constructive concentration. This is visualizing, or in other words, using mind to produce something under the direction of the will.

The third aspect of concentration is improvising. If a poet is asked to write a poem on the rosebud, the poet begins to improvise. The poet brings a dewdrop there and produces the picture of dawn; and the poet brings a gentle stream of water there and builds a beautiful background to it. This is the third kind of concentration.

Very often what people think about concentration is closing the eyes and sitting quiet in church, and that only once in a week. And while doing it they don't know where their mind is going. They themselves are in the church, but they don't know where their mind is.

There is a story of a teacher. He had many disciples working under him. He taught them concentration. To each he gave a different work. A new disciple came, a good and simple and innocent sort of man. The others thought, "What can he learn in the spiritual path?" And when the teacher asked him, "Is there anything you like, that you can call your favorite?" "Yes," he said, "There is a cow in my house." "Yes," the teacher said, "then think about that cow. The other pupils are sitting in their rooms. You have a room, sit there and think about it." The other pupils closed their eyes for five minutes, ten minutes. Then they were annoyed and went away. This man sat for a very long time. The pupils could not understand why they did not see this new man in all their games, conversations, and plays that they had around there. One day the teacher asked, "Where is that new pupil? Where is he gone?" They said, "We have never seen him, only the first time he came." The teacher said, "See in his room." They went. But they got no answer. The door was closed. The teacher went there, and what did he see? This pupil was sitting concentrating on the object given to him. The teacher called him by his name. He answered in the tone of the cow. The teacher said, "Come out." He answered, "My horns

220

are too large to come out of the door." The teacher said to his pupils, "That is called concentration."

The Bible speaks of self-denial. People think that it means not to eat, not to drink, to give up all that is beautiful and good in life, to go somewhere in solitude never to appear again. It is a wrong interpretation of a true teaching. Self-denial is self-effacing; it comes from self-forgetting. If you study the people in your surroundings, you will find that those who are happy are happy because they have less thought of self. If they are unhappy, it is because they think of themselves too much. One is more bearable when one thinks less of oneself, and one is unbearable when one always thinks of oneself. There are many miseries in life, but the greatest misery is self-pity. Such a one is heavier than rock, heavy for oneself and heavy for others. Others cannot bear it, and one cannot carry one's own self. When this disciple thought of the cow he had no thought of himself, there was nothing other than the cow. It is no easy thing to do, to forget oneself to that extent. If one did what a wonderful power one would be created within. It is a great mystery. It gives power over heaven and hell. Omar Khayyam says in his *Rubaiyat* that, "Heaven is a vision of fulfilled desire; hell is the shadow of a soul on fire."[2] Where is that shadow? Where is that vision? Is it not within ourselves? It is we who hold it. Therefore, heaven and hell are what we have made for ourselves. And if this can be changed, it cannot be changed by anything else but concentration.

But there is even a greater significance to concentration than this. It is that creative power which a human being possesses and has as a heritage from God, and it is creative power that works wonders. For instance, when a person thinks that, "I should like to eat fish for dinner," that person comes home to find the housekeeper had cooked fish that evening. And when a person was thinking of apple pie, came home to find it; it was already there. That is the phenomenon of concentration.

2 See *The Rubaiyat of Omar Khayyam*, trans. Edward FitzGerald.

That person may not know it, but it worked in that way. The one who thought of those dishes, that person's thought struck the mind of the housekeeper, and the housekeeper brought it for that person. Imagine what great power it is. One need not even think about one's desires. The very fact of having the desire—concentration works it out and materializes it.

I knew a person in India, a sage. Many people used to go to him, and he would treat them so coldly that they would go away, because he did not want publicity. Nevertheless people went. And someone would say, "I have got a case in the court, and I have no money. I am in great distress. I am a poor man." The sage says, "Tell me all about it." The man told him everything about it. There was a pencil and paper. The sage wrote, "I don't see any fault of this person. Therefore, the case must be dismissed." The sage said to this man, "Go." This man was surprised the sage did not say any prayers for him, that he did not bless him, but that he sat there and wrote down a sentence and then told him to go away. And when this man goes to the court, to his great surprise, what does he find? That the judge says the same words this man had written. The words were written in the *akasha*, that means, in the spheres.

Such is the power of concentration. There are many stories told in the East about fakirs, dervishes, sages, mahatmas. Many ask if they are all true, and if they are true, how it can be done. They want a scientific explanation, and maybe one day science will discover it. Nevertheless, one finds as much truth as falsehood in these things, because anything can be imitated. There is gold and there is imitation gold; there is silver and imitation silver. So there is imitation truth also. Therefore, all that one sees as most wonderful and surprising may not all be so wonderful. But at the same time there are things which are more wonderful than one can imagine. And where does it belong? It belongs to the power of mind. And where does it come from? From the source of all things. It is the power of God.

But even in the attainment of union with God it is concentration which helps. There is a story of a boy who was sent to school. And the teacher gave him the first lesson, which is writing the figure 1. In [Arabic] it is called *alif*, which means "one" and "a." The other students learned it and many other letters, but the boy kept drawing the same figure all the time. The teacher saw him do it for three days. The teacher was surprised. On the third day the teacher asked, "Now have you finished the lesson? Shall I give you another lesson?" But the boy said, "It is not yet complete." The teacher was annoyed with him. He said to his parents, "This boy will never learn. It is better to take him away. He is stupid. He continues to write the same thing for three days, and he refuses to learn further." The parents brought him home. They were very annoyed with the lad. When the lad saw that the parents were so annoyed and displeased with him, he escaped and ran away. He did not show himself for a very, very long time. And one day he appeared in the same school where he had learned his first lesson. He said to the teacher, "You don't recognize me. Now you will be surprised that I am still writing the same first lesson. I have not yet taken the second lesson. But I come for it now. I have been practicing the first. Shall I write it?" When he made the sign, the wall split. The teacher said, "For God's sake, don't write again!" The meaning is that he contemplated on that form. And he saw that form in the tree, in the plant; in the whole of nature he saw that one figure. By that his concentration became perfect, and his power became so great that there was nothing he could not do. Very few know what secret is hidden behind the power of concentration.

And now we come to contemplation, which is the second stage of concentration. Contemplation is the repetition of a certain idea, and this repetition produces the materialization of that idea; in other words, it materializes that idea. Those who have been able to make great works in the world have been contemplative people, and often they don't know it. It is a continual repetition of a certain idea which creates that idea, which brings it about in the physical world. For instance, those who can contemplate on health can bring about that perfect health which no medicine, nothing can give. Those who contemplate upon inspiration will show great inspiration. Those who contemplate upon strength and power develop strength and power. One cannot arrive at this stage unless one has accomplished concentration, because concentration is the first stage. And one must proceed gradually to the stage of contemplation. The idea that Coué now preaches about, saying that, "In every way, every day, I am getting better," is something which has been known to thinkers for thousands of years. Upon this the whole method of mysticism has been based. And he skips the first part, concentration, because contemplation is the second part.

One might ask to what extent contemplation can help? In answer to that, I will say nothing in the world is impossible for the contemplative person to accomplish if only one knew how to contemplate. No doubt it is gibberish to those who don't understand the subject. People say, "What relation does the mind have with affairs outside? Perhaps one can heal oneself from illness, but if there is an affair outside which is going wrong—a monetary affair or a business or industry—what connection does that have with the mind?" And my answer is that all that exists, whether it is business or commerce, all that is visible and invisible, all that seems to be outside is, in reality, in your mind. It is outside because your eyes see it outside, but it is within you because your mind surrounds it. It is accommodated in your mind. Mind is an accommodation of the world that is outside.

A Hindustani poet speaks wonderfully about this. He says, "The land and sea are not too large for the human heart to accommodate." In other words, the human heart is larger than the universe. If there were twenty thousand universes, the human heart could accommodate them. But human beings, unaware of their inner being, impressed by outer limitations, remain under the impression of their weakness, limitation, smallness. And that keeps them from using that great power which they can find within themselves, this great light with which they can see life more clearly, only because they are unaware of themselves.

And the third stage is meditation. This stage has nothing to do with the mind. This is the experience of the consciousness. Meditation is diving deep within oneself, and soaring upward in the higher spheres, expanding wider than the universe. It is in these experiences that one attains the bliss of meditation.

And one might ask, "By attaining all these things, what benefit do we get by it?" Perhaps we are more concerned with benefit than ever before. In no age have people been as anxious about gaining benefit as today. They say, "Time is money. If there is a benefit, I will give my life to defend a piece of ground, sword and gun. I will take the life of my fellow human beings to save a little ground under their feet. That is a tangible benefit. It remains for my children to hold, to touch, to feel that it is there." They will give their life for it. Tell of something which is beneficial and everyone will listen, but if it is in the clouds they do not know it. Time is precious. Something they don't know, they can't believe in. It does not mean that a human being today is less inclined to make a sacrifice. It is not so. A person is as ready to make sacrifices as a thousand years ago, or to make even greater sacrifices that one can make today. But one must be sure what one can get by it. One is so concerned with gain. One always has gain before one's view. Concerning that which does not show immediate gain and about which one does not know properly what it is and how much it is, one thinks, "Well, perhaps there is something without sacrifice. I shall get it."

It is strange. When people go to the voice producer in order to develop a tenor voice, they work six or nine years and listen to everything the voice producer says. They make grimaces, everything, all sorts of noises they will make in order to develop a tenor voice. But when they come to a spiritual person, they ask whether the spiritual person can speak of concentration at the tea table. Taking tea they ask, "What about meditation?" In one sentence they want the answer. I have seen it, traveling all these years. They consider it like a newspaper talk. It is not gained in this way. This knowledge is attained in accordance with one's ideal about it. It is greater than religion, more sacred than anything in the world. The knowledge of self is like union with God. Self-realization is spiritual attainment. Can this be gained by having a light conception of it? It is the deepest thing one can get, the highest thing one can reach, the most valuable thing to attain to. It is therefore that in the East a person does not look for these things in a book, nor does a real teacher write a book on these things. Yes, a real teacher writes philosophy and prepares minds to appreciate it, but does not say how to do it.

To my greatest surprise I saw, while traveling in the United States, people looking for books of this kind, wanting to buy books about Yoga, Yogis, some attainment. Many lost their head by reading such books. They cannot keep balance. They try to do what is in the book. It is just like going to the drug-store to get some Yoga pills to attain spirituality. There are also many who look in the mirror to be clairvoyant, who look into a crystal or something in order to see the depth of life. They make light of the highest and best and most sacred things.

This path is only pursued by those who are serious. The ones who go to this society, that institute, that occultist group, they don't know what they are doing and what they are looking for. High knowledge is not to be got from going to twenty places, and those who do will be disappointed in the end, because they went into it lightly. They came in foolish and went out foolish.

There is a story of a Brahmin to whom a Muslim said, "I am a worshipper of God who is formless, and here you are praying to this idol of God." The Brahmin said, "If I have faith in this idol, it will answer me. But if you have not faith, even God in heaven will not hear you." If we don't attach ourselves seriously to things, then those things laugh at us. Even with the things of the world, if we take them seriously, we will gain serious results.

There cannot be anything more serious than spiritual attainment. If that is taken lightly, one does not know what one is doing. One must not go into these things and come back empty-handed. To come back disappointed from the spiritual path before reaching the final goal, to come back from that power, is the worst possible thing. To go bankrupt does not matter. One can pick up again what one has lost of the world. It does not matter. But the one who has gone on the spiritual path and has turned back, that one is to be pitied. It is the greatest loss, a loss that can never be repaired.

MAGNETISM

As interesting as the subject of magnetism is from a scientific point of view, it is even more interesting from a mystical point of view.[1] For in the first place, a magnet and something which is attracted to the magnet have a relation. The magnet represents the essence, a part of which is held by that object which is attracted. Very often one does not find the trace of that essence in the object that a magnet attracts, but at the same time the essence is there, and that is the logical reason that it is attracted: because its essence is there. And what they used to call, among the ancient people, a blood relationship is an influence of that kind recognized by them. In the East this blood relationship was always signified by the [magnetism] which exists between two persons who have the same blood. And the deep study of this fact will certainly prove that there is an unknown attraction between two people having a blood relationship.

Lately I had a similar experience, something that a friend was telling me in Stockholm. This friend was visiting London where he thought that he had no relations, or that if there were any relations, they were perhaps a century ago. And while walking in a part of London, he met someone who called him by his name. When he turned back, this person excused himself, saying, "I am sorry, I have made a mistake." But this man asked, "How did you know my name, that same name is mine?" And when they spoke together, they found that they were cousins,

1 Lecture, Sorbonne, Paris, March 25, 1925.

228

but cousins only if they studied their genealogy. We do not give much attention to this subject, but the more we give attention to it, the more proof we can find of this element which is drawn to its similar. And Sa'di, the great poet of Persia, says that, "Element attracts element as eagle is attracted to eagle, and a dove is attracted to a dove." But do we not find the same thing in life every day? A gambler who goes to another country, by the help of providence—one does not know how—attracts another gambler very soon. It will not take much time for a person who is a thief to find another thief in a country where that thief arrives. It is not only that when two persons of a similar element see one another that they are attracted to one another, but even conditions, life itself, brings about their meeting; life itself draws them together. And therefore, it is natural that a person who is very sad naturally attracts a miserable one to join up with. The one with joy, the one with happiness, naturally attracts happiness. And in this way magnetism is working throughout the whole creation, and in all aspects you will see the phenomena of magnetism in the physical world as well as in the mental spheres.

No doubt one cannot always say that it is the element which attracts the same element, for the element also attracts what it is lacking, what is opposite to it. And when we think of friendship, that to some we feel inclined to be friends, and with others we feel inclined to keep away, the most interesting part is that those whom we feel disinclined to be friends with, they also have some who are drawn toward them in friendship. And this takes us to the truth which lies in musical harmony: how two notes have a relation with one another, and the combination brings about a harmony.

And now coming to the question of the practical use of magnetism. Whether you are in business or in industry, whether you are in domestic work or political work for the state, in whatever situation, you will always find that magnetism is the secret of your progress in life. And you will find at the same time that with regard to qualification, to which we give such great importance, that there are numberless people who are most qualified who do not make their way through life because of lack of magnetism. Very often one is most qualified, but before speaking of one's qualification, the person to whom one has gone has had enough of one. And personality holds such an important place in life that even the absence of qualifications is tolerated when a personality has magnetism, especially in these times, when materialism is so much on the increase that personality is given much less importance in society. And at such a time when heroism has no place in life, magnetism automatically works and proves to be the most essential thing even now, and it will always prove to be so. But when it comes to the question of magnetism, people do not go deeper into the subject and only recognize personal magnetism by the attraction that they feel.

When we think of personal magnetism, we can divide it into four different classes. The first kind, the ordinary kind of magnetism, is what is concerned with the physical plane. And this magnetism has to do with nourishment, with hygiene, with regular living, and with right breathing. This magnetism also depends upon the regularity of action and repose. Besides, this magnetism works with age, as the ascending and descending of notes in an octave; this magnetism may be likened to the season of spring which comes and goes. And at the same time this magnetism is dependent upon all things of this physical world, since this is a physical magnetism.

And now we come to the magnetism which can be called mental. Naturally, a person with a sparkling intelligence becomes the center of that person's society. The one who perceives well, the one who conceives well is liked by everyone. For the person who has wit, the person who can express freely, the person who can understand quickly, that is the person who always attracts others. The person who has knowledge of human nature, the person who knows of things and conditions, is that person who naturally draws others. And in reality this is the qualification, if there is any qualification; and without this qualification, no other qualification can be of very great use. But this sparkling condition of intelligence is born with a person. It is this person who becomes a genius, and it is this person who accomplishes something, if ever anyone accomplishes anything. And it is this person who helps others to accomplish something, for others depend on this person's mind. It is this one who can guide one's own self and direct others. And with all our thought of equality in which we are so much absorbed, we shall find that it is this person who will win the battle in life. And it is this person who stands above the masses, and it is this person who leads; and without this person many are lost.

And now, we come to the question: How can this magnetism be developed? This magnetism is developed by study, by concentration, by keen observation of life, and by the knowledge of repose. Very many intelligent persons, without knowing how to concentrate and how to take repose in their lives, in time blunt their intelligence, because there is a certain fund of energy which is reserved and which is limited. And when there is too much pressure put upon that limited energy, in the end what happens? A person becomes less and less intelligent, and the power of mind becomes less every day. And whenever you find a most intelligent person becoming duller every day, that always proves that the amount of energy that has been there has been spent. Therefore, when one knows how to reserve one's energies by repose, and when one knows how to concentrate and sharpen one's intellect, then that magnetism remains in a right condition. What generally happens is that it is the intelligent person on whom a great responsibility falls. Much more is asked of the intelligent person than of the others who lack intelligence. If one does not give a rest to the mind by knowing the manner of repose, and if one does not concentrate and thereby sharpen the intellect naturally, then, just like a knife which is always used, it will become blunted; naturally, the continual use of intellect will make one short of [mental] funds.

And now we come to the third aspect of magnetism. Perhaps this aspect of magnetism may be called a higher kind than the two which I have already explained to you. For this magnetism is more profound, and it touches another person more deeply. This is the magnetism of love, of sympathy, of friendliness: a person who by nature is sympathetic; a person who tolerates, who forgets, who forgives; a person who does not keep bitterness or malice against anyone; a person who admires beauty, who appreciates beauty, who loves it, who loves it in art, in nature, in all its forms and who goes out to friend and foe, to an acquaintance, to a stranger, to all. The person who can endure and who can suffer and who has the power to have patience through all conditions of life, who feels the pain of another in the heart and who is always willing to become a friend, it is that person whose magnetism is greater than all other magnetisms that we know of. We do not need to go far to see this. If only we were to look for good things in others, we shall find this, for among our surroundings we can find many people in whom we can appreciate this quality.

One day a man who had traveled very much saw me and said, "We heard so much and we have read so much about the saints and sages and mahatmas and masters that lived in India, but after having gone there, I found no one." And I told him, "You need not have gone so far. The souls who are worthwhile, the souls who love one another, they are to be found everywhere. What do we seek saints and sages for? It is for this that we seek; they are to be found everywhere." I said, "I am here, away from home for all this time. Do I not find them? I find them everywhere." If we can appreciate them, we can find them. But if we cannot appreciate them, even if an angel came we could not find these qualities. Nevertheless, call it a saint or a sage, call it a prophet, or a mahatma, if there is anything that draws one person toward another, it is the love element that a person pours out.

And now the question is: How can one develop this quality? And my answer will be by one thing: by studying, by knowing, by practicing, and by living the life of a friend. By contemplating this thought from morning till evening: "To everyone I meet, those who love me and those who hate me, do I practice in my life that thought of friendliness, that outgoingness, that pouring out of sympathy and love? If I do it, that is quite enough." And besides this, apart from the magnetism that one gets from it, when we consider life as it is, with all its limitations, with all the pain and troubles and responsibilities it gives us, if there seems to be anything worthwhile, it is just this one thing. And that is the thought and impression that we have done our best to be gentle, to be tender to those whom we meet in our everyday life. If there is any prayer, if there is any worship, if there is any religion, it is this, for there is no one there to please. If there is anyone to be pleased and whose pleasure it is worthwhile to earn, it is here, it is a human being; and it is in the pleasure of a human being that—if one understands it—there is the pleasure of God.

And now we come to the fourth aspect of magnetism. And this aspect is magnetism itself. The lack of magnetism means that this aspect is hidden. This magnetism is the human soul. And if I were to define what the soul is, I would say the soul is the self of a human being. But if you asked which self, I will say that self which one does not know.

There is a humorous story from India about some peasants who were traveling, but it was the first time in their life that they went traveling. And being worried about one another, the next morning they thought they should count if they were all there. And they were very disappointed after having counted, for they counted nineteen, and it was understood that twenty peasants had left home. And so each peasant counted, and each said nineteen; and they could not find who was missing, for everyone was there. In the end they found that those who counted forgot to count themselves. That is the condition of the soul. It sees all selves, but it does not see itself. And the day when the soul realizes itself, that day a new life begins, a new birth. And it is the self-realized soul which grows, which expands. So long as the soul has not realized itself, it does not develop, it does not grow. Therefore, the moment the soul begins to realize itself is the moment that a human being really begins to live in the world. But it must be understood that the magnetism of the self-realized soul is greater than any magnetism one could ever imagine. It is power, it is wisdom, it is peace, it is intelligence—it is all. It is this magnetism that heals, heals bodies and heals minds. And it is this magnetism that raises those fallen into difficulties, in pain and sorrows. It is this magnetism that brings others out of confusion and darkness. It is by this magnetism that the illuminated souls spread out their love, attracting thereby all beings. It is for this magnetism that Christ said to the fishermen, "Come hither, for I will make you fishers of men."[2] It is with this magnetism that the great ones—such as Buddha, Moses, Muhammad, Christ—came, who attracted humanity; and humanity for ages has not forgotten. It is with this magnetism that they, after having gone to the other side, have held millions and millions of people in one bond of kinship, sympathy, friendship. The immense power that the soul magnetism gives shows it is a divine magnetism. It is a proof of something behind the seen world.

---

2 Mark 1:17.

THE POWER WITHIN US

One reads in books from the East about the different wonders performed by great souls, and one wonders if there is some truth in them.[1] One hears that there are people who know what is going on at a distance, that there are people who can send their thought from a very far distance, that there are people who can create things in a moment, produce things in a moment without having anything else there, that there are people who can make things disappear. One even reads and hears that there are some who can command the rain to fall and who can make the multitude move according to their commands and by their will, and who can inspire the multitude in a flash, who can prevent plagues from coming, and who can perform wonders in war.

No doubt there are many jugglers among them, for whenever there is truth, there is falsehood on the other side to laugh at it. Nevertheless, the truth remains just the same. There are stories of the wonder workings and phenomena in the East. Many of those stories no doubt are of the jugglers who, by some sleight of hand or hypnotic influence, can perform wonders. But there are others who are real and not performers. They perform wonders during their lives, and those who see their wonders are seen by others. But the real ones never say that they can perform wonders; neither do they pursue such powers. But these powers come naturally, because one is generally not conscious

1 Lecture, Engineering Societies Auditorium, New York, May 20, 1926.

of the power one has. When one becomes conscious of that power, one is able to do things which people ordinarily cannot accomplish.

There are two powers: one is called in [Arabic] *qaza'* and the other is called *qadr*. One is individual power, and the other is God's power. The individual power can work and can accomplish things as long as it is working in consonance with God's power. But the moment the individual power is working opposite to God's power, one realizes that one's strength diminishes and that one cannot accomplish anything. Therefore, the first thing that masters seek is the pleasure of God, to be in consonance with the will of God. And just like a person who has practiced the game of gambling or any other sport and has become accustomed to knowing the manner in which to handle it, so the one who is constantly in the thought of doing everything in consonance with God's power is helped by the will of God.

Very often people have misunderstood the will of God. They think that what they consider good is the will of God, and what they consider not good is not the will of God. But their ideas of good and wrong have nothing to do with the power of God, because God's outlook is different from the human outlook. We only see so far and no further, whereas God sees all things.

But one wonders, if we all belong to the body of God, if we are all as atoms of God's being, why do we not understand, why do we not readily know what is in consonance with the will of God and what is not? And the answer is that each atom of our body is conscious of itself. And if there is a pain in the finger, the ear does not feel it. If there is a pain in the toe, the nose does not feel it, only the toe feels it. But in both cases, either in the case of the toe or of the finger, the person feels it, because the person possesses the whole body.

Such is the narrow world of humanity, that each one lives in a small world that one creates according to what one sees as right and wrong and one's interest in life. Therefore, one is not always able to work in consonance with the will of God unless one makes a habit of working in consonance with God's will.

And now we come to understand the question: What is a human being? Is a human being only the body? No. A human being is the mind; a human being is the soul. And therefore, the power of a human being is greater than the power of the sun, because the sun is only a body, but a human being has a body, mind, and soul. Once a person has become conscious of the body, mind, and soul, that person's power becomes greater than the power of the sun, because the sun is the material manifestation of the light, but a person has all lights within. The human body is radiance, a radiance which is so great that all invisible beings which live in space are hidden by the glow of the human form. Nothing exists which is not visible, but one thing which is most visible hides the other thing which is not as visible. Therefore, it is the glow and radiance of the human body which is so great that it hides the beings in space. In reality they are all visible, but the radiance of the human form stands out and hides all that is less visible compared with it. And when we look at life from this point of view, there is nothing that is invisible, it is only that there are things which our eyes have no power to see, which does not mean that they are formless. All things that have existence have form.

Besides, the human mind has a still greater power, and that is the power of will, of mind, that can bring about change in conditions, in environments; it can have power over matter, over objects, over affairs; it can even work so wonderfully that one cannot explain it. The power of mind can work on the multitude. Not long ago there was a sage living near the palace of the maharaja of Kashmir, Ranjit Singh. Many thought this man was insane, that he was not in his right mind. Still the maharaja had great respect for him and allowed him to wander about in the court garden of the palace. And there was a miniature gun kept in the garden of the palace. There used to come a time, perhaps once a year, that this man at the palace, just like a child, would play with the cannon, turning to the east, west, south, and would become very excited, playing with that gun, making gunfire noises. The maharaja said, "Whatever he does, tell me." [The sage] would say that from the north or south, from that side, will come an invasion, and he must be ready for it. And the maharaja was ready in time to face it.

The story of Muhammad is not a tradition; it is history. Muhammad being the last prophet, Arabia has his history. In one of the great wars that Muhammad had to fight, the whole army was defeated. And there only remained ten or fifteen friends of Muhammad by the side of the Prophet and all others ran away or were dead or wounded. And the Prophet turned to his people and saw that they were all downhearted and disappointed. And he said, "Look, before us there is an army and here we are fifteen persons." They said, "Yes." The Prophet said, "You do not see any hope, now you must go back. But I, I will stand here, whether I will come back victorious or lose my life here on this battlefield. Now you go. As many of them have gone, you should go also." They said, "No, Prophet, if your life will be finished here on this battlefield, our life will be taken first. What is our life, after all! We shall give our life with you, Prophet. We are not afraid of this army." And then the Prophet threw down the arms that he had in his hand and bowed down and took a few pebbles from the earth and threw them at the army. And the army began to run for miles and miles. They did not know what was behind him. It was only a few pebbles, but what they saw were bullets, and they began to run.

That is called power, that is human power. It is not only that a human being has power over objects, but a human being has power over beings. It is only a little touch of power that the master of the circus uses to make the elephants work and tigers and lions dance. When that power is greater, the master has only to look at them to make them work as the master wishes them to work.

When the story is told of Daniel, who went in the caves of lions and found them all tamed at his feet, that again is spiritual power. That only shows what power a human being has. At the same time, not knowing of it, not being conscious of it, not trying to develop it, one debars oneself of that great privilege and bliss that God has given, and with limited powers one works in the world for pennies. In the end no pennies remain, nor has the person ever known power.

Power depends greatly upon the consciousness and the attitude of mind. A guilty conscience can turn lions into rabbits. They lose their power once they feel guilty, and so it is with a human being. When one is impressed by what others think, if that impression is one of disappointment or distress or shame, then that diminishes one's power. But when one is inspired by a thought, a feeling, or by one's own action, then one is powerful. It is the power of truth that makes one stronger. Those who know truth, even those who do not know truth but think they are in the right, even they have some power—the power of sincerity. Very few realize what power sincerity carries. A false person, however physically strong that person may be or how great in willpower, if there is falsehood, it will keep that person down. It never allows the false person to rise; it eats at the false person because it is a rust. Those who have done great things in life, in whatever walk of life it may be, have done them by the power of truth, the power of sincerity, of earnestness, by conviction. When that is lacking, power is lacking. What takes away human power is doubt. As soon as a person thinks, "Is it so or not?" or "Will it be or not be?" or "Is it right or not right?" then that person is powerless. And this is such a disease that every mind catches it. You can go to a doubting person when you have great enthusiasm and hope, and the doubting person may so impress you with darkness that you end up in the same boat. Doubt takes away courage and hope and optimism.

There are three grades of evolved human beings. In Sanskrit they are called *atma, mahatma,* and *paramatma,* an illuminated soul; in other words, a holy person, a divine soul, and an almighty soul. In the case of the first, an illuminated soul can show five different powers. These powers are magnetic powers. The first one is the revivifying of the physical body. The next is brightening the intelligence. And the third is deepening the love element in the heart. The fourth is etherealizing and deepening insight. And the fifth is uniting with God. With the fifth aspect, the illuminated soul shows great power. This power can be divided into two parts. One is the power of insight; the other is the power of will. The power of insight does not construct, does not make anything. It only sees; it is a passive power. The one who has the power of insight can see into human nature, and has an insight into the heart of another person, into the soul of another person, into the life of another person, into the affair of another person, into the past, present, and future of another person. And one might say, "What inspires such a person in that way? What is it that person sees?" The one who has the power of insight seems to understand the language of nature, the language of life, and seems to read the form, the feature, the movement, the atmosphere, the thought, and feeling. Everything has certain vibrations, a certain tendency, and therefore, to have insight is to know the language, to know the language of life which is without words. This can be seen even to the extent that the one who has insight knows more about another person than even that person does. For everyone is blinded by one's own affairs, although when one is told one knows it, but if one is not told, one does not know. It seems as if the knowledge of one's own being is buried within oneself.

Where does science come from? Also from the knowledge of insight, at least in the beginning. Other things improve upon it, but this science begins in intuition; it is insight. The great inventors of the world have insight into things. They may not believe it, but they have it just the same. They penetrate through the object to its purpose, and they utilize it toward its purpose. In that way they make use of insight's knowledge for scientific inventions. If they knew, they could make use of the same insight a thousand times better. From where does the science of medicine come? From insight. And those who have studied the lives of animals in the forest found out that the bear knows more about herbs than any other animal, and whenever it is ill, it knows what herb to take and cures itself by taking that herb. And ancient people who investigated nature invented medicine by seeing this tendency of animals, and they cured themselves. This shows that humanity has not only invented medicine but has also come to it by intuition; and it is the same with all other sciences.

And when we come to mahatmas, they are different. It is not only that they have a magnetic power but they have divine instinct, divine inspiration. There are stories told about the constructive power of mahatmas. And one is very interesting, which shows what this power can do. Once a prince was sent away from his country, his father having disapproved of his conduct. And he went and lived in the forest for a long time under the training of a guru, a teacher, and developed spiritually. And when the time came that he should be given initiation into the higher power, the guru asked, "My *chela*, have you any relatives?" He said, "Yes, my father and mother." The teacher said, "You must go to them and ask them first that you may take the initiation, because once you take it, you will have to live the life of solitude." The teacher thought that, "It is better that he went first to his people and saw all the possibilities of worldly life. If he does not want it, then he can come back." And the *chela* was so developed by that time that he had no desire to go to his parents in that kingdom and see them again. But since the guru told him, he went. When he reached his kingdom, he went to the garden where he lived first and which was neglected for many years. And there was nothing left in the garden. He went there and sat, and was very sorry to see his garden so neglected. He took out some water from his pitcher and threw it to both sides. And the garden began to flourish.

And so it was made known to the whole kingdom that there was a sage there, and the place where he stayed for a few days began to flourish. The story goes on to say that the king knew that his son was there, that he came and wanted him to take over the kingdom, to take up the work of the country. But [the son] refused and went away.

This story is an example of the constructive power of the sage, that the soul of the mahatma is constructive. And it is not true, as people say, that mahatmas can only be found in the caves of the Himalayas and that one cannot see them in the midst of the world. They can be found anywhere. They can be found in a palace, in the midst of riches, of comfort, and in remote places. They can be in any situation, in any position—they can be a mahatma just the same. But what comes out of a mahatma is a continually spreading constructive influence. They are a protection from illnesses and plagues, wars and disasters. The mahatma's constructive power is working and helping people to flourish today. And people are ready to believe that a minister or prime minister or a great person in the country can be such a help, can raise up the country, can put the finances of the country in good order, or can guard the country against other nations. They can believe that, but not if told that a hidden soul, who is not known, can have a greater influence still on the whole country. It has been known and seen by millions of people in the East at different times when divine souls lived, that their influence spread through the whole country and lifted it.

And now we come to the third aspect of sages, which is the *paramatma*, the almighty one. The *paramatma* is still greater in that the *paramatma* is no longer a person; the *paramatma* is God-conscious. We all are that of which we are conscious. A person in prison is conscious of the prison. A person who has a lot of money in the bank and is not conscious of it is poor in spite of that person's wealth. We can have anything and yet we only have that of which we are conscious. Therefore, our greatness or our smallness and our reach, high or low, depends upon our consciousness. Even to become an illuminated soul is only a difference of consciousness. It is not how much good a person has done. There are perhaps many good people, but they do not know what they themselves are and may be quite content with the good they have done.

Besides, there are some who believe in God and others who love God. And there are others who are lost in God. For those who believe in God, they are on earth and God is in heaven. For those who love God, God is before them; they are face-to-face with their Lord. And those who are lost in God have gained their real self. They are God themselves. I know of a God-conscious soul who was once moving about in the city of Baroda, where the rule was that no one should go about after ten o'clock at night. And this sage was wandering about, not knowing time. A policeman asked him, "Where are you going?" But he did not hear. Perhaps he was far away from the place where he was wandering. But when he heard the policeman say, "Are you a thief?" he smiled and said, "Yes." And the policeman took him to the police station and made him sit there all night long. In the morning the officer came and asked, "What is the report?" This policeman said, "I have caught one thief. I found him in the street." When the officer went and saw this man, he knew that he was a great soul and that people respected him very much. He asked his pardon. "But," he said, "when the policeman asked you the question, why did you say that you are a thief?" The answer was, "What am I not? I am everything."

We try to become spiritual, to raise our consciousness. But when it comes to an insult, we do not own it, we do not like it. As long as everybody flatters us, we are glad to attribute those things to ourselves. But as soon as it comes to an insult, we do not like it. Then we say that, "It is not me." But the *paramatma*, the high soul, is united with God, and is God-conscious, all-conscious. Everyone is the *paramatma's* own self. Whether it is a good person or a wicked person, whether one is right or wrong, one is the *paramatma's* own self; the *paramatma* looks at that person as the *paramatma's* own self. Even if it were the name of a thief, the *paramatma* can say, "Yes. All names are my names."

In conclusion, spirituality is not a certain kind of knowledge. Spirituality is the expansion of consciousness. The wider the consciousness expands, the greater is one's spiritual vision. And when once the consciousness expands so much that it embraces the whole universe, it is that which is called divine perfection.

THE SECRET OF BREATH

It is very little known in the world what mystery lies in breath.[1] Since the last religious conference which took place in the Chicago exhibition, and following the lectures of Vivekananda, people have inquired and want to know what is meant by Yoga.[2] And some who were uninitiated and who did not know the importance and sacredness of the idea, put out books, put something in the form of books which cannot be given in books, which has been taught for thousands of years in the East, handed down from teacher to pupil, trusted to those who were initiated. Initiation means a trust. Therefore do not, please, think that I am speaking this evening on the subject of the science of breath. I am speaking on the subject of the mystery of breath.

In the first place, it is clear even to those who do not know medical science that the whole mechanism of the body becomes a corpse when the breath departs. That means that, however perfect the mechanism of the body may be, in the absence of breath the body is a corpse. In other words, what is living in the body, or what makes it living, is breath. And how few of us realize this fact. We go on day after day working, busy with everyday life, absorbed in the thoughts we have before us, occupied with business, pursuing motives, and yet ignoring the principle upon which the whole life is based. And if one

1 Lecture, Sather Gate Bookshop, Berkeley, California, February 27, 1926.
2 The World's Parliament of Religion, where Swami Vivekananda spoke, took place as part of the Columbian Exposition of 1893 in Chicago.

comes out and says, "Prayer is a very important thing," people begin to think, "Yes, perhaps." If one says, "Meditation is a great thing," people say, "Yes, it is something." But when one says, "Breathing is a great secret," one says, "Why, I have never thought about it. What is it, after all?"

As far as science goes, breathing is known as air breathed in and breathed out. When it is breathed in, one gets oxygen from space, and when it is breathed out, one throws carbon dioxide into space. When one goes still further one knows that breathing keeps the lungs' capacity and the organs of breath going, that digestive gases are drawn in, and that one gets a greater digestive power. On the basis of that principle people are now beginning to use breathing in physical exercises. Also the latest discovery is that physical exercises together with breathing exercises make the body healthier, and there is a greater profit in doing physical exercises together with breath. For some years now, voice producers have given greater importance to breath. In reality, breathing itself is voice, and the whole voice construction depends upon breathing.

Then again, some physicians begin to see that many different illnesses of nerves, character, or of lungs or different nervous centers can often be helped by breathing. This is coming out as something new. There seems to be a general awakening toward the science of breath. And those who have practiced breathing in connection with physical culture or for the improvement in their particular condition, illness, or weakness, have found wonderful results; every day they are finding wonderful results. As a new invention, they say that breath is connected with everything on earth: with voice production or healing or curing of nervous conditions or developing the muscular and nervous system. And that is as far that the science of breath has reached.

But when we come to the mystery of breath, it is another domain, altogether different. In order to come first of all to the meaning of breath according to the mystic's point of view, the perceptible breath which the nostrils and hand can perceive as air drawn in and air going out—this breath is only an effect of breathing. It is not breath. For the mystic, breath is the current which takes the air out and brings the air in. The air is perceptible, not the current. The current is imperceptible. This is what the mystic calls *nafs*, which means the "self." It is not called breath; it is the self, the very self of a human being. Besides, *atma* is the soul and means "soul." In German the same word is used for breath: *atem*. They do not know, but it is the same word. The word of the mystics for the self, the soul, in Germany is used for the breath without them knowing; still it is the soul. That shows, if there is any trace of the soul, it is to be found in breath.

Naturally, breath, being the self, is not only the air which one exhales but it is a current which, according to mystics, runs from the physical plane into the innermost plane, a current which runs through the body, mind, and soul, touching the innermost of life and at the same time coming back: a continual current, perpetually moving in and out. This gives quite a different explanation of the breath and shows you the importance of something which very few people consider important. And it makes you understand that the most important part of being is breath, a being which reaches the innermost of life and reaches outward to the surface, which means touching the physical plane. But the direction of breath is in a dimension that today's science does not recognize, a dimension that is recognized by mystics, the dimension which is meant by mystics when they say "within."

The other day I was lecturing in England, and to it came a very wonderful scientist who heard the lecture and was very interested. He came to me and asked, "I am very interested, but there is one thing that puzzled me very much." He said, "I cannot understand the word *within*. What do you mean? Within the body? We can only understand inside the body." This shows the difficulty of reaching a common understanding between science and mysticism. It will come; it is only a momentary difficulty. It will only take a few years more.

To offer a philosophical explanation of this dimension, I would give as an example the simile of the eyes: what is it in these eyes of ours that can accommodate the horizon of so many miles? The size of the eyes is so small, and yet they can accommodate such a large horizon. Where is it accommodated? It is accommodated within. That is the only example one can give. It is a dimension which cannot be measured, but which is accommodating, which is an accommodation. The accommodation of the eye is not a recognized dimension, yet it is a dimension, the same way there is a dimension of mind. One can think deeply, feel profoundly. One can be conscious of life and be more deeply conscious still, but one cannot point to it, because it is abstract. If there is any word to describe this dimension, it can only be called *within*. And through that dimension, a current runs from the innermost plane to the physical plane, and there it keeps life living. And therefore, if I were to say that breath is the soul and soul is the breath, there would be nothing wrong in doing so.

The picture of God and of souls is that of the sun and its rays. The rays are not different from the sun, the sun is not different from the rays. Yet there is one sun and many rays. The rays have no existence of their own; they are only an action of the sun. They are not separate from the sun, and yet the various rays appear as so many different things. The one sun gives the idea of one center. So it is with God and humanity. What is God? The spirit which projects different rays, and each ray is a soul.

Therefore, the breath is that current which is a ray, a ray which comes from that sun which is the spirit of God. And this ray is the sign of life. And what is the body? The body is only a cover over this ray. When this ray has withdrawn itself from this cover, the body becomes a corpse. Then there is another cover, which is the mind. The difference between mind and heart is as the surface and the bottom. It is the surface of the heart which is the mind, and it is the depth of the mind which is the heart. The mind expresses the faculty of thinking, and the heart, of feeling. This is a garb within, a garb worn by the same thing which is called breath. Therefore, if the ray which is the breath has withdrawn itself from the body, it still exists, because it has another garb, it has a garb within. The outer garb was the body, the inner garb is the mind. It still continues to exist. And if it is lost in that garb which is called mind, then there is another garb, finer still, called the soul. Because breath runs through all three: body, mind, and soul.

The Yogis, they say, have learned very much about the secret of breath from the serpent. This explains how the custom of calling the serpent a sign of wisdom came to be. Shiva, the lord of Yogis, has a serpent around his neck as a necklace. It is the sign of mystery, a sign of wisdom. There are cobras in the forests of tropical countries, especially in India, who sleep and rest for six weeks. And then one day the cobra wakens, and it breathes because it is hungry, it wants to eat. And its thoughts attract food from wherever it may be. From miles away, food is attracted by its thoughts. The breath of the cobra is so magnetic that its food is helplessly drawn; a doe or deer or any animal is drawn closer. A fowl can be so strongly drawn that even from space it comes down out of the air, helplessly drawn, and falls into the cobra's mouth. The cobra makes no effort. It just breathes, it opens its mouth, and its food comes into its mouth. And then it rests for six weeks again. Besides this, it shows such a might in its construction that without wings it flies, and without feet it walks. And if there is any animal which can be called the healthiest animal, it is the serpent. It is never ill. Before it is ill, it dies. And if there is any animal that lives long, it is the serpent.

And it is said by those living in tropical countries, that a cobra can take revenge after twelve years. It remembers. If you once hit a cobra, it always remembers. That shows its memory, its mind. It has a mind. It knows the person. Besides, music appeals to the cobra, and music appeals to intelligent people. The more unintelligent the person, the less music appeals to that person; music has such a relation with intelligence. This shows that every sign of intelligence, of wisdom, of power is to be seen in the cobra. The mystics have studied the life of the cobra, and they have found two wonderful things. One thing is that it does not waste energy. Birds fly until they are tired. Animals run here and there. The cobra does not do so. It makes a hole where it lives and rests. It knows the best way of repose, a repose which it can continue as long as it wishes. We cannot do this. We human beings, of all creatures, know least about repose. We only know about work, not about repose, because we attach every importance to work, never to rest. Because we do not find anything in rest but everything in work, the work of rest we do not see.

Besides that, the natural breathing capacity of the cobra is such as no other creature shows. That capacity goes as a straight line throughout its body that gives it energy. The current, which it gets from space, runs through it and gives it all the light and energy and radiance and power. And compared with the cobra, all other creatures are awkwardly built, but the cobra is a straight line.

The skin of the cobra is so soft and of such a silky structure. And in a moment's time it can come out of its skin and be new, just as if born anew. The mystics have learned from it. They say, "We must go out of the body just as the cobra goes out of its skin; we must go out of our thoughts, ideas, feelings, like the cobra does with its skin." They say, "We must be able to breathe as rhythmically, to control our breath as the cobra does. We must be able to repose and relax in the same way as the cobra can. And then it will be possible to get all we want." As Christ has said, "Seek ye first the kingdom of God and all things shall be added unto you."[3] The same things that are added to the cobra, all that it needs, could also be added to a human being if

3 Matthew 6:33.

only one did not trouble about it. As Sa'di, our great poet, has said, "My self, you worry so much over things that you need, but know that the one who works for your needs is continually working for them. But you worry over them because it is your disease, your passion, that makes you worry all the time." And when we look at life more keenly, it is the same thing. Our worry about things, it seems, is our nature, our character; we cannot help it. It becomes such a part of our nature to worry, that if we had no worry, we might doubt if we are really living. Mystics, therefore, have for thousands of years practiced it, practiced the control of breath, the balance of it, the rhythm of it, the expanding of it, the lengthening of breath, the broadening of it, the centralizing of it. By this, great phenomena have been accomplished. All the Sufis in Persia, in Egypt, in India, have been great masters of breathing. And there are some masters who are conscious of their spiritual realization at every breath they take in and take out. With every breath, the consciousness of their plane of realization is attached.

For a person who really knows how to work with breath, if that person is not lazy, there is nothing that person cannot accomplish. That person cannot say of anything that it is impossible. It only requires work; it is not only a matter of knowing the theory, but it requires the understanding of it. The adepts, mystics, therefore do not consider breathing as a science or as an exercise; they consider it as the most sacred thing. It is like religion. And if in order to accomplish that practice any discipline is given by a teacher, they obey it, do it.

But there is a great difficulty. I found sometimes in my travels and teaching, when I had been speaking about these things, that people come with preconceived ideas. They are willing to learn, but they do not want any discipline. But to work in the military there is a discipline, in the factory and in the office there is a certain discipline, in the study at the university, everywhere there is discipline. But a person will have discipline everywhere, but not in spiritual things. If the voice producer says to make such grimaces, such faces—"Open your mouth so much, stand before the mirror and make this terrible face or not"—people will do it. But when it comes to spiritual attainment they make difficulties. They think so little of it that they do not want to make any sacrifice. Because they do not know where it leads to, they have no belief. On top of it, there are false methods which are taught here and there, and people are commercializing that which is most sacred and beautiful and joyous.

Today there is much talk that people in America are longing for truth. There is no doubt about it, because people in America have so much materialism that they are already tired of it and want to experience something else. At the same time there is greater demand for what is new, but the spiritual is only a business, and in that way the higher ideal is brought down to the lowest depth. And this is the time that the real thing should be introduced, seriously studied, experienced, and realized by practice.

A great service to humanity can be done here, in this land of America, if a few people came with a real sincere desire for searching, with patience, with endurance, with full confidence in esoteric teaching. It would be of such great use to the whole land, a service to God beyond price. And the one who seriously does it, to that one the doing of this service would be a greater pleasure than anything in the world. And I do not think that it would be a small number of people who would be quite willing to give their lives, their thought, and their time if they knew what they could accomplish. But to make them know is the difficulty, to have that confidence and trust in the study of breath. It wants only patience. And it wants, before all else, confidence. The real faith is confidence; when a person has confidence, that is faith. No medicine from any doctor would be taken if there was no confidence in the doctor. In the East, the secret of spiritual attainment is to have great confidence. In other things, yes, people will doubt—in business, and in industry.

But in spiritual things there is no question. In the mind of the wise and of the foolish there is no question about the value of spiritual attainment

And what is necessary today, in order to have first awakened, is confidence. When a person comes with doubt and confusion and suspicion, that person does not know what is true and what is not. Of fifty books read, perhaps five are of some use; all are not. The mind is confused. A book about Yoga at a drugstore—you can buy it anywhere, like a bottle of something, or so many bottles. Perhaps one has gone to twenty different societies, perhaps visited six or ten mediums, but there is such confusion about it all. One does not know which to believe, which are not true. One's mind is not yet clear. When there is confusion, when twenty or a hundred thoughts are muddled up, nothing is clear.

The Buddhists, for thousands of years, have taken one line, studied it with patience, with endurance. The Hindus have done the same thing. What is required today is a constant effort on a single line with patience and endurance to attain to the realization of truth.

THE MYSTERY OF SLEEP

It is very difficult to point out what condition it is that may be called sleep.[1] For, on consideration of this subject, one finds that one is always asleep and always wakeful. The difference is that of the particular sphere of which we are conscious when we are awake. In one sphere we think, "I am awake," and when that sphere is not before our consciousness we think, "I am asleep." Therefore, sleep and the wakeful state are nothing but the turning of the consciousness from one side to the other, from one sphere to the other sphere—in other words, from one plane to another. And therefore, according to the mystical idea, we are never asleep. Although the soul is much higher than the physical body, it is the character and nature of the soul which the physical body expresses.

When we are looking at one side we are unconscious of the other. This shows that the faculty of seeing and being conscious of what one sees, can only engage itself fully with one thing at a time. A conception of musical sound which has been held for a long time in the East, and which is today recognized by the scientists in the West, is that the human ear can hear fully one sound at a time, not two or three. This shows that every sense is capable of looking at one side only, and therefore the other side is absent from consciousness. And in order to see a particular side, one has to turn one's face; in other words, one has to expose one's faculty of seeing to that side.

1 *Sufism* magazine, June 23, 1922, 4–10.

This is not only the nature of the body, but also the nature of the mind. The mind cannot think of two things at the same time. Also, when the mind is at work, and when mind is fully absorbed in a certain thought, a certain imagination, the outer senses may be opened but they are not fully at work. When poets are thinking of a verse, the verse is before their mind. Their eyes are open, but they do not see; and if it happens that they see at the time they are thinking, then it is just like a film of moving pictures. It is so many different pictures coming one after the other, and so it seems that they are continuous. When the mind stops, the eyes work; and when the eyes work the mind stops. And in the end it seems to make one picture, but it is a separate action of the mind and senses. Besides that, the wakeful state of every individual is different and peculiar to that person, as the sleep of every individual is different and peculiar to that person. One person will be what is called fast asleep, that is, in deep sleep. There is another person who says, "I was half asleep." Still others know what is going on around them, and yet are asleep. This shows that the extent of sleep is different in every experience, and no one can define this extent of sleep.

Also the wakeful state of every individual is different. Many people may be sitting in the room, but one is more conscious of what is going on in that room than another. Five people may be hearing music, and each will apply consciousness differently to what each one hears. And therefore, each one will enjoy and will receive the effect of the music differently, and this shows that the body or mind are vehicles or instruments through which the soul experiences life. And in explaining what the soul is, I should say it is that part of our being which is capable of being conscious by means of the mind and body. Therefore, to the mystics it is that part of one's being which witnesses life through vehicles such as the mind and body which is the real being. And it is that part of their being which they call themselves or their soul. To the Sufis it is called *ruh*, and in the Sanskrit and Vedantic terminology it is called *atma*, the real being of a person. By experience in life, with the help of the mind and body, this *atma*, or soul, becomes deluded. And the delusion is that it loses consciousness of its pure self, as it is natural that when one is poorly dressed, one thinks one is poor; one never thinks one's dress is poor. When one is moving in a beautiful palace one is a big person. One does not think it is the palace which is big instead of oneself.

This shows it is not what one is, but what one believes one is, that one is related to. The soul is never ill, but when it is conscious of the illness of the body, the person says, "I am ill." It is the same with a person's garment being torn. One thinks, "I am torn," instead of the garment. And the reason is that one cannot point out to one's own consciousness one's own true being. As the eyes cannot see themselves but can see the whole world, so the soul cannot see itself except when it is conscious of all which is reflected in it. The soul is neither poor nor is it rich; it is never sorrowful or joyous. These are reflections which fall into it. And as it cannot realize itself, it considers itself to be that which is reflected in it, and therefore, one lives one's life in one's consciousness. One is, at every moment, what one is conscious of. In cheerful surroundings, one is pleased. In miserable surroundings, one is sad. There is nothing of sorrow or joy which can make an everlasting impression on the soul, because the nature of the soul is like a mirror, and all that stands before the mirror is reflected in it. But nothing can stay in the mirror; no reflection can remain in the mirror. When the person who stood before the mirror is removed, then the mirror is as clear as ever; and so it is with the soul.

For convenience, the mystics have divided that which consciousness experiences into five different phases and distinguished them as different from one another. The particular phase that consciousness is most familiar with is the wakeful state in which the soul experiences through mind and body. This state in Sufi terms is called *nasut*, and in Vedantic terms it is called *jagrat*. As the soul considers what it experiences through the senses with the help of the mind, the reason that there are many souls who are not ready to believe in the soul or in the hereafter or in God, is that the soul is acquainted with only one sphere, and that is the sphere which it experiences with the help of the body and mind.

An intellectual person also develops consciousness of another sphere, which is called *malakut* in Sufi terminology and *swapna* in terms of the Vedanta. This state is experienced when one is absorbed in a thought and is not aware of one's surroundings, and all one knows at that moment is the imagination in which one is absorbed. The state called *malakut* is not dependent upon the body for its joy or its experiences of sorrow. One who can experience joy and sorrow by raising one's consciousness to that plane can make heaven in oneself.

The great poets, thinkers, writers who have lived through difficulties, through poverty, through such conditions that people did not understand them, opposed them, and even despised them, have lived a most happy life, for the reason that they had been able to raise themselves to that plane where they could enjoy all the beauty, comfort, and joy that ordinary people can only enjoy if it is given to them on the physical plane. And when the key of this plane has come into one's hand, one is then the master of one's future life. As Omar Khayyam says in his *Rubaiyat*, "Heaven is the vision of fulfilled desire and hell the shadow of a soul on fire."[2] In this he shows that when the consciousness has heaven reflected in it, then we are in heaven; and when we are conscious of torture and pain and suffering, we are in the place of suffering. We make our heaven or our hell for ourselves. You will find many in this world who keep their illness by thinking about it all the time, by being conscious of it. And one sees others who might become well after having suffered a pain for some years, but the consciousness of the pain is held by them, not as something new but as something

2 See *The Rubaiyat of Omar Khayyam*, trans. Edward FitzGerald, verse 67.

which has always been there and is reflected and held in their consciousness. Nothing belongs to one unless one is willing to hold it. But when one becomes accustomed to holding a certain reflection, not knowing the nature of it, in time that reflection becomes one's master and one becomes a slave to that reflection. And so it is with the worry and anxiety and sorrows which people have on their mind. Many say "I cannot forget," because they imagine it. It does not mean that that one cannot forget but that one is holding something which one does not wish to throw away. There are many people who say "I cannot forget it," but if they only knew that it is not that any other person is holding something before them, it is they themselves who hold it. Some memory, something disagreeable, something sorrowful, some severe pain, anxiety, worry—all these things one holds in one's own hands and are reflected in one's consciousness. The soul, by nature, is above all this. This is an illusion whose place is beneath the soul, not above, unless we, with our own hands, raise it and look at it.

When we consider the psychology of failure and success, failure follows failure. And why is that? Because the consciousness reflecting success is full of success, and the activity which goes out from the consciousness is creating productive activity. And if the consciousness has success before its view, then the same reflection will work and bring success; whereas if the consciousness is impressed with failure, then failure will work constantly, bringing failure after failure. Very often pessimistic people speak against their own desire. They want to undertake some work, and they say, "I will do this, but I don't think I shall succeed in it." They thus have hindered themselves in their path. One does not know that every thought makes an impression on the consciousness and on the rhythm with which the consciousness is working. According to the rhythm, that reflection will come true and happen, and one proves to be one's own enemy by one's ignorance of these things. The mistake of one moment's impulse creates a kind of hindrance in one's path through all of life.

This state of consciousness is also experienced in the dream, for the dream is the reaction of one's experiences in a wakeful state. The most wonderful thing which one can study in the dream is that the dream has a language, and a true knowledge of dream experiences teaches one that every individual has a separate language of the dream peculiar to one's own nature. The dream of the poet, the dream of the person who works with the hands, the dream of the king, the dream of the poor—all are different. There are many differences, and one cannot give the same interpretation to every person for a dream. You must first know who has dreamed it. It is not the dream which has its interpretation, it is the person to whom the dream came that one must know. And the interpretation is according to one's state of evolution, occupation, ambitions, and desires, to one's present, past, and future, and to one's spiritual aspirations.

Thus the language of dreams differs, but there is one hint which may be given, and that is that in the wakeful state a person is open to outward impressions. For instance, there are moments when the mind is receptive, there are moments when the mind is expressive. And during the moments when the mind is receptive, every impression which comes forth, sent intentionally or without intention from any person, becomes reflected in the consciousness. Very often one finds oneself depressed and cannot find a reason, and then one finds oneself in a mirthful attitude and one cannot find the reason. As soon as one has a certain feeling, one at once looks for a reason, and reason is ready to answer, rightly or wrongly. As soon as a person thinks, "What is making me laugh?" there is something which reason offers as the reason why that person laughed. In reality, that impression came from someone else. What one thinks is the reason is different, and so very often in the dream it happens that the reasoning faculty answers to the demands of the inquiring mind, and frames and shapes the thoughts and imaginations which are going on so freely when the will-power is not controlling the mind in sleep. It is producing at that time, just like an actor on the stage: free, without control of the will. And therefore, if it happens that, at a certain moment when the mind is in a receptive condition, it receives the impressions coming from other persons, from those who are friends or from those who are enemies, all those who think of the dreamer or with whom the dreamer is connected in any way. Those who are spiritually inclined or who are connected with souls who have passed away, also feel the impressions reflected upon their souls, sometimes as guiding influences, sometimes as warnings, sometimes as instructions. They also experience what are known as initiations, and sometimes have deluding, confusing experiences; but it all takes place on that particular plane where the consciousness is experiencing life, independently of the physical body and of the senses.

The third experience which the consciousness has is called in Sufi terms *jabarut*, and in Sanskrit and Vedantic terms *sushupti*. In this state, as consciousness is not accustomed to this world very much, it does not bring its experiences to the world, except that it brings a feeling of joy, of renewed strength, or health, and all one can say after this experience is, "I have had a very good sleep and feel very much better for that." The real cause is that the consciousness was freed from pain and worry and any activity or any limitation of life. And even prisoners can enjoy the blessing of this state when they are fast asleep; they do not know whether they are in a palace or in prison. They reach the experiences of that plane which is better than a palace.

People do not realize the value of this state until the time comes when, for some reason or other, they cannot receive this blessing. They cannot sleep; then they begin to think there is nothing they would not give to be able to sleep soundly. This shows that it is not only the sleep which they need, but the blessing behind it. It is something which the soul has touched which is much higher and deeper, for this experience is greater than one can imagine. In this experience, consciousness touches a sphere whence it cannot get an impression of any name or form. The impression it gets is a feeling, a feeling of illumination, of life, of joy. And what message does it give? It gives a message of God which comes directly to every soul. And what is this message? God says to the soul, "I am within you, I am with you, I am your own being, and I am above all limitations, and I am life." And you are more safe, more living, and more happy, and more peaceful in this knowledge than in anything else in the world.

Besides these three experiences, there comes a fourth experience to those who search after it. Why does it not come to everybody? It is not that it does not come to everybody, but that not everybody can catch it. It comes and slips away, and one does not know when it came and when it went. In the life of every person there is a moment during the wakeful state, a moment when one rises above all limitations of life; but so swiftly does it come and go in the twinkling of an eye, that one cannot catch it, one does not know it. It is just like a bird which came and flew away, and you only heard the flutter of its wings. But those who wish to catch this bird, those who wish to see where this bird goes, and when it comes and when it goes, look out for it. They sit waiting and watching for the moment when it comes, and that watching is called meditation.

Meditation does not mean closing the eyes and sitting. Anyone can close the eyes and sit, but one may sit for hours or sit all one's life and still not know what came and what went. It is looking out for what comes, and not only looking out for it, but preparing oneself by making one's senses keen, by making one's body and mind a receptacle for the vibrations, so that when the bird makes a vibration one feels that it has come. And it is this which is expressed in the Christian symbology of the dove. In other words, it is the moment, which approaches one's consciousness rapidly, of such bliss that one, so to speak, touches the depth of the whole life, reaches above the sphere of action and all that, even above the sphere of feeling.

But now you will ask, "What does consciousness receive from it?" It receives a kind of illumination which is like a torch lighting another light. This inner life, touching the consciousness, produces a sort of illumination which makes our life clear. Every moment after this experience is unveiled because of this moment. It charges our life with new life and new light. And therefore, in the East, Yogis sit in samadhi or in a certain posture for so many hours or go into the forest and sit in the solitude; they have always done so to catch this light, which is symbolized by a dove.

And there is one step even higher than this, which in the terms of the Sufi is *hahut*, the fifth sphere which consciousness experiences. In this consciousness touches the innermost depth of its own being; it is like touching the feet of God. That is the communion which is spoken of in Christian symbology. It is just like touching the presence of God, when one's consciousness has become so light and so liberated and free that it can raise itself and dive and touch the depth of one's being.

This is the secret of all mysticism and religion and philosophy. And the process of this experience is like the process of alchemy, which is not given freely, except to those who are ready and who feel there is some truth in it. It takes time for a person to become familiar with things of this nature, even to think there is some truth in them and that it is not only talk and imagination. Even one who has felt the truth of the mystical state may question if it is worthwhile to go on this quest, but if one does so, one must take the guidance of someone who has knowledge of this path, in whom one can put trust and confidence. But it must be understood that the path of discipleship, which in mystical terms is known as the path of initiation, is not such that the teacher gives to the pupil some knowledge, tells something new which the pupil has not heard, or shows the pupil some wonder; and the teacher who does that is not the true teacher. Each one is one's own teacher; in each one is the secret of one's being. The teacher's word is only to help one find oneself. Nothing you can learn in words, nothing that can be explained in language, nothing that can be pointed out with a finger, is truth. If one is sure of oneself, one can go further. But when one is confused in oneself, one cannot go further, and no teacher can help. Therefore, although in this path the teacher is necessary and the teacher's help is valuable, self-help is the principal thing. And one who is ready to realize one's own nature, and to learn from oneself, it is that one who is the true initiate. And it is from that initiation that one will go forward, step-by-step, and will find the realization and conviction that one seeks. And all that comes throughout that person's life will but deepen that realization of truth.

SILENCE 1

I ask your indulgence for my discourse this evening on the subject of silence.[1] There is a saying that words are valuable, but silence is precious. This saying will always prove true. The more we understand the meaning of it, the more we find its truth. Sufism is quietism. It is not a particular sect, a dogma, or a doctrine. It is an art, the art of silence through which beauty is produced. And before going further into this most serious subject, I would like first of all to consider what our relation is with daily life. How many times we find during the day that we have said something which would have been better left unsaid. How many times we disturb the peace of our surrounding, without meaning it, by lack of silence. How often we make our limitations, our narrowness, our smallness come out, which we would rather have covered, because we did not keep silence. How very often, desiring to respect others, we cannot manage to do so because of not keeping silence. And that great danger awaits us in the life of the world, the danger of confiding in a person in whom we did not wish to confide. One jumps into that danger by not keeping silence. As the great reader of life, the Persian poet Sa'di, says, "What value is that sense, if it does not come to my rescue before I utter a word?" This shows to us, friends, that in spite of great wisdom we may have, still, if there is no control over our words, we can make a mistake. And we shall find examples of this truth. Those who talk much have

1 Lecture, Kunstgewerbehaus, Munich, Germany, March 16, 1925.

264

less power than those who talk little. For a talkative person may not be able to express an idea in thousand words, which those who are masters of silence express in one word. Everyone can speak, but not every word has the same power. Besides, what a word says is much less compared to what silence expresses. If one asked me for the keynote of harmonious life, I would answer, "Silence."

There is a mirthful story told in India. The story tells of a woman who went to a magnetizer and asked for a remedy for every day having disagreement in her home. "Don't be afraid," the magnetizer said, "that is the easiest thing to cure. I shall give you some sweets. Eat them, and do not speak a word while they are in the mouth. They are magnetized sweets; there will be no more inharmony in your home." And so it happened. All the days the lady had the sweets there was no disagreement. Naturally, the poor husband, nervous and rigid after a whole day's labor, found no stimulant, no bad temper from his wife, just one or two words and then silence. The lady came one day to the magnetizer and asked him, "Please give me more of those sweets." The answer was, "There is no need to have more sweets. Only think of them; that is enough."

We can learn much from this story. In everyday life we are confronted with a thousand troubles that we are not always evolved enough to meet, and only silence can help us. For if there is any religion, if there is any practice of religion, it is to have regard for the pleasure of God in regarding the pleasure of human beings. The essence of religion is to understand. And this religion we cannot live without having power over the word, without having realized the power of silence. There are so very many occasions of repenting after hurting friends which could have been avoided if there had been a control over words. Silence is the shield of the ignorant, the protection of the wise. For the ignorant do not prove their ignorance if they keep silence, and the wise will not throw pearls before swine if they know the worth of silence.

Now, coming to the question: What gives power over words? In other words, what gives the power that can be attained by silence? The answer is that it is willpower which gives the control over words; it is silence which gives one the power of silence. It is restlessness when a person speaks too much. The more words are used to express an idea, the less powerful they become. What a great pity that a person so often thinks of saving pennies and never thinks of sparing words. It is like saving pebbles and throwing away pearls. An Indian poet says, "Pearl shell, what gives you your precious contents?" And the answer is, "Silence. For years my lips were closed." For a moment it is a struggle with oneself, it is controlling an impulse; but afterward the same thing becomes a power.

And now, coming to the more scientific, metaphysical explanation of silence. There is a certain amount of energy spent by words; and breath, which has to bring new life in the body, is hindered from its regular rhythm when a person speaks all the time. Therefore, it is not that a nervous person speaks too much, but much speaking makes a person nervous. The great power of which you have heard attained by Yogis and fakirs—where did their power come from? It was gained by having learned and practiced the art of silence. And that is the reason why in the East, at the court and in the houses where fakirs meditated, there was silence. There were times in the world during different civilizations that people were taught, whenever they were collected together for a feast, to keep silence for a certain time. It is the greatest pity that at this time we have so neglected that question, we think so little about it. It is a question which affects health and which is related to the soul, to the spirit, to life.

The more one thinks about this subject, the more one sees that we are involved in a kind of activity. Where does it lead us? And what is the result of it? As far as we can see, it leads us to greater struggle, competition, disagreeableness. If we think of the result, we see that it leads us to greater care, worry, and struggle in life. There is a saying of the Hindus: the more one seeks for happiness, the more unhappiness one finds. And the reason is that when happiness is sought in a wrong direction, it leads to unhappiness. Our experience in life is sufficient to teach us this, yet life is intoxicating; it absorbs us in action so that we never stop to think of it. This has been my own experience while traveling for some years, that it seems as if the world is wakening to spiritual ideals, and in spite of this, there is more activity—not only outer activity, but also activity of the mind.

In reality, humanity has shattered its nerves by the lack of silence, by the activity of body and mind. When the body is resting one calls it sleep, but one's mind is going on the same record as during the day. Then there comes a time when one can say, "I am really restless." No doubt, life just now in the world is [busy]. In this competition one is a hundred times more busy than one ever was. Naturally one needs rest and quietude and peace more than those who live in the forest and who can call all the time their own. When activity is increased and the art of silence is lost, then what can we expect?

Now, coming to a metaphysical question: Where do we learn thoughtfulness? In silence. And where do we practice patience? In silence. Silence that one does as meditation is something apart, but we should consider silence at every word, in every action we do; that is the first lesson to learn. If there is a meditative person, naturally that person has learned to use that silence in everyday life. Who has learned silence in everyday life has already learned to meditate. "Besides," a person may say, "I have appointed a time when I meditate for half an hour." But when there is half an hour of meditation and twelve or fifteen hours of activity, the activity takes away all the power of the meditation. Therefore, both things must go together. A person who wishes to learn the art of silence must decide, however much work it may be, to keep the thought of silence in mind. When one does not consider this, then one will not get the full benefit out of meditation. It is just like a person who goes once to the church and the other six days keeps the thought of church as far away as possible. A Persian king was advised by his prime minister, who said to this most devout king, "You are spending most of the night in meditation and all day long you do the work. How can that go on?" The shah said that, "During the night I pursue God; during the day God follows me." I would say the same in connection with silence: "Who seeks silence, silence follows." So it is with all things we wish for. When we seek after them sufficiently, they naturally follow us in time.

There are many who do not mind if they hurt anyone as long as they think they have told the truth. For then they feel so justified that if the other one cries or laughs, they say, "I don't mind." But friends, there is a difference between fact and truth. Fact is that which can be said; truth is that which cannot be put in words. The claim, "I tell the truth," falls flat when the difference is realized between fact and truth. People discuss dogmas, beliefs, and moral principles as they know them. But there comes a time in life when one has touched truth which one cannot speak in words. And at that time all dispute, discussion, and argument finishes. It is then that a person says, "If you have done wrong or if I have done wrong, it does not matter. What I want just now is to right the wrong." There comes a time when the continual question which arises in the active mind, "What is what, and which is which?" finishes, for the answer rises from the soul and is received in silence.

Friends, there is an audible voice and an inaudible voice, from the living and from those who are not living, from all life. What a person can say in words always expresses little. What can one say about gratefulness, about devotion, about admiration? One can never say it. If there is profound devotion, admiration, or gratefulness, one never can say it, there is a lack of words. Every feeling, every deep feeling has its own voice; it cannot be expressed in outer words. This voice is coming from every soul, and every soul is only audible to the heart. And how is the heart prepared? Through silence.

We need not be surprised to think that some have sought the mountains and the forest and preferred the wilderness to the comforts of worldly life. They sought something valuable. They have given something of their experience gained by their sacrifice. But it is not necessary to follow them to the forest or to the cave of the mountain. One can learn that art of silence; throughout a busy life, one can maintain silence.

SILENCE 2

Apart from meditative silence, even in our everyday life silence is the most essential thing.[1] There is an energy that gets accumulated, functioning in the innermost of our being, and it is in speech that one gives outlet to that energy. And that energy may best be called magnetism. It is inspiration and it is wisdom. It is therefore that you will always find in the less talkative person a greater wisdom than in the one who is talkative. Apart from wisdom, from a physical point of view, a talkative person is all the time giving out an energy which, if one conserved it, would make a great vital power in oneself. With some persons it becomes a passion to speak without purpose, without a reason to speak, because they like to speak. If one knew what the Bible says about the word, that first was the Word and the Word was God,[2] if one only knew what the tradition of humanity has been—it is the word. Those who have the esteem of the word, those who value the word, their word becomes precious. Their word is worth millions, and even millions are less than the price of their word.

The great teachers of humanity have come and passed away, and what they have left behind them, which the world prizes more than anything, is their word. If we keep anything as most sacred just now, whatever be our faith or religion, it is the word that has been given to us, it is the word which we keep as the

1 Lecture, 451, rue de Loxum, Brussels, December 8, 1924.
2 John 1:1.

270

most precious thing in the world. The moment that we begin to value our word, from that moment we begin to think about what we say. Those who have no value in their word are of little value themselves. The greater ones are those who stand for their word. However great some people may be, if they have no honor of their word, they cannot really be great. It is such a pity that, in this time of materialism, we are losing the idea of the most valuable thing we have; and we have got it from the heavens, for the word is heavenly and what is in the word is the soul, the spirit. And when that word is uselessly used, life is abused by it. Do we not see that there is a person who comes and speaks perhaps a thousand words to us, and not one word strikes us? There is another person who comes and speaks one word to us, but it penetrates, it makes an impression. That word is of value, for there is a living word and there is a dead word. A living word has a life, it acts chemically; the dead word has no life, it is only a corpse. The living word will go and float in space, it will go into the hearts of human beings and work. And the dead word will drop from the mouth on to the earth and will be buried in the dust.

And very often a person speaks because of weakness. That person is weak, cannot control the idea, the thought, and helplessly drops a word that should otherwise have been kept and not spoken. A gossiping person, a person who criticizes another, you will always find, is a person of weak character. It is not that they like to speak, it is because they cannot help speaking. It is just like a person who eats, but cannot digest. When one cannot keep one's own secret, when one cannot keep the secret of one's friend, one has no power of digestion, one's conscience will always feel guilty, and one's heart restless. There is another person who goes on like a machine, a machine which is hearing from the ears and speaking from the mouth, and it is going on all day, and it goes on like a machine. Is it not the experience of many of us that very often we think, "Oh, I wish I had not said that to that person"? Is it not the experience of many of us when we think that, "I should not have spoken so rudely with the other person?" Is it not the experience of many of us to think that, after having spoken, "Oh, what a terrible thing I have done. I have opened my heart to that person, I do not know what will become of it!" Sa'di, a great Persian poet, says in his poem that, "My intelligent friend, what use is your repentance after once you have dropped the word out of your lips?" To control the word is more difficult than controlling the most energetic horse. The one who controls one's word, controls one's mind.

There is another way of looking at this subject. When a person is talking to those not yet evolved to one's own grade of looking at things, one may say things of a greater wisdom which will prove to be as pebbles in the place of pearls. It is a loss of words of a higher ideal, of some greater truth, to a person who is not capable of understanding or appreciating. You have given something to the hand of another who will ridicule it, who will mock it, and to whom it is of no use. You would find it more thoughtful, more wise, that you did not speak the word at that time, but prepared the person to hear that word, even if it wouldn't be for ten years.

And then there are times when you meet with an evolved person to whom your words are of little importance; you are just like a child speaking to a grown person, which means very little. But the thing is this, that in doing so you will spoil that person's time as well as your own. Besides, many well know that many disagreements between relations, between friends, are brought about by useless talking. The talking had no importance whatever, but it has culminated perhaps in a great disharmony or separateness.

There is an amusing story that a woman went to the house of a healer, a magnetizer, and she asked him if he would tell her something, for she was in great distress. This distress was that every day she had a disagreement with her husband. The healer said, "It is very easy. I will give you some sweets, and you will put them in your mouth and keep your lips closed. Every time when your husband comes home, you put them in your mouth." The remedy proved successful. And the woman came after the sweets were finished to thank him and to ask for some more magnetized sweets. He said, "My dear lady, you do not need any more bonbons now. Just think that you have them and close your lips, and all will be all right." This example is for us all to learn, whether wise or foolish. For the wise it is the most beautiful thing; for the foolish it is the only dignified thing possible.

And now, coming to a still deeper side of silence. What is silence? Silence is something which we consciously or unconsciously are seeking every moment of our life. We are seeking for silence and running away from it, both at the same time. Where is the word of God heard? In silence. The seers, the saints, the sages, the prophets and masters, they have heard that voice which comes from within by making themselves silent. I do not mean by this that if one maintains a silence, one will be spoken to. I mean that one will hear the word which is constantly coming once one is silent. Once the mind has been made still, a person gets in communication with every person one meets. One does not need too many words; when the glances meet, one understands.

Two persons may talk and discuss their whole life and they will not understand one another. And two persons with still minds look at one another, and in one moment there is a communication. From where come the differences between people? It is by their activity. And when does agreement come? It comes by the stillness of mind. It is the noise which hinders a voice that we hear from a distance. And it is the troubled waters of a pool which hinder us seeing our own image reflected in the water. When the water is still it makes a clear reflection. And when our atmosphere is still, then we hear that voice which is constantly coming to the heart of every person. We are looking for guidance. We, all of us, search for truth, we search for the mystery. The mystery is in ourselves. The guidance is in our own soul. Besides this, very often one meets a person who makes one restless, nervous. The reason is that the person is not restful, not tranquil. This shows that being restless makes others restless, being calm makes others calm. And it is not easy to stand calm and to keep one's tranquility in the presence of a restless, agitated person.

The teaching of Christ is, "Resist not evil."[3] And that means: do not give in to that troubled condition, or do not respond to the troubled condition of a restless person. It is just like partaking of the fire that will burn oneself. And now how can one develop that power in oneself to stand, in everyday life, against all disturbing influences? For our life is exposed to this atmosphere every moment of the day. The answer is that one has to quiet oneself by the way of concentration. And now you may ask what I mean by concentration. Our mind is like a boat, a boat which is in the water, subject to being moved by the waves and subject to being influenced by the wind, both. And the waves for this boat are our own emotions and passions, our own thoughts and imaginations; and the wind is the outer influences which we have to meet with. And in order to stop the boat you ought to have the anchor to put in the water, and that anchor makes the boat still. And that anchor is the object which we concentrate upon. If this anchor be heavy and weighty, then it will stop the boat. But if this anchor is light, the boat will move and not be still, for it is in the water, it is in the air.

But now, coming to the question that by this we only control the boat, but utilizing the boat is another question again. The boat is not made to stand still, it is made for a purpose. To make it stand still is only to control the boat first. Although all of us may not know this, at the same time, at the end of the examination, this boat is made to go from one port to another port. Now, sailing the boat needs different conditions. And

3 Matthew 5:39.

those conditions are that the boat must not be more heavily laden than the weight that it is made to carry. And so our heart must not be heavily laden with the things that we attach ourselves to, because then the boat will not go. The boat must not be tied and chained to this one port, for then it is held back and will not go to that other port for which it is made. The boat may be tied to one port for a thousand years, but the boat is not doing its work then. In the first place it must have that responsiveness to the wind that will take it to that port. And that is the feeling that a soul gets from the spiritual side of life. That feeling of the wind helps one to go on, to go forward to that port to which we are all bound. The mind which is once concentrated fully must become a compass, as they have in the boat, which always points to the same side. A person who has a thousand different sides of interest, that person is not ready to travel in this boat. It is the one who has one thing in mind, all other things being secondary, who travels from this port to that port. It is this journey which is called mysticism. It is this journey which is called Sufism.

The efforts of the Sufi message is to give the opportunity to those serious seekers after truth that they may come in touch with the deeper side of life. No doubt, truth is never taught. Truth is discovered. It is not the wonderworking, it is not the love of phenomena that is the sign of the seeker. For it is in the search for truth that God is found, and it is in the finding of God that truth is realized. But where is God to be found? God is to be found in the human heart.

DREAMS AND REVELATIONS 1

When considering the idea of the dreams one finds that although it is something which is known to everybody, this subject leads to the deeper side of life, because it is from the meaning of dreams that one begins to realize two things: something is active when the body is asleep, and to the deep thinker this gives faith in the life hereafter.[1] For the dream is the proof that when the body is not active, the person is still active and seems to be no less so than in the physical body. And if one finds a difference, it is a difference of time. For here one may pass from one land to another in two hours instead of doing it in a month. In no way is one hindered with the hindrances of the physical plane. From England to America, one jumps in one moment; one flies there. The facility of the plane of dreams is much greater. There is no difficulty in changing one's condition, from illness to health, from failure to success, in one moment. People say yes, yes, but it is imagination, a working of the mind. But what is the mind? The mind is that in which the world is reflected; heaven and earth are accommodated in it. Is that a small thing? What is the physical body compared to the mind? It is a world in itself. The physical body is like a drop in the ocean. It is nothing other than ignorance that one does not know there is a kingdom in oneself, if only one were conscious of it. Why is one not? Because one wishes to hold something; only then does it exist. One does not wish to

1 Lecture, 44, blvd. des Tranchées, Geneva, Switzerland, April 3, 1924.

276

confess to oneself the existence of sentiment, for then they say it is of no account, it is nothing. The same about thought: it is only imagination, it is nothing. But science and art come from imagination, from the mind, not from a rock, not from the physical body. The source of all knowledge is the mind, not an object. Mind means "I." It is the mind with which one identifies. The body is an illusion. When the mind is depressed, we say: "I am sad." Not the body, but the mind was depressed. So the real identification is the mind, not the body.

If in a dream one is able to see oneself, what does that show? That after what is called death one is not formless, that nothing is lost, that only the freedom is gained which was lost. The absence of this knowledge makes one afraid for this physical body, makes one have a horror of death. But what is death? Nothing but a sleep. A sleep of the body which was a cloak; one can take it away and yet be living. One will realize, after all the talk about death, that one is alive and has not lost but gained. The human being is in the physical world to learn, and the dream teaches that a law is working, that all that seems surprising, accidental, a sudden happening, was not sudden and was no accident. It seemed accidental because it was not connected with the conditions. Nothing happens which does not go through the mind. One has turned one's back on it and is open only to the manifestation. It was no surprise, it was only preparing. Did they not say in all the countries when the war came: "We did not know"?[2] Yes, it was so to those who slept, but the awakened had seen the preparation. In all things we see this. Every accident, pleasant or unpleasant, has a long preparation before it. First it exists in the mind, then on the physical plane.

A dream shows the depth of life; through a dream we see things. One may ask: What is the meaning? Has every dream a meaning? The only thing is this: there are those in a country who do not know its language, and so it is with minds. Some

2 World War I.

minds are not yet capable of expressing themselves, so the dreams are upside down, a chaos. They see a goat with the ears of an elephant. The mind wanted to express itself. There is a meaning in what the child says, but it has not yet learned, it has no words; it can only cry or make a sound, yet this has a meaning. So it is with dreams which are not expressed correctly. But you may say: How can the mind learn to express itself? It has to become itself. Often the mind is disturbed, inharmonious, restless. When a person is drunk, and wants to say yes, that person says no. So is the expression of the mind in a dream.

It is a marvelous thing to study the science of dreams. How wonderful that a dream of the poet is poetical, of the musician harmonious. Why is this? Because their mind is trained, their mind has become focused. Their mind expresses itself in the realm of art. Sometimes one marvels at the dreams one hears of experienced by poetic souls. You will see the sequence from the first act till the last. You will see that every little action has a certain meaning. More interesting still is the symbolical dream, to see the meaning behind it. It is a wonderful thing that to the simple person comes a simple dream, and when a person is confused then the dream is confused. So you see the person in the simple dream, in the dream with fear, with joy, with grief. Then the dream shows the sadness. But this is not small, this is not past, it was not a dream. It is as real as life on the physical plane. Is this life not a dream? Are the eyes not closed? The king has forgotten his palace. A person says: "Oh, it is a dream, it is nothing." But this dream can be the whole life of the past. This dream can be tomorrow. It is only on the physical plane that it was a dream. The condition into which the mind has passed makes it only a dream. But a person says: "Yes, but when we awake we find a house, therefore this is reality. If we dream of a palace, we find no palace." This is true and not true. The palaces which are built in that world are as much our own, are much more our own. As soon as the body dies, this is left, and is always there. If it is a dream of pleasure, the pleasure will come.

If it is a dream of light, of love, then all is there. It is a treasure you can depend upon; death cannot take it away. It is of a glimpse of that idea which the Bible says: "Where your treasure is, there is your heart."[3] We can find glimpses of that by comparing dreams with the wakeful state. Whatever we hold, the longer we have held it, the more firmly it is established, and it can be more firmly established than what we hold in our hand. Then we create a world for ourselves to live in. This is the secret of the whole life. How can words explain it?

Now, a question arises: Where does inspiration come from? Is it the work of the mind? Is it produced as in a factory? No. There is a storehouse of all knowledge that has ever been or ever will be. What is it? It is the divine mind. Where is the divine mind? It is in the depth of your being, far and yet so near. If someone is in front of you, you might see that person, even at a distance of hundred miles. But if you are close to that person, and your back is turned, you cannot see. But if you look at that person, there is communication. If only there is a will to reach, then it is possible. What is it that gives inspiration to the musician? It is the fairy, the ghost, pictured in a thousand forms, and yet it is a voice from the depth of one's own heart. The mind begins to call out. When the heart's ears are open, then comes perfection. Then the composer conceives in one moment what will be perfect a hundred years later, what will be perfect in any age. After the death of the heart of the composer, this will be living. This comes not from the brain, it comes from the fountain at the bottom of the heart, from the divine mind. One may study counterpoints and notes, and be puzzling for a whole year and never come to the right point. Poets may be working for years, and only at that moment reach the divine mind. They dug to the depths, till they reached the living water. In some parts you have to dig a little, in some parts much, but in the bottom of the heart is inspiration. What the brain makes is mortal. One can easily see this by an example. There

3 Matthew 6:21.

are two ways: the way of heritage, and the other way of making. Most depend on heritage; some few make. Medicine, when it is inspiration, is a divine heritage. But where does the divine mind collect the knowledge of all minds? This knowledge is in the divine mind, as all the heat is in the sun, its origin is in the sun. So one can never say: "I have invented, I have discovered." It all comes from one source.

There are different forms of inspiration. The beginning is impression. By what a person sees, that person is impressed. One can be impressed by kindness, by goodness, and that is the beginning. For this, no clairvoyance is necessary; everyone has that gift to a certain extent. For people who already have experience in life, this is more difficult than for children who really get an impression of people. Some make them afraid, some annoyed, others pleased or joyous. This is the way of children. Grown-ups often cannot partake in that impression, the direct and natural impression of children. Besides, there is the link of love and sympathy. Words are not needed to express it, only a little light or shade. You do not need to say or to do anything to express the increase of love; by impression one feels it. What does this show? That the world of the body is dead, and that the world of the heart is living. Who is conscious of the body is dead. Alas, how many dead persons live, and their number is increasing—the number of those who do not believe in the existence of the mind.

Then there is intuition, a further step. This step is like a voice that tells one, that warns one, the voice of the heart that says: "No, do not do it." Or "Do it." It is this voice that decides. Many say: "But very often it was not the right intuition." But if they study it they will find out it was right—but you must hear the voice at once. It rings once, not twice. Besides, the doubting person says: "Which was the right one? The first or the second voice?" They mix them up. The more they doubt, the more they become confused. A person may blame intuition, but in doing so one fools oneself, not intuition. In the form of warning, in the form of suggestion, intuition comes.

Then there is a further manifestation that is inspiration. The heart becomes absorbed in art, in poetry, in beauty. The whole phrase comes as a stream; it comes in one stream. What it was not possible to make in six months, comes in one moment's time. You have only to get it down. There is a great delight after this has come. The one to whom this comes does not give the credit to oneself, but gives the credit to the king of all beauty.

And another step further is the inspiration in the form of a dream, the vision. What a person sees clearly will happen perhaps after twelve years; that is a vision or knowledge of the past. It is like a flash. One sees the whole series like a moving picture. Where does one get this? When the heart is focused on the divine mind, all is there as a moving picture. There was a poet of Persia, Firdausi. He was asked by the king to write the history of the land. This king promised that he would receive a gold coin for every verse. After this promise Firdausi went into solitude and wrote the traditions of centuries: characters, lives, deeds, he saw it all as a play, and he wrote of it in verse. When he returned to the court, the king was most impressed; he thought it wonderful. But there are many in the world who will always refute. The truth is only accepted by the few. Many made a bad expression, many showed skepticism. They went so far as to tell the king that it was all Firdausi's imagination. It hurt him terribly. He took a person who was skeptical and put his hand upon his head, and said to him: "Now, close your eyes and look." This person saw it like a moving picture and exclaimed: "I have seen." The poet's heart was struck, and he would not accept the gold coins. The message given by the great ones, by the prophets and masters, by Rama, by Krishna, what was it? Not imagination. It was that record which can be found by diving deep, that prophecy given to the world as a lesson, living in the world, like a scripture. It is a direct communion given by all masters.

Then there is another step forward, and that is revelation. When one has come to this degree of revelation, then every thing and being is living; a rock, a tree, is living; the air, the sky, the stars, all are living. One communicates with everything. Nature, characters—one reads their history. Wherever the glance falls—on nature, on characters—one sees the future. That is revelation; that is the magic lantern of Aladdin. Once discovered, it throws its light to the right or to the left, and all things become clear.

DREAMS AND REVELATIONS 2

I will speak about revelation, when awake and when asleep.[1] It wants a certain amount of spiritual progress in order to believe in such a thing, in order to believe that there is such a thing as revelation. Life is revealing, its nature is revealing, and so is God. Therefore, in the Persian language God is called *Khuda*, which means "self-revealing." All science and art and culture known to humanity has originally come by revelation, and even today every invention, every improvement in science or art comes by revelation. Human beings do not only learn art or science by study; there is much that they learn by revelation. A scientist, an artist who may only learn by study, is not a true scientist or artist but only a machine. No doubt modern life seems to have covered that revelation side of culture by pushing forward mechanical culture.

Now, putting this in plainer words, I should like to say that one does not only learn by one's own study, but one also draws, so to speak, knowledge from the multitude. In other words, I may say that a child does not only inherit its father's or its ancestors' qualities, but also the qualities of its nation. If this is true, then it can be also true that one inherits the qualities of one's race, and also that one inherits the qualities of the whole human race. Therefore, if one realized profoundly that storehouse of knowledge that exists behind this veil, one will find that one has a right to this heritage. And this gives one a key, a

1 Lecture, Brussels, May 24, 1924.

283

key to understand the secret of life: that knowledge is not only gained from outside, but also from within. Therefore, knowledge that one learns from outside life, one calls that learning; but the knowledge that one draws from within, that knowledge is called revelation.

There are different degrees of revelation. In the first place one sees, to a small or greater extent in every person, a capacity for impression. Every person more or less feels, in the presence of a new person who is met, whether to trust that person or not to trust that person. If you ask this person: "What makes you think like this?" This person does not always have a reason to tell you, but can only tell you: "I feel that way." Women sometimes are more impressionable than men, for the reason is that woman by nature is responsive. But then among two men, the more responsive man is the more impressionable. But besides the impression of a person, there are some who easily get an impression of a place. Any place they walk or they sit, they feel whether there is something agreeable or disagreeable, if something sad or something joyful has happened there. There are some who are so very impressionable that they can see not only the condition of a few years back but even of many years back. And very often in the East they take a person, an impressionable person, to find out where they can easily get water, and that person begins to feel where the water is closest. And after digging in that place, they find out that it was true. This I am not telling as a great spiritual power, but as an ordinary simple thing of everyday life. Because impression only depends upon that responsive attitude, and one gets an impression from everything that one responds to.

And now going a little further, one finds another aspect of revelation that may be called intuition. Before beginning to start a business or a certain affair, one feels a kind of feeling. One may go against it. One may not believe in it. But one feels a feeling that, "I may not have a success in this"; or when joining forces with another person in business, one might feel that it may not endure long. Also, sometimes a person feels that, "I might see a friend, a particular friend," and then sees that same friend has come without any arrangement between them. It is intuition. There are many intuitive people but they do not know it, because intuition is the portion of a person with gentle feelings. As one goes a little further into the subject one finds that there is another aspect of it, and that aspect is vision. A vision is more clear in the sleeping state than in wakeful state. The reason is that when one is asleep, one lives in the world of one's own, but when awake one is partly in that world but mostly in the outer world. Every phenomenon wants accommodation. It is not only the sound that is audible, but it is also the ears that make it possible to hear the sound. The mind, therefore, is the accommodation to receive the impression, just like the ears are the accommodations to receive the sound.

Therefore, a natural state of sleep is like a profound concentration, like a deep meditation. And therefore, what comes like a dream has a significance to it. But one might ask: "Are all dreams significant of something?" Yes, I should say, everything in the world has significance. Why must a dream not have significance? There is nothing without meaning; it is our lack of understanding its meaning that keeps us in a darkness. But, one might ask: "There are sometimes quite meaningless dreams one has—what about that?" It is the condition of mind. If the condition of mind is not harmonious, if the rhythm of mind is not regular, then the real thing is so mixed up that you yourself cannot read it. It is just like a letter written in darkness that a person did not see while writing. But at the same time, it is a written letter, it has an idea behind it. Even if the very person who has written it in a dark room may not be able to read it, yet it is a letter. When one cannot understand the meaning of one's dream, it is not that the dream has no significance. It only means that the letter has become so mixed up that one cannot read one's own letter. But the most interesting thing to study in the dream is its symbolical expression. The more subtle the mentality of the person is, the more symbolical will be that person's dreams. The dreams of the poets, the dreams of the prophets, have been so significant that they are just like a beautifully written novel.

Sometimes the symbology is so subtle that it seems an art in itself, nature's art that produces such a dream. No doubt, if a simple person has a silly dream, it is not a thing to be surprised at. But, going further, one reads from the dream something of the past, something of the present, something of the future. And one might ask when does the past end and the future begin? And the answer is: when one's mind is focused on the past one sees the past; if upon the future, one sees the future; if one's mind is concerned with the present, one sees the present. But a still greater phenomenon of the dream is that sometimes a dream proves to be a medium of communication between two souls. And this communication is not limited only to this world, but this communication extends even to the next world.

Then there is another side of revelation which is expressed by a poet, a musician, and a philosopher, a thinker. And this is called inspiration. A person may try to write a piece of music, perhaps for a whole year, and may not succeed in creating it. And there might come in one moment a whole symphony that the writer has no power to alter; it is perfect in itself. By altering it the writer would be committing a fault to the harmony of the inner life, because it is given as something already made. No real poets, no real composers, no true thinkers will deny for one moment that it is not their own experience. It seems that these things they cannot create from their brains; there is a factory already creating these things. By their communication with this factory, they get things ready-made. Once I asked a poet who had shown me a most beautiful poem he had written: "Will you kindly explain to me the meaning of a certain line in that poem?" The radiance of the poet's face became pale because he had not thought about it, but after seeing this line, he found he did not know himself the meaning. I said: "You need not trouble about it." It is that which is called inspiration, and it is this phenomenon that makes the creative soul, like that of a poet, a prophet, or a composer, to bow the head to something higher, to something beyond comprehension. To the extent that a poet, an artist, or a thinker has not come to this stage, when one's own creation surprises one so much that one no longer can own one's creation, to that extent one has not really been a real genius. Besides, inspiration does not want pleading. A diamond does not want bugles and trumpets to call it a diamond; its light calls it a diamond. And so is true inspiration. The great composers, the poets who have written real inspirational things—of them the world will never be tired. After millions of years, what they have written will still be alive, it will still make the same impression upon the world.

And when we go further than this, we find that the highest aspect of revelation, which alone can be called a revelation, is that which comes from within. It makes the heart self-revealing. It is just like a new birth of the soul. It is just like the waking of the heart. And when such a thing has begun, one begins to feel a communication with all things and all beings. Every person one meets, before one has spoken a word with that person, one begins to communicate with that person's soul. Before one has asked anyone a question, the soul begins to speak its own history. Every person stands before one as an open letter, and every object is like an open book. Then that continual "why?" that you see in different people no longer exists. "Why?" no longer is there because one finds the answer to every question in oneself; and as long as that answer is not created, with all the learning that exists in the world and has been taught to humanity, that continual "why?" will exist.

Now, the question is how one arrives at this revelation. And the answer is that there is nothing in the whole universe which is not to be found in us if we only care to find it out. But if we will not find out, no one will give it to us. For truth is not learned. The truth is discovered. It is with this belief that the sages of the East went into solitude and sat with their meditations in order to give that revelation an opportunity to come up, to arise. Of course, as life is in the present day, there is hardly time for a person today to give to such solitudes. But that does not mean that we must keep ignorant of the best that is in ourselves. For when we compare all other treasures of the earth with this great bliss which may be called revelation, they cannot be compared. Therefore everything that occupies humanity in earning the things of the world cannot be so important so as to sacrifice that privilege of having revelation.

Considering this, the Sufi Movement gives a facility to those who wish to take the path of meditation. There is no pretense on the part of this movement to teach anyone. For God alone is the teacher, and God alone can teach, and it is by the grace of God that revelation comes and not by the teaching of human beings. The service that people can give to their fellow human beings is in helping them to prepare for that bliss which can only come by the grace of God.

INSIGHT 1

Insight is likened to a telescope.[1] From a distance you can get a wide horizon before you, and when you are close to things you get a limited horizon. By getting a smaller scope of horizon things are clearer because you see things in detail; and when there is a larger horizon then things are not seen in detail, but then there is a general outlook. And the same law must be considered with insight. When you look at a person you get a glimpse of the person's character, and when you look at an assembly you get a feeling of the assembly. And as both long sight and short sight can be developed in a person, so there are persons who have one of these two qualities. There is one who sees deeply into the character of a human being, and another who gets a general feeling. And those who can get a general feeling, they have only to visit a country, a city, a place, and the vibrations of the whole city can be felt by them. But a balance can be achieved by developing these two views: the closer examination of persons and objects, and a general idea of things.

The heart is the telescope of the soul, and the eyes are the telescope of the heart. Just like when seeing through the spectacles it is the eyes which see, not spectacles, so when seeing through the heart and through the eyes, what sees is the soul. The eyes have no power to see; the eyes have the power to help the soul to see. The moment the soul departs, the eyes do not see. And so even the heart is a telescope which helps one to

1 Lecture, Sufi Center, San Francisco, February 23, 1926.

289

perceive, to conceive all that one seeks. But at the same time the heart does not see; it is the soul that sees.

The faculty of seeing needs direction. For instance, in order to look at the right side or left side or before or behind, you need to direct the eyes. And this directing is the work of the will. In the twenty-four hours of day and night, it is perhaps five or fifteen minutes at the most that we see under the direction of the will. All the other times we see automatically. In other words, our eyes are open, our heart is subject to all that can be seen, and we unknowingly catch the different things that attract our eyes and mind. All we see during day and night is not all we intended to see, for we are compelled by the life around us to see. This is, therefore, why the thinkers and sages of the East in ancient times used to have mantles put over their heads. And they did not see anything or anybody in order to control the sight. The Sufis of ancient times used to keep their heads covered for many, many years. And in doing so they developed such powers that their one glance would penetrate rocks and mountains. This is only the control of the sight. Yogis in all ages have worked not only with their mind but even with their eyes to attain to a stability of glance, so that they could direct their sight to anything they wished to examine, they wished to penetrate. Eyes, therefore, are the representatives of the soul at the surface; and they speak to a person more than words can speak, and they are signs one can read as to what plane of evolution the person is. A person does not need to speak with you. A person's eyes tell you whether that person is pleased or not, willing or unwilling, whether favorably inclined or unfavorably inclined. Love or hate, pride or modesty, all can be seen in the eyes, even so much that wisdom and ignorance—anything— manifests through the eyes. The one who can trace the condition and character in the eyes certainly communicates with the soul of another person.

Not very long ago in Hyderabad there was a murid, a rather intellectual pupil. And he liked to talk, and the teacher was interested in his intelligent inquiries. And so the teacher helped him to talk, whereas it is the custom in the East that the pupil holds one's tongue before one's teacher. One day the teacher was in a condition of exaltation, and this pupil, as usual, wanted to discuss and argue, which was not agreeable to the teacher at that time. He said in the Persian language, "*Khamush*," which means "silence." And the pupil became silent. And he went home from there and was silent, and week after week was silent. And no one heard him speak after that, no one in the house, or outside—nowhere did he ever speak. Years passed by, and the man still kept silent. But there came a time when his silence began to speak aloud. His silent thought would manifest, and his silent wish would become granted; his silent glance would heal, his silent look would inspire. His silence became living. It was the spoken words which kept him dead all that time. The moment the lips were closed, the silence in him began to live; his presence was living. In Hyderabad people called him Sheikh Khamush, the king of silence, or the silent king.

By this I wish to say that everyone has eyes, but to make the eyes living, it takes a long time. For eyes see so far and no further. It is the heart connected with the eyes that can see further still. If the soul sees through them, it sees still further. But now how to get them focused?

And now, coming to an entirely different question. If you wish to look at the moon you must look at the sky instead of looking on the earth. And if one wants to look at heaven, one must change the direction of looking. That is where many make a mistake. And today in the United States, where a very large number of students are seriously engaged in finding the truth, many among them are mistaken in this particular thing: that in order to see what can be seen within, they want to look without. And that is a natural tendency. When one looks without for anything one wants, one naturally looks for inner attainment also on the outside. And one will say, "How can we look within, and what shall we see?" In the first place, to a material person, *within* means in the body, inside the body. In reality, *within* means not only inside but also outside the body, both. This can be seen by the light inside a lamp. The light is inside the globe, and it is outside the globe too. So is the soul: it is inside and outside too. So is the mind: it is inside and outside too. It is not restricted inside the body. In other words, the heart is larger than the body, and the soul is larger still. Still the soul is accommodated within the heart, and the heart is accommodated within the body. That is the greatest phenomenon, which it is very difficult to explain in words.

There are intuitive centers, and in order to see into the intuitive centers one has to turn the eyes back, to turn the eyes within. Then the same eyes which are able to see without, they are able to see within. But that is only one phase of seeing. The other phase of seeing within the eyes cannot see; it is the heart that sees. And when you are able to see that way, the pain and pleasure and joy and sorrow of every person that comes before you manifests in your own heart. You actually see it. You see it even more clearly than your own eyes can see. But that is the language of the heart. The eyes do not know it.

Besides, when once the heart begins to live, another world is open for experience. For generally what one experiences in one's everyday life is all that the senses can perceive but not beyond it. But when once a person begins to feel and experience subtle feelings of the heart, one lives in another world, walking on the same earth and living under the same sun. Therefore, be not surprised if you find any beings walking on this earth, living in another world. It is as natural as anything can be for one to live in one's heart instead of only living on the earth. The people in the East call it *saheb-i-dil*, that is, "master mind."

And then if one goes still more within, one begins to live in the soul. Inspiration, intuition, vision, revelation are natural to this person. The soul begins to become conscious of its own domain. And it is the same kingdom of which is spoken in the

Bible, "Seek ye the kingdom of God first."[2] It is the soul which begins to see. Seeking further, what enables one to attain to this stage is the way of meditation under the guidance of the right teacher.

The first thing to do is to get control of the glance. The next thing to do is to get control of the feelings. And the third thing to do is to get control of the consciousness. If these three things are attained, then one begins to look within. Looking within helps very much for a person in looking without, in that the same power with which the heart and eyes are charged begins to manifest outward. And the one who looks within, when that one looks without, all that is within manifests without. The influence of such a one is healing and consoling, uplifting and soothing. Besides, the sight becomes penetrative, so that not only human beings but even objects begin to disclose to this person their nature, character, and secret. As Sa'di says, "Each leaf of the tree becomes a page of the sacred book the moment your vision is clear and your eyes can read."

* * *

Question: *What is psychism?*

Answer: These are new terms: *psychism*. And therefore in making use of this term, myself I do not know. Very often people claim that being clairvoyant, seeing spirits, is psychism. If I were to give my explanation I would say that [psyche] is the soul bound to the earth, longing to free itself. Psychism therefore, if I were to give an explanation of it, would be the process by which a soul can unfold itself, that its wings may no longer be bound but become free to fly upward.

Question: *Why is it that psychic people are mostly negative people?*

Answer: The idea is this, that generally a person is coarse and dense on this earth. That is the general type. And in that coarseness and denseness there is no inclination for spiritual

2 Matthew 6:33.

attainment. If a person is not coarse and dense, then perhaps that person is only ignorant of the other path. That person is capable of something, but has not yet taken a step in that path. Then there remain some who are not coarse and dense but who are fine, fine by nature, nervous temperaments, keenly intelligent. Well, such persons are called negative, especially when they become gentle. Either they are self-assertive, powerful, or they are gentle. But if only one understands what power there is behind gentleness and what mastery in fineness. It is the sharpness that makes the soul a sword. The power of the sword is that it is fine and that it is sharp.

Question: *When the eyes are not in good working order, does that hinder the development of the soul? Have any Sufi practices a connection with the cure of the eyes?*

Answer: It deprives the soul of free expression. Just like the body is a vehicle for the soul to experience life, so the eyes are the vehicle to direct itself. Suppose if the pen of the writer is blunt, it is not the writer's fault; it does not make the qualification of the writer any less if the pen is blunt. Especially, for the development of spiritual attainment, the practices which are given have no connection with the cure of the eyes. That is another department.

Question: *Is your object to make all those who come to you your pupils, and to gather them in your movement?*

Answer: When I look at the world with the idea I have these goods to sell, I see that everyone in the world is my customer. There is not one person who is not. That is the first thing. The second is this: the psychology of different persons. There comes a person who says, "Well, that is something very beautiful which concerns the deeper side of life. I would like to be benefited by it. But I do not wish in any way to be affiliated with you or with the organization. I am against societies and organizations." The most wonderful thing is that this person could be against something that I, with my spiritual attainment, would not be promoting if a society was such a bad thing. I would be the first to run away from it. Besides that, it is a little vanity for people to think that, "I am free." They do not know the sense of freedom. If they knew what freedom is! The very fact that you cannot attach yourself is a lack of freedom.

I will tell you my story. I was invited to speak at a church. When I went in that church the priest of that church thought it the best occasion to advertise his church; he thought it was a better advertisement than anything else. Because he thought, "I can say my word in the conversion." So he said, "Will you be anointed?" I asked, "What is it?" He said, "To put on some oil." I said, "Put some oil or water or anything." So oil was put on my head, and I was confirmed in that particular religion. This man was pleased because he gained his object, and I thought, "I have not joined a new church, I am a member of all churches." Can anyone change us if we do not change? What can join us if we do not want to join? We are at the same time joined with heaven and hell both, with the worst and the most virtuous person. We are linked with one another. If the races and lands are different, what does it matter? In spirit, in consciousness, we are all one. We cannot be different. Those who say, "I do not want to join, but I want to get all the benefit," it is [just] unfriendliness. We cannot help them. They are not ready to be helped. Besides, if they do not want to join, what do I care if they joined a society or class? I come to gather people, not for the sake of society but for humanity. If I gather them in a society or movement, it is that it may spread throughout the whole world. For the same reason the ship exists, and the post office and the telegraph and the radio. All these things help. It is all organization. And the East has understood and it will understand more and more the benefit of it, the benefit of broadcasting the teaching. That is the idea of a society. We who are working to try to make the different creeds meet, we do not want to form another creed to add to the many. That would be lost work if we did worthless things, or we meant or thought to do business or money-making, but did not do the higher things. And not doing the higher things is the worst thing possible.

Besides, there are murids who come to a teacher and then think, "It is very interesting, but shall I or shall I not join?" And then some have said, "Yes, I am very interested in your lectures and I have read your books, but I am not yet sure. I want to read more of it in order to become your pupil." That surprises me more than anything else. That a dead book will convince them more than my living self, than my presence. The dead book will one day convince them, but not before I am gone to another country. Besides that, the one who does not trust in the living person but in the book, this person is not yet deep enough. I think—spiritual teaching apart—even in friendship, if there is anything that binds two persons it is trust. In order to trust you do not need to be acquainted for six months. Then you can wait for the whole life. Real friends are friends in one moment's time. That is the way friendship is. Spiritual guidance is a friendship too, however, it is a spiritual teaching journey. Once my murshid told me, "There are many things that cause friendship between different persons. But the friendship in the spiritual path is the greatest friendship. It cannot be compared with anything else. It is above all things of the earth, and it will always last." If one does not take it in this way, then a spiritual teacher is like a professor in the university who is there for a certain time. There is not that sacred, deep feeling. For a deeper character and nature, there is a deeper friendship connection. Therefore, in the East they look at it from a different point of view.

There is a story of a pupil in the East who was a villager and who was very interested in spiritual things. He was the pupil of a teacher. One day another teacher came into that village, and it was made known to the villagers that, "Those who come to hear this teacher, they will have the doors of heaven open for them." This wonderful young man did not come. All the others came to see this new teacher. This teacher was wondering why this young man did not come. He said, "I would like to see him." And he says to this young man, "You are very interested in this idea, and you did not come to see me." He said, "Teacher, forgive me. It is not antagonism toward your teaching. Only that my teacher has passed away from this earth. I do not know yet if he is in heaven or in hell. If by your kindness I went to heaven, and if I did not find my teacher, heaven would be hell for me. Whatever that place would be, it would become my hell." If there were not that confidence and faith, then a person may read many books and discuss them for a whole life till becoming deaf and dumb, and not arrive at that stage. It is easy and yet so difficult.

INSIGHT 2

As there are some who have short sight and others who have long sight, so there are some who see things at a far distance with the eye of their mind but who cannot see what is near them.[1] They have the long sight. And then there are others who have the short sight; they see all that is near them, but they cannot see further. As they say, there is a third eye that sees. It is true, but sometimes that third eye sees through these two eyes, and, therefore, the same eyes see things more clearly than they would see otherwise. With the help of the third eye, our eyes can penetrate through the wall of physical existence and see into the minds of people, into the words of people, and even further. When one begins to see, the first thing is that everything one's eyes see has a deeper meaning, a greater significance than one knew before. Every movement of the person, every gesture of the person, the form, the feature, the voice, the word, the expression, the atmosphere, it all becomes a narrative of the person's nature and character. Not knowing this secret, many want to study what they call physiognomy or phrenology or handwriting or palmistry. But in comparison to the clear vision, all these different sciences are limited. They have a certain meaning, but at the same time, when you compare these limited sciences with the insight that a human being has, they prove to be too small. Besides, character reading is not learned,

1 Lecture, Sufi Center, Steinway Hall, New York City, May 26, 1926.

it is discovered. It is a sense that wakens. You do not need to learn it, you know it.

That is one kind of insight. Then there is another insight which is in affairs. Be it a business affair, a professional affair, a condition, a situation in life, once the insight is clear one has the grasp of the situation. Because what makes things difficult in life is lack of knowledge of things. There may be a small problem, but when you do not know, it becomes the heaviest and worst problem. It is because one cannot understand it that it makes it worse. And you may analyze a problem and reason it out, but without insight it will always be puzzling. It is the development of insight that gives you a clear vision in affairs, conditions, and in the problems of life. There is impression, there is intuition, there is inspiration, there is dream, and there is revelation. In these different aspects insight shows itself.

What do I mean by impression? When one gets an impression of a person, one need not wait and see how the person comes out. One knows it instantly. And very often many have a feeling at the first sight of a person, whether a person will be their friend or be unfriendly. When someone comes and tells me, "I am very interested in your philosophy, but before I take it up, I want to study it," I tell you that person may study it for a thousand years, and will go on studying it and not get to that insight. It is the first moment—either you are my friend or not my friend. For friends it does not take many years to develop friendship. When two persons meet, a confidence is established; you do not need years in order to become a friend. It is foolish. Besides that, one gets an impression if one makes a person one's business partner or professional colleague. If, in that impression, one feels that it will not go right and one does not listen, in the end it is a failure. And if one listened to impressions first, one would be really safe.

Intuition is deeper still, because by intuition you get a warning. Intuitively you feel this person will one day deceive me, or turn against me, or else prove faithful to me, is sincere, someone to rely upon. Or in this particular business I will have success or failure. One knows it. But the difficulty is in distinguishing the right intuition. That is the great question. Because as soon as intuition springs up, reason, its competitor, rises also and says, "No, it is not so." And then there is conflict in the mind, and you cannot distinguish, because there are two feelings at the same time. If a person makes a habit to catch the first intuition and save it from being destroyed by reason, then intuition is stronger and one can benefit by it. There are many intuitive people, but they cannot distinguish between intuition and reason. And sometimes they muddle them, because very often the second thought, being the last thought, is more clear to one's vision than the first. Therefore, the intuition is forgotten and the reason remembered. And then a person calls it intuition, and it is not so.

Besides, those who doubt intuition, their intuition doubts them. In other words, the doubt becomes a wall between themselves and their intuitive faculty. And there is a psychological action: as soon as intuition has sprung up, doubt and reason have sprung up too, so that their vision is blurred.

The intuition of dogs and cats and of horses and cows sometimes seems to be more clear than in a human being. They know if there is going to be an accident, if death is going to occur in the family or disease or a fire in the house or any such thing. They know beforehand and give people warning. But people are so busy in their daily occupations that they do not respond to the intuition of the animals. People believe in the East that small insects know about happenings and give a warning to those who can understand it. And it is true. Besides, birds always give a warning of the storm and wind, and of the rain and of the absence of rain.

Inspiration comes to some few, especially those who are artists, painters, sculptors, singers, poets, musicians, thinkers, writers, inventors. Inspiration is a gift. It is like a room opened before a person in which all beautiful things are to be found.

Everything one wants to have is at hand. And therefore, for a poet or musician to get an inspiration, no striving is necessary. There is no effort needed. One must only feel inclined to it, and then one just reaches it. And you might ask: What is this storehouse where inspiration comes from? It is the divine mind, which has in it all knowledge. One has only to reach it, and the knowledge comes in one's grasp. A person may make an effort toward producing something worthwhile for a long time and not accomplish it, and yet, by the help of inspiration, one can accomplish it at once. One may not be able to finish a poem in six months' time, and yet, in an inspirational mood, it is finished in a moment. And that which is made inspirationally is greater than that made by effort. And all things made in inspiration have made the greatest impression upon people. They are living things, any things produced through inspiration, and they have their charm forever. Inspirational poetry and music—one is never tired of these things.

Now, we come to the aspect of dreams. We have different kinds of dreams. There is one kind which is an automatic action of the mind. Whatever one experiences in the day, the mind goes over the same line at night, and therefore, it is reproduced in the dream. And then there is another kind of dream that is the contrary to what must happen. If one is going to be happy, one sees oneself unhappy; if one is going to be successful, one sees oneself fail. It is contrary to everything that is to happen. It is a kind of upset condition of mind, just like those mirrors where one who is thin looks and sees a stout person, and one who is thick looks and sees a thin person. It is the same thing. Everything looks contrary to what it is.

And the third kind of dream is the symbolical dream, and this is the most interesting dream. The greater the person, the subtler the symbolism of that person's dream. With the grossness of the person, the symbolism is gross. The more evolved the person, the more fine, artistic, and subtle the dream. For instance, to a poet there will be poetic symbols; and the dream

301

of a musician will have musical symbols; in the dream of the artist there will be symbols of art.

And then there is the realistic dream in which one sees actually what is going to happen. That also gives us insight into what we call fate, that all we call accident is only our conception. Because we did not know it before, we call it accident. But there is a plan; it is all planned out and known beforehand to the spirit and those who know it. There are sages who know of their death a year before. So there is no such thing as accident. When a person does not know, it means one does not see. But it is there.

Revelation is still greater. It is the perfection of insight. It is a higher development when one has revelation. It begins when a person feels in tune with everybody, everything, and every condition. But in order to come to that stage one must develop it. The heart must be tuned to that stage, to that pitch, where one feels at-one-ment with persons, objects, and conditions. For instance, when one cannot bear the climate, it only means that one is not in harmony with the climate; when one cannot get on with people, that one is not in harmony with them; and when one cannot get on with affairs, that one is not in harmony with affairs. If the condition is hard, one shows that one is not in harmony with the condition.

Sages in the East used to be called *balakush*, which means one who took the draught of all difficulties. They called life's difficulties a wine to drink; once you drink, it has gone. They were not afraid of it, they did not want to keep out of it. They said, "If we keep out this moment, next moment it will meet us. It will meet us one day. If we escape one moment, it will meet us in the other moment. So let it come such as it is, and let us drink it as a wine." The principle of *mahadevas*, of the dervishes, and of great fakirs, of all sages, is this one principle: to drink all difficulties as a wine. Then there is no more difficulty. When one is in tune with life, then life becomes revealing, because then one is a friend with life. Before that, one was strange with it. Attitude makes such a difference. And it is the difference of attitude that makes a person spiritual or material. Nothing need be changed, only the attitude.

Very often people ask, "What is Sufism? Is it a religion? Is it a philosophy?" I say, "It is not a religion, because it does not have any dogmas. It is not a philosophy because it has no particular theories." They ask, "Then what is it?" I say, "It is an attitude, it is a certain attitude toward life that makes you a Sufi. It is not holding a theory or being subject to a certain dogma." One might ask, "What attitude?" And in answer I will say, "A friendly attitude to friend and foe alike, to things agreeable and disagreeable, to all conditions. When you are rising and when you are falling, when you are successful and when you have failed, in pain and in comfort, to be in tune with it all." The great person is the one who is always inclined to be friendly to all persons and to all conditions that one meets in life. That develops the revelation. Then things and beings in life begin to reveal themselves to a person, and one gets a greater knowledge.

And now, what lesson do we learn from this, to develop insight? The lesson we learn is this: not to become excited by any influence that tries to take us out of tune, but to keep in tune under all conditions of life; to keep one's equilibrium, one's tranquility under all conditions of life. It is sometimes very difficult to keep one's equilibrium when the influences of life are shaking us, and to keep one's poise through it all; it is difficult in the face of opposing influences to keep a friendly attitude. But at the same time, because it is difficult, it is a great attainment. To attain anything valuable and worthwhile one has to go through difficulty. But one does not pay for it. One learns without paying for it. It is something that one can practice in everyday life, because from morning till evening we are continually among jarring effects from all sides. Therefore, there is plenty of opportunity for practicing this lesson of keeping a friendly attitude toward everyone, and meeting courageously every condition, and taking upon oneself all influences that come along. It is in this way that a greater insight into life is attained.

* * *

Question: *When a person is killed by a train, was it that person's destiny to die?*

Answer: Yes.

Question: *When a person is guided by reason in life instead of being guided by intuition, what becomes of intuition?*

Answer: Reason and intuition are two competitors, and yet both have their place, their importance, and their value. And the best thing would be first to try and catch the intuition, and to distinguish and know and recognize it as intuition, and then to reason it out.

Question: *Can one attain unlimited knowledge without a scientific foundation?*

Answer: Scientific knowledge is never a foundation. Scientific knowledge is always an outcome of intuition. It is a seeming foundation, but it is never a foundation. Science has never been learned from science; it has been learned from intuition. On the foundation of science, other science has been formed, but the foundation is intuition. No doubt, what is built today as something higher is built upon science, but the foundation is not science. The foundation is a human faculty.

Question: *How is stability of mind to be attained?*

Answer: By the love of all that is stable. A person without a stable mind is worthless. It does not matter what capacity one has, what quality; the one whom you cannot rely upon, whatever that one be to you—your friend or your companion or your assistant or your servant or your master. In any capacity, one is worthless if one's mind is not stable. Therefore, stability is the sign of the everlasting life shown in the midst of this life of changeability.

Question: *If all is mapped out, how does free will come in?*

Answer: It is always mapped out by the free will.

Question: *Are accidents prepared by unseen teachers or by our own karma?*

Answer: Unseen teachers are not interested in accidents. Why should they be? If you say, "our own karma," yes, but even I would not emphasize that. I would give the words of Christ in answer to this question, that all is done in this way so his actions may be known.[2] In other words, if one says, "Why should there be a drum in the orchestra? Why should there be a flute in the orchestra?" I should say, "In order that the music may be played as the composer wished it to be played." Maybe it is disagreeable from our view, but the composer has written music which requires the drum and the flute. In the same way, all that seems useless was all there for some purpose, all making the divine symphony. We say, "Why is this?" But it is our limited mind which says that. In reality, everything has its place and its purpose. Someone asked in jest to the Prophet "Why were mosquitos created?" And the Prophet said, "That you may not sleep all night but devote some of your night in prayers."

Question: *How to distinguish between automatic and other forms of dreams?*

Answer: By the dreams themselves.

Question: *Is it true that with the evolution of the race, the physical sight will disappear?*

Answer: No, it should not necessarily disappear. On the contrary.

Question: *What about being in tune with bad habits?*

Answer: One could not correct bad habits if one were not in tune with them. The one who speaks to a person who smokes cannot correct the person of that habit. But the one who sits with the person who smokes and tells that person naturally to

2 See John 3:21.

get rid of this habit can correct that person. The woman who says, "My husband drinks, I cannot go near him," will not cure him. But the one who will go in the street and pick him up and not feel ashamed of it, it is she who is in tune with him and will raise him and will cure him and help him toward evolution. It is not by thinking that, "Because it is a bad habit, or the person is bad and wrong, I have nothing to do with such a person." It is by our friendliness, by our sympathy, by our understanding that we get closer with the person.

Question: *Please explain more fully the three methods of concentration.*

Answer: The one method of concentration is to make the mind as a mirror and let the object one sees reflect in it. Another method is like little children do. They take bricks and tiles and make a little house—that is, to take different impressions and build a thought. It is constructive thought. And a third method is to take one thought, one form; and that form is fixed and unchangeable, but the background is improved. This is another kind of concentration.

Question: *How can one develop intuition without reason interfering?*

Answer: As I have already said, one must develop self-confidence and trust in one's intuition. And even if it proved wrong once or twice or thrice, still to continue. In time one will develop trust in one's intuition, and so intuition will be clear.

THE EXPANSION OF CONSCIOUSNESS

My subject this evening is the expansion of consciousness.[1] Consciousness is the intelligence, the intelligence is the soul, the soul is the spirit, and the spirit is God. Therefore, consciousness is the divine element. Consciousness is the God part in us, and it is through consciousness that we become small or great, and through consciousness either we rise or fall, and through consciousness we become narrow or we expand. You have perhaps seen in Greek mystical symbology the two wings of the eagle, two wings always taken as a mystical symbol. That symbol is the symbol of consciousness, and when the wings are open it is the expansion of consciousness. What is called the unfoldment of the soul is the expansion of consciousness. Therefore, anything in the way of religion, occultism, philosophy, mysticism—any path you take—when you wish to go further in the spiritual journey to attain to the spiritual goal, you have to come to the expansion of consciousness.

And now I will come to the word *consciousness*. What is consciousness? When we say a loaded gun, we mean that there is a bullet in it. *Consciousness* means the loaded intelligence, intelligence charged with knowledge, with impression, which is carrying an idea in it. This means consciousness. In other words, we say *moving picture*. But what is it? The screen. But we do not see the screen, we see moving pictures.

---

1 Lecture, Sufi Center, Steinway Hall, New York City, May 29, 1926.

When we say *consciousness*, what is it? It is pure intelligence. Intelligence impregnated with some idea is consciousness because it is conscious of something. And what is intelligence? Intelligence is the soul. There is no other trace of the soul to be found except the intelligence. And very often people, not understanding, say the seat of the soul is in the heart or in the right or left side of a human being. But really speaking, there is something more expressive than any side in the body, and that is intelligence.

Now I will demonstrate the idea of the universal or general consciousness, of consciousness apart from individual consciousness, by telling a little story. There was a magician who imagined that he was fluid—liquid, moving, rising, and falling, and turning into the sea. But then he imagined, "But I am solid." Atoms grouped together, froze, and turned into ice. But then he thought, "I am not so cold. I can try and be stable and will not melt. And he turned into stone. Then he said, "And I want to come out. I do not want to remain stone, I want to come out." And he came out as a tree. "But," he said, "still I am not moving, not working," and he twisted and turned, and turned into an insect. But the magician thought, "How helpless it is to live as an insect. I should like to play and sing." And he turned into a bird. But then he said, "I want to be more gross and dense, and feel myself more intelligible." And he turned into an animal. He said, "I want to stand on my hind legs, to stretch my spine." And he turned into a human being. This is the phenomenon of one magician who wanted, who imagined something, and became it.

And now we shall think of this idea in connection with the scriptures. In the Qur'an it is said, "Be, and it became."[2] It was the magician's work: what he was conscious of, he became. First was consciousness, and the idea it held turned into something.

But now, coming to another question. If the magician was so powerful as to think and turn into something, then why

2 Qur'an 19:37.

did the magician himself become obscured? The idea is this: that when one says, "I would like to rest, to go to sleep," naturally one has lost one's action. Turning into something naturally made that consciousness, which is divine or universal consciousness, limited; and this limitation robbed it of its own consciousness. That is the deepest point of metaphysics. For instance, when the consciousness thought, "I will turn into a rock, I am a rock," it became a rock. The consciousness did not lose its fluid substance, but intelligence no longer knew its own existence. And yet when the magician thought, "I will turn into a rock," what went into the rock? Just one little thought of the magician. But, through that thought, he could not express himself, not feel as he felt in the condition of being a magician. When he turned into a rock, he did not feel through this thought; he felt nothing.

The more we understand this idea, the more we shall see that consciousness is to be seen in two different aspects. In one aspect the consciousness is buried under the dense aspect of creation such as mountains, rocks, trees, plants, earth, and sea. And yet the tendency of consciousness is to come out, even through those dense aspects, to express itself. And we can see that tendency by getting in touch with nature. For instance, those who sit before the rocks in caves in the mountains, in the midst of the forest; and those who get in touch with nature and whose minds are free from the worries and anxieties and troubles of the world, get a sort of peace first. And having experienced peace and rest, the second thing that comes is a kind of communication between themselves and nature. And what does nature express to them? With every action, with the rising and falling of the waves, and with the upward-reaching tendency of the mountains, and with the moving of the graceful branches of the trees, and with the blowing of the wind and the fluttering of leaves, every little move of nature seems to whisper in their ears. That is the consciousness that wants to come out; through trees and rocks, water and plants, it wishes to unfold itself, wants to express itself, because it was not dead but living, buried in the rock, in the tree, in the plant, in water, and in earth and air. That living being tries to make itself audible, intelligible. It wants to communicate, trying for years and years and years to break through this dense imprisonment, to come out to its original source. Just like the magician who wanted to break through, to come out and see himself. And what did he turn into? He turned into a human being.

There is a saying of the Sufis that God slept in the rock, God dreamed in the tree, God became self-conscious in the animal, but God sought for God's own divine self and recognized the divine self in the human.[3] Therefore, that denotes clearly life's main purpose: that whatever be one's occupation, whatever may please one, engage one through life, whatever one may admire, there is only one motive. That one motive is working for one's unfoldment, again to recognize, "What I have made, how great it is and how wonderful, how beautiful it is to recognize it, to see it." It is that inclination which is working through every soul, whether a person wants to become spiritual or not. Yet, unconsciously, every soul is striving toward the unfoldment of the soul.

And now on the topic of human consciousness. Naturally, when consciousness has turned into something, it has limited itself. Although in comparison with trees and plants and rocks and mountains, human consciousness is fully wakened, yet every human being is not wakened but is still in captivity. As Rumi said in the *Masnavi*, humanity is captive in an imprisonment, and humanity's every effort, every desire, is to break through in order to realize inspiration, greatness, beauty, happiness, and peace, independent of all the things of this world. One comes to this sooner or later, but there is a continual yearning; wise and foolish, everyone is striving for it, consciously or unconsciously.

---

3 This saying is often attributed to Jalal ad-Din Rumi.

There are some who are perhaps very interested in themselves, their health or mind or thoughts or feelings or affairs or families. Their consciousness does not go any further than that little horizon. It does not mean that in that way they are not right. They occupy that much space in the sphere of consciousness, as much as they are conscious of. There are others who have forgotten themselves, who say "There is my family, my friends, and I love them," and then their consciousness is larger; or "For my citizens, for my country, for the education of the children of my country, for the good health of the people in my town," their consciousness is larger still. It does not mean that their consciousness is larger, but that they occupy a larger horizon in the sphere of consciousness. And so do not be surprised when a poet like Nizam says, "If the heart is large enough, it can contain the whole universe." That consciousness is such that the universe is too small compared with it; the sphere of that consciousness is the absolute.

There is no piece of consciousness cut out for a human being, but the human being occupies a certain horizon, as far as it can expand. For the whole absolute can be one's consciousness. Therefore, on the outside a person is an individual, but in reality you cannot say what a person is. It is this idea that is hinted at in the Bible when it is said, "Be ye perfect as your father in heaven."[4] What does it mean? That the absolute consciousness is the sign of perfection, and you are not excluded from it. All move and live in it. But we occupy only as much horizon as is within our consciousness, or as much as we are conscious of. This shows to us that each individual has its own world, and the world of one individual is as tiny as a lentil, and of another is larger than the whole world. And yet on the outside all human beings are more or less equal in size, one somewhat taller than the other; in size every person is about the same. But in one's own world there is no comparison of how different one

4 Matthew 5:48.

311

can be from another. There can be as many varieties of worlds in human beings as there are of creatures from ant to elephant.

And now, coming to the question of what has been called in scriptures heaven and hell. What is it? It is our world, our consciousness, that in which we live day after day, and year after year, and what continues in another world is heaven or the other place. Whatever we have made of it, it is this we are experiencing today. And what is said by the prophets, that after death we will be brought to something, only means that in all this earthly plane we are so little conscious of our world, so absorbed in the outer world, that we do not know what world we have created within ourselves. We are occupied and absorbed so much in the outer world, in our desires, ambitions, and strivings, that we hardly know our own world. One who works in the factory is tired at night, comes home and reads the newspaper. The same is true with everyone. So much of the outside world attracts us all day long: everything outside, thousands of advertisements, shops sparkling with electricity.

And there will come a time when one's eyes will be closed to the outside world that occupies all one's mind, and one will become conscious of the world created within. That is what is said in the scriptures: one will find what one has made. One need not say, "What will become of me tomorrow?" If one can direct one's mind into oneself, one can see what is within the consciousness, what it is composed of, what it contains. Then one will know the hereafter today.

Sufis have in all ages tried their best to train their consciousness. How did they train it? The first training is analysis, and the second training is synthesis. The analytical striving is to analyze and examine one's own consciousness—in other words, one's own conscience. To ask one's conscience, addressing it, "My friend, all my happiness depends on you and my unhappiness also. If you are pleased, I am happy. Now, to tell you truly, what I like and what not, is what is in consonance with your approval." One should speak to one's conscience, as a person goes to the priest to make confession, "Look here, what I have done or said, maybe it is wrong, maybe it is right, but you know it. You have your share of it, and the influence of it, and your condition is my condition, your realization is my realization. If you are happy, I alone can be happy. Now I want to make you happy. How can I make you happy?" At once a voice of guidance will come from the conscience, "You should do this and not that, and say this and not that. In this way you should act and not in that way." And the conscience can give you better guidance than any teacher or book. It is a living teacher awakened in oneself, one's own conscience. The teachers, the gurus, the murshids, their way is to awaken the conscience in the pupil, to awaken it by making clear that which has become unclear or confused. And sometimes they adopt such a wonderful way, such a gentle way, that even the pupil does not know it.

There is an amusing story of a teacher. A man went to a teacher and said, "Will you take me as your disciple?" The teacher first looked at him and then said, "Yes, with great pleasure." But the man said, "Think about it before you tell me yes. First thing, I am a difficult subject. There are many bad things in me." The teacher said, "What are these bad things?" The man said, "I like to drink." The teacher said, "That does not matter." "But," the man said, "I like to gamble." The teacher said, "That does not matter." "But," he said, "There are many other things, there are numberless things." The teacher said, "That does not matter." The man was very glad. "But," the teacher said, "Now that I have agreed with all the bad things you have said about yourself, you must agree to one condition." The disciple said, "Yes." The teacher said, "Do not do any of these things which you consider wrong in my presence." The pupil said, "That is easy," and went away. And as the days passed and months passed, this pupil, who was very deep and developed and keen, came back beaming, his soul unfolding every moment of the day and happy to thank the teacher. The teacher said, "Well, how have you been?" "Very well, thank you," he said. The teacher said, "Have you done your practices which I gave you?" "Yes," he said, "very faithfully," "But what about the habits you had of going to different places?" the teacher asked. "Well," he said, "I very often tried to go to drink, gamble, but wherever I went I saw you; you did not leave me alone. Whenever I wanted to drink, I saw your face before me. I cannot do it." That is the gentle way that teachers handle their disciples. They do not say, "You must not drink, you must not gamble." They never do. The wonderful way of the teacher is to teach without words, to correct a person without saying. What the teacher wants to say, the teacher says without saying. When we put something in words, it is lost. You can teach and correct and help as much as you can without words. That is fine. That helps much more.

Now, coming to the most important subject of the expansion of consciousness, there are two directions in which to expand. In other words, there are two dimensions in which to expand. The one is outward, the other is the inner dimension. The outer dimension is pictured as horizontal, the inner as a perpendicular line. These two dimensions are pictured as a cross, the symbol of the Christian religion. But before the Christian religion existed, in Egypt and Tibet, in different forms it existed, and in the ancient pictures of Buddhist and Tibetan symbols you will find the symbol of the cross.

One direction is inner, and the other direction is without. And what is represented by the horizontal line is without, what is represented by the perpendicular line is within. The way of expanding within is to close your eyes and mind from the outer world and, instead of reaching out, one should reach within. The action of the soul is to reach out and upward and straightforward, or sideways or backward or in an ellipse. It is like the sun: its light reaches out, it sends currents out, and so the soul sends currents out through the five senses. But when the five senses are controlled, when the breath is thrown within, the ears do not hear any more and the mouth does not speak. Then the five senses are directed within. And when once these senses are

314

closed by the help of meditation, then the soul, which has been accustomed to reach outward, begins to reach within. And in the same way, as one gets experience and power from the outer world, so one gets experience and power from the inner world. And so it can reach further and further and further within, until it has reached its original source, and that is the spirit of God.

That is one way, the way of reaching within. And then there is the way of reaching without, and that is expanding which comes by changing one's outlook. Because we are narrow, by the narrowness of our outlook we think, "I am different, she is different." We are making barriers out of our own conceptions. If we lived and communicated with the souls of all people, of all beings, our outer horizon would naturally expand so much that we would occupy the sphere unseen. It is in this way that spiritual perfection is attained. Spiritual perfection, in other words, is the expansion of consciousness.

* * *

Question: *Is it helpful to close the eyes when meditating? What is the best method?*

Answer: Meditation is prescribed individually. A method for one may not be good for another. But at the same time, there is a Japanese symbol, a kind of toy of these three monkeys, one holding his nose, the other his ears, and the other his mouth. This is the keynote to meditation; this is the key to the expansion of consciousness, this is the key to inner expansion. But in everyday life we can see that ethically, from a moral point of view, and that is to hear no evil, see no evil, and say no evil. And if we can take that oath, it can do a great deal and can take one very far on the way, if these three things are practiced in everyday life: never speak against anyone, never [hear] about anyone or against anyone, and never see any evil. If we close our eyes without closing our ears and without closing our lips, we cannot accomplish anything.

Question: *How can one recognize the state of cosmic conscious-ness? What is the nature of that state?*

Answer: It is a state which cannot be explained in words very well. And if I tried, I will only say that when we see, we do not hear, and when we hear fully, we do not see. In this way, every sense is doing its work fully when only that sense is doing work. When we are seeing something, if somebody is speaking to us, we do not see fully. I have seen a child most interested in music who closed his eyes; then alone can the hearing enjoy it fully. But to hear music while drinking lemonade and eating ice cream or anything is something different. But the condition of meditation is different from what I have said. It is not limited to a rule. When meditating, at that time every sense is evenly balanced. Therefore, meditation [is apart] from the human life that is outside, uneven, unbalanced. But in meditation every sense is wakened and yet every sense is asleep. To be closed from outside and yet to be wakened evenly, that experience is something which cannot be said in words; it must be experienced.

Question: *Are not persons more often interested in removing limitations?*

Answer: We live in world of limitation and sometimes have need of limited help. And we are helplessly limited because the first thing is that for our sustenance we need food, which is outside of ourselves. For our living we need something which is not within us. That makes us dependent. And today, under different circumstances, other things become necessary. We use electricity and X-rays for the benefit of our maintenance—it is just as well to make use of anything that is there. But as much as one can be independent of outside things, one must try and do it. Life in India teaches this, life as it has been for thousands of years. How more evolved they are in science, in mysticism, in philosophy. The Hindus had one motive especially, and that was to be as independent as possible of all things outside. You will see evolved Hindus, great thinkers, drinking water from their hands like this. It does not mean they do not know about the cup. No. They drink like this for two reasons: the cup may have been used by fifty persons; their hands are their own, with their own magnetism, no other person's magnetism has gone into it. They do not know of plates and saucers. They eat on leaves from the banana tree. It makes life so simple. At the same time, once they have eaten on the leaf of the banana tree, it is thrown away, and is not like a plate washed with other dishes and wiped with the same towel. Perhaps it looks very uncivilized when one eats with one's hands, but it is much purer. One's hands are only used by oneself.

We have forgotten simple life today. And home life, we do not know it. The pleasure and comfort and happiness of home, they are forgotten. What we know today is life in the world. Home was something apart, something sacred, something like a temple, a sanctuary where one keeps one's own atmosphere. Today, when we eat in a restaurant there is no consideration for sacredness and no thought as to the purity of the food. Therefore, anything regarding eating or dress or the home that we can get on without is just as well, for without those things we become less dependent. Today we are very dependent on things, and unthinkingly so. We have so many things in the house that the house would be much cleaner and clearer without. The more things we have in the house, the better it looks. But the more there is in the house, the worse it is. We bring so much care and worry and so much more anxiety into a house which is growing and growing for the sake of conventionality, till life becomes so difficult because there is so much money needed to live. Otherwise with so little one could be contented. One does not need to have much money in the bank, and perhaps without it one is happier than with it. But life today is difficult. One cannot move without money. And one cannot be happy because there is never enough. One has to decorate the house, one has to have so many dishes for dinner, all clothing

317

should be according to this and that fashion, that life becomes heavy for everybody, married and unmarried. What we should do, before striving for spirituality, is to change our outlook in life, to know that to become dependent on outside things is to lessen power, mastery, honor, and greatness. It does not matter if we are in a lesser position compared with others. If we are contented, we are just as happy and even more so than others.

Question: *Does the development of the inner consciousness tend to personal isolation that diverges from the world?*

Answer: We are in the world, and therefore, however much we may try to run away to spiritual spheres, it does not go easily, for again we are thrown on the earth. We are bound here as long as we have this earthly body. And so the best way is to do the process in another way, to have inner expansion of consciousness. And in doing so, no doubt one must go within and close oneself to the outer world, but at the same time one must strive to practice the outer expansion of consciousness. And in this way there is balance. And those who do not keep this balance only evolve spiritually, become one-sided: they expand inner consciousness and but do not expand outwardly. Then they become unbalanced. Maybe spiritually they have extraordinary powers, but they do not have balance. For this reason many people think of a spiritual person as somebody who has something wrong with the brain. If that is the condition of the world, we should be most conscientious in order not to give the world a wrong impression. If we have a profession, if we are in business, in industry, we should do it fully, proving to the world to be as practical as everybody else, most economical, regular in every way, systematic, persevering, enthusiastic. All these qualities we must show and at the same time evolve spiritually. But that must give the proof.

THE MIND WORLD

The contents of "The Mind World" were compiled from lectures given by Inayat Khan during the Summer School in Suresnes from June 18 to September 8, 1924.

THE MIND WORLD 1

Mind world, in the terms of the Sufi poets, is called *a'ina khana*, which means "the palace of mirrors." One knows very little of the phenomena that this palace of mirrors has in it. Not only among human beings, but also in the lower creation, one finds the phenomenon of reflection. In the first place, one wonders how the small germs and worms, little insects who live on other small lives, reach out to their food, attract their food. In fact, their mind becomes reflected upon the little lives, which then become their food. The scientist says that animals have no mind. Yes, it is true to a certain point. They have no mind—what the scientist calls mind according to scientific terminology. But according to the mystic the same intelligence as in humankind, to a smaller degree, is to be found in the lower creation. They have a mind, but it's not as clear; and therefore, comparatively, one might say it is like having no mind. But at the same time for the mystic—who calls the mind a mirror—the mind, even in the lower creation, is also a mirror. It may not be so clear, yet it is a mirror.

Friendship, hostility, the fights which take place among birds and animals, their becoming mates—all this takes place not as thought or imagination, but as a reflection from mirror to mirror. What does it show? It shows that the language of the lower creation is more natural than the language humans have made and gone far from that natural, intuitive way of expression.

You may ask any horse rider about the joy of horse riding, which the rider considers greater and better than any other form of enjoyment in sport. The rider may not be able to give the reason for it, but the reason is the phenomenon of reflection. When the reflection of the rider's thought has fallen upon the mind of the horse, then two minds have become face-to-face, and the horse knows where the rider wishes to go. And the more there is sympathy between the rider and the horse, the greater joy one experiences in riding. After having ridden upon a horse, instead of feeling tired, one feels exalted. The joy is greater than the tiredness, and the more communication there is between the mind of the horse and the rider, the greater the joy the rider derives from it and so does the horse. In time the horse begins to feel a sympathy with its rider.

There is a story of an Arab, a rider who fell on the battlefield, and there was no one near to take care of his dead body. And the horse stood there three days without having eaten anything, in the hot sun, till people came and found the dead body. It was guarding its master's body against vultures. I know of a dog that cried three days after the death of its mate and died at the end of the third day. That is the reflection by which they communicate with one another.

Often one sees in the circus horses and other animals working wonderfully according to the instruction given to them. Is it their mind? Have they learned it? No, they have not learned it. It is not in their minds. It comes at that instant when the trainer stands with the whip. Where does it come from? From their mind; it is mirrored upon their mind. If they were left alone they would not work, they would not think about it. Elephants in Burma work in the forests, bringing the logs of wood. But the one who trains them—it is the trainer's thought mirrored upon them that makes them do the work. When one studies it minutely one finds that it is not a training, it is a reflection. Always, the animals are doing what the humans are thinking in their mind. They, so to speak, become the hands and legs of their master. Two beings become one in one thought. As in the Persian verse, that when two hearts become one they can remove mountains, there can be a relation established between a human being and an animal when they can become one. But it is difficult to establish that oneness among human beings.

The story of Daniel, who entered in the cave of the lions and the lions were tamed instantly—did he will them to do so? No. Did he teach them to be calm and quiet? No. It was the calm and peace of the heart of Daniel reflected upon the lions that made them quiet like him. His own peace became their peace. They became peaceful. One might ask: "After Daniel left the cave of lions, did they remain the same?" I have doubts about it. It does not mean that there is not some remnant left there, but that the predisposition of the lions wakened. No sooner was Daniel out of the cave than the lions woke to lionhood again.

Very often birds and pet animals give one a warning of death in the family. One might think that they know from somewhere, or they have a mind, they think about it. No. The condition is reflected upon them. The condition of the person who is dying, the thought of those around that person, the condition of the cosmos at that time, the whole environment there is reflected upon their mind, and they know. They begin to express their feeling, and that becomes a warning of the coming death

One might ask: "If it is a palace of mirrors, do animals project their thought or feeling upon a human being? Does a person reflect the feeling of an animal?" The answer is yes. Sometimes human beings who are in sympathy with a pet animal feel its pain without any other reason. The animal cannot explain its pain, but they feel to what degree the animal is suffering. Besides, a most amusing thing is that on farms one sees shepherds reflecting the feelings of the animals, making noises, singing or dancing in the same way as the animals would do, and showing in many ways the traits of animals.

It is most interesting to watch how the phenomenon of reflection between an animal and a human being manifests to the view of one who sees it keenly, and it explains to us that language is an external means by which we communicate with one another. But real language is always this reflection which is projected and reflected between one and another, and this is the universal language. And once this language is understood, not only with human beings, but even with the lower creation, one can communicate. It is not a story when people said that the saints in ancient times used to speak with animals, with birds—it is the truth. Only they did not speak in language such as we use in our everyday life, but in that natural language by which all souls communicate with one another.

Furthermore, with the bullfight that takes place in Spain and the elephant fights which are known in India—it is not often that the elephants fight in the forest—it is the mind of the spectators who wish the bulls to fight or the elephants. It is this mind which gives a stimulus to their fighting nature, and their desire reflects upon the animals, making them, the instant they are free, inclined to fight. Thousands of persons who watch these sports all expect them to fight, and this expectation of so many minds being reflected upon these poor animals gives them all the strength and desire for fighting. Besides, there are snake charmers who are supposed to attract snakes from their holes. Yes, it is music of the flute, but it is not always the music. It is the mind of the snake charmer reflected upon the snakes that attracts the snake out of the hole. The music becomes an excuse, a medium.

And again, there are some who know a magic to drive certain flies from a house or from a garden, and it has been experienced that in one day's time they were able to drive all the flies from a place. It is mind reflecting upon their little insignificant minds. There is so much that we could learn in little things which can reveal to us the greatest secret of life, if only our eyes were open and if we were keen to observe the phenomena.

* * *

Question: *The mind of the insects—would that indicate a greater mind or just that the fly controllers developed a side of their mind? The fly-side of their mind, is it the evidence of mind or . . .?*

Answer: It is the evidence of mind, not a peculiarity of mind. The human mind is incomparably great in power and concentration, and naturally it projects thought upon the object it chooses to project. It is only the one who knows how to focus the mind, the one who drives away flies from a place. It does not mean that one has in one's mind a fly element, only that one can focus the mind upon flies, which another would not be able to do. Because a person does not generally give thought to it, cannot imagine that such a thing can happen or that there would be an effect of it; and because one does not believe it, one cannot concentrate the mind. And even if one concentrates the mind, one would have no result. It is automatic reflection.

The reason is that, as it is said in the Qur'an, "We have made the human being chief of creation."[1] This means that all beings around humans, large or small, are all attracted to human magnetism; they all look up to the human being, for the human being is the representative of [the Creator]. They unconsciously know it and surrender to it.

Question: *Can that power of projection be increased?*

Answer: Yes, it can be increased with the increase of willpower. It can develop by will, by thought, by deepening the feeling, by the power of concentration.

Question: *Should it not be a great danger if everyone knew it?*

Answer: I think the less a person knew, the better. It is just as well that everyone does not know it.

Question: *That person has willpower to affect the snakes or the flies. It takes a long time to acquire it; it is a special thing trained in one's nature that willpower only works in that direction. Has*

---

1 Qur'an 2:30.

that person not acquired a special power at the expense of other powers?

Answer: Yes, one develops, by focusing one's thought on a certain object, one's concentration; and therefore, one can do that particular thing better than any other thing by one's willpower. Then willpower, once developed, will be useful in any other direction. Those who play the brass instruments in the military band naturally develop the power of blowing instruments, and they will be able to play the wood instruments, clarinet or flute. But if they once have practiced the horn, they can blow the trumpet better than the flute. They are accustomed to that one thing, and they are unaccustomed with other instruments. So it is with concentration. If the snake charmer went near the bank and wanted to attract a purse, the snake charmer cannot very well do it. The snake charmer can attract snakes, but not very well a purse. No doubt, once willpower develops, it will be useful in all things one does.

Question: *Horses are reported to have solved extremely complicated mathematical problems . . . ?*

Answer: It is the reflection of the teacher's mind projected upon the mind of the horse, for a horse is not capable of mathematics, nor can it be. It is a kind of mediumistic process in which, upon the mind of the horse, a mathematical idea is projected. It is possible that even the person who does it does not know it, but that person's very effort of making the horse do it has shown the success.

Question: *How can we make our mirror clearer and keener?*

Answer: By living a life of kindness.

Question: *Is this mirror clear in childhood?*

Answer: In childhood it is clear. But then as one grows it becomes corrupted; it has to be made clear afterwards.

Question: *I have seen an exhibition of animals, sheep, and so on. The shepherds had faces like sheep, and the keepers looked like sheep in their features.*

Answer: It is natural.

THE MIND WORLD 2

This [mind world] phenomenon differs in its nature and character, especially by reason of the nature of different personalities. In the first place, the person whose thought becomes reflected in the heart of another may have a concrete form in thought, may be able to hold it as one design or a picture. In that case the reflection falls on the heart of another, clearly. But if the mind is so weak that it cannot hold a thought properly, then the thought is moving, and it cannot reflect in the mind of another properly. If the memory of the person is not in good condition, then the picture there is not clear. If a person's mind is not clear, if it is upset, if it is too active, then that mind cannot convey the reflection fully.

The mind is likened to a lake of water. If a wind is blowing and the water is disturbed, then the reflection will not be clear; but when the water is still, the reflection is clear. And so it is with the mind. For the mind which is still is capable of receiving reflection. For the mind which is powerful, capable of making a thought, a picture, holding a thought, its thought can project beyond any boundaries that may be standing there to hinder it. Nothing can come between the mind and another mind if they are really focused.

No person with an affectionate heart, of tender feeling, will deny that two sympathetic souls communicate with one another. Distance is never a barrier to these phenomena. Have we not seen in the recent war[1] how the womenfolk of the soldiers, their mothers, their wives, their little children, were linked with their dear ones fighting at the front and felt their dear ones' conditions and knew when a soldier was wounded or was dead?

Many will say that it is the thought which reaches, but at the same time, even the thought vibrations are, in their profound depth, a picture; they are a design. One thought is one particular design, one particular picture; it becomes reflected, and by being so mirrored the other person feels it in an instant. The reflection is not like a conversation. In conversation, every word unfolds the idea, and so the idea gradually becomes manifest. But in the reflection of thought, in one instant the whole idea is reflected, because the whole idea is there in the form of a picture, and it is mirrored in the mind which has received it.

It is this theory which opens before us the mystery that lies in the communication between the living and the dead. The idea of obsession may be thus explained that a reflection of the thought of someone on the other side, held fast by a living creature on the earth, becomes an obsession. Very often a young anarchist may assassinate someone, and in the end you will find that there has not been such a great enmity between the anarchist and the person whom the anarchist has killed— the mystery was behind it. Some enemy of the person who was killed, on the other side, has reflected a thought in the passive mind of one who, through enthusiasm and strength, feels inclined to kill someone without knowing the reason, and has caused someone's death.

Especially among anarchists one finds such cases, owing to their extreme point of view. Their heart is in a condition to be receptive. They can receive a good reflection or a bad reflection and act accordingly. But you might ask, "Is it possible that a person living on earth would be able to project a thought on those who are on the other side?" And the answer is that every

1 World War I.

religion has taught this lesson, but the intellectual evolution of humanity at this time has not grasped it fully. For instance, among Hindus there exists a custom today to offer to the dead all that the dead person loved in the form of flowers and colors from the natural environment and the river, the stream, and the mountains behind. All this that their dear one loved, they make it all an offering to that dear one.

Among some people there is a custom of bringing delicious dishes, burning incense, flowers, and perfume; and then, after having offered it to the dead, they partake of it. But even if they partake of it, it may appear amusing, and yet it is their experience which is reflected. And therefore, it is right for them to partake of it though it is offered to the dead, because it is through them that the dead experience it. They are the medium for the dead to receive that offering. Therefore, if they partake of it, it means they give it to the dead. That is the only way that they can give it. This teaches us another idea: that those who mourn after their dear ones certainly continue to give those who have departed pain. Because from this world, instead of having a better experience and reflecting it to them, they gather pain and offer it to their dead. The wisest thing that one could do for those who have passed is to project the thought of joy and happiness, the thought of love and beauty, the thought of calm and peace. It is in this way that one can help the dead best.

At the present time, when materialism is growing prevalent, very few recognize cases of obsession. Very often those obsessed are sent to the insane asylum, where they are given medicine or different treatments, physicians thinking that there is something wrong with the person's brain, with the mind, that something has gone wrong with the person's nerves. But in many cases, that is not the case—that is the outcome of it. When once one is obsessed, naturally one has lost one's rhythm, one's tone, and therefore does not feel oneself—one feels queer. A continual discomfort causes a disorder in one's nervous system, thereby causing different diseases. But at the root of it there is obsession. In short, either a communication between living beings, or a communication between the living and those who have passed from this earth, is in the reflection, a reflection which depends upon the power and clearness of mind.

* * *

Question: *Could there not be some obsessions which would be beneficial to the ones who receive them?*

Answer: Yes, it is possible. But what generally happens is this, that the souls who are attached to the earth are either earthbound or the inspirers or protectors of the earth. Those inspirers and protectors of the earth, their love comes like a stream. No doubt it would come to the individual, but at the same time it is mostly for the multitude. Therefore, it cannot be classed with what we call, in general terms, obsession. It can be called bliss. But then the other souls, who are earthbound, when those souls reflect, it is for the reason of a want. And however great a reason or a want it be, it is an imperfection, because it is limited. Besides, the creation is a phenomenon where every individual must have freedom, to which one has the right. When that freedom is deprived by obsession, however much it may help, that person remains in a limited condition. Furthermore, it is possible that obsession might become most interesting to those obsessed, and if they were cured from the obsession, they would not feel themselves. They feel that some life that they had experienced for a long time was taken away from them.

Question: *Would you explain the strong concentrated effort for automatic writings and the appreciation of it?*

Answer: The inclination for automatic writing comes from a mediumistic tendency. A person who has a mediumistic tendency is naturally inclined to automatic writing. The reason is that, by automatic writing, one begins to feel in connection. One forms a connection with some souls floating in the air. It does not matter whichever soul one contacts. From that soul one begins to take reflection and then begins to put it on paper. There are some who, if they once become interested in one soul on the other side, and the soul on the other side becomes interested in that particular soul, then there is formed a continual communication. Then it is natural that day and night, or often in the day or night, a communication is established; but there is a danger in this play. It is interesting to begin, but then it could be most difficult to get rid of. I have seen a person who had put himself in spirit communication so profoundly that the spirits would not leave him alone one moment. It was just like a telephone ringing every moment of the day, and the most amusing thing is that he used to live with them. The thing that amused me most was: "I do not want you! Go away!"—but they came again, day and night. Poor man, exposed to the telephone's ringing, could not protect himself. Once he laid himself open to them, he focused himself on the other world, and then he could not close the doors.

Besides this, it is a great strain on nerves, for the reason that the nerves must be very fine in order to get the communication. The intuitive centers in the body are made of fine nerves, finer than one can imagine. They are not matter, they are not spirit—they are in between. When once these fine nerves have become sensitive, then the communication is open with the other side. But then the difficulty is this, that the gross vibrations of this earth are too hard on the nerves, and the nerves cannot answer the demands of this gross world, this material world; they become too fine. The result is that a nervous illness comes from it. It is for the betterment of some mediums who were used by the great explorers of spiritualism that I showed my disapproval to that line, not as an unbeliever nor as someone who makes fun of these things, but only for the welfare of these simple ones who are made use of and whose lives are ruined in order that the others may find out some secret of it. But what secret do they find after all? Nothing. It is not the spectator who will find the secret of the play. It is the players themselves. If they want to experience, they must experience themselves—this is where the joy is—and take the consequences. But this way of taking an innocent young person, a weak person, a mediumistic person, putting that person into a trance and profiting out of that person's ruination, neither brings a blessing, nor brings that knowledge which illuminates the soul.

Question: *When a person dies insane, does that condition of confusion last a long time after death?*

Answer: It depends. As on the earth, some patients, soon after having a disease, find a physician, a healer who has healed a condition and that has helped them to be cured. Then there are others who go on for some time before they are cured, and so it is in the hereafter. Nevertheless, perfection belongs to the other world; imperfection to this. And as the soul approaches perfection, so it is gradually made free from all limitation and imperfection that the soul had experienced when on the earth.

Question: *Is there any risk, when one is treading the spiritual path, of obsession?*

Answer: I do not know what connection there is between the spiritual path and obsession. They are two things: either you exist, or someone else exists in you. They are two things. In the spiritual path it is that you exist in God. God exists in you, and you exist in God. It is the oneness between yourself and God that is the spiritual path. In the other you are apart from the spirit that obsesses you. That is a different path altogether. It is no path; it is an idleness, a chaos.

Question: *Can we influence a soul that has passed beyond this world to such an extent that we can make it commit any special action on the mind of another person on earth?*

Answer: It is a thing possible in theory, but I should say: "Why trouble that spirit? If you are able to influence that spirit, why not influence that person on earth?"

Question: *Is it not painful for the dead to know the beloved ones left behind dress in black as a sign of mourning?*

Answer: It is as we look at it. It is true that this impression is bad, and yet there is that feeling that so many sympathize with one. There is that happiness. There was a great thinker, and he was sitting in his house, and a maid came and said to this man that, "I saw a funeral of someone, he must be received in heaven." The thinker was very amused; how did she see him in heaven? He asked her, "How did you see him in heaven? How do you know that he will be received there?" She said, "I did not see him in heaven, but I saw some in the funeral who were wiping their eyes with the handkerchief. This made me think that he will be received in heaven." What we learn from this is that it is sure that if he lived in life and won the sympathy of some few, certainly there must have been something good in him and he must be received in heaven.

Question: *An artistic mind visualizes easily. But for those who do not visualize or hold mental pictures easily, is mind communication more difficult?*

Answer: Yes, for them it is difficult to project their thought but not difficult to reflect thought.

Question: *Can one focus one's mind on an unreceptive, distant mind?*

Answer: Receptive or unreceptive—the one who can focus the mind can. Of course, the receptive receives sooner and with less difficulty.

Question: *Can obsession only be caused by the dead, or also by a living person?*

Answer: By both. Only in the case of the former it is called obsession; in the case of the latter it is called impression.

THE MIND WORLD 3

A thought may be compared with the moving picture projected upon a curtain. It is not one picture, but it is several parts of the same picture changing every moment that completes the picture, and so it is with the thought. It is not always that every person holds a picture in mind. As a rule, a person makes a picture by a gradual process of completing it. In other words, the thought picture is made in parts, and when the thought is complete, all the parts form a picture. It is according to this theory that the mystics have made *mantra shastra*, the science of the psychical phenomenon of words, which the Sufis have called *zikr*. For a concentration of thought, the holding of a thought in mind is not sufficient. In the first place it is impossible for every person; only for a certain person is it possible to hold a certain thought as a picture. If there is any possibility of completing a thought, it is only by repetition. It is therefore that the Eastern art also shows the same tendency. If a border around a wall is made of roses, it is a rose repeated twenty thousand times, that the picture of a complete rose may be made at the end of one glance cast over it.

If there are many objects before one, there is no object that one can hold in thought. Therefore, the best way that the mystics adopted of contemplation was to repeat a word suggestive of a certain thought, a word that caused the picture of a certain idea by its repetition. Yet one repetition cannot suffice for the purpose. In order to engrave a certain figure upon a stone, a

335

line drawn with pencil is not sufficient. One has to carve it. And so, in order to make a real impression of a thought, of an idea, deeply engraved on the subconscious mind, an engraving is necessary. That is done by the repetition of a word suggestive of the desired idea. No repetition is wasted, for every repetition not only completes it but deepens it, making thereby a clear impression upon the subconscious mind.

Apart from the mystical process, one sees those in one's everyday life who have perhaps repeated in their minds the thought of pain, of hatred, of longing, of a disappointment, of admiration, of love, unconscious of the work it has done within themselves. And yet a deep impression of it has been produced in the depths of their hearts, and that becomes projected upon every person they meet. One cannot help being drawn to a loving person, and therefore, one is unconsciously drawn to an affectionate person. One cannot cover one's eyes from the feeling of hatred that comes from someone. One cannot ignore the feeling of pain that comes forward from a person, for the pain is engraved in that person's heart. This is the phenomenon of reflection, reflection of one mind upon another. There are those who may sit together, who may work together, who may live together for their whole life, and yet they may be closed to one another. It is the same reflection. If the heart of one person is closed, its influence is to close the heart of another. A person with closed heart will close the hearts of others everywhere that person goes. Even the most loving people will helplessly feel the doors of their hearts close, to their greatest regret, not knowing what has happened. It is an unconscious phenomenon.

Therefore, the pleasure and the displeasure, affection and irritation, harmony and agitation, all are felt when two persons meet, without speaking a word. It is our words which hide reality. If they did not, it would seem as if the phenomena of the mirror-land are such that the whole universe is nothing but a palace of mirrors, one mirror reflecting the other mirror. If we do not see it, it does not mean that we cannot see it. It only means that our eyes are not always open, so we remain ignorant of the condition.

If this is true, there is nothing in this world which a person can hide. As the Qur'an says, on the Day of Judgment your hands and feet will give evidence of your doings.[1] But I declare that every moment of the day is a judgment day. We need not wait till Judgment Day for this phenomenon. We see it, we experience it always, yet we do not pay attention to it sufficiently, that never can we have a kind feeling and goodwill toward another, an irritation, an agitation and antagonistic feeling, or hostile inclinations which we can keep from another.

And this is sufficient for us to know that main truth, that absolute truth of the whole universe: that the source is one, the goal is one, the life is one, and the many are only its covers.

* * *

Question: *Is subconscious mind non-individualistic?*

Answer: Not necessarily. The surface of the subconscious mind is non-individualistic, but the depth of the subconscious mind is universal, absolute. In the depth of the subconscious mind every person can find the ultimate mind, absolute mind.

Question: *Could one in reality call subconscious mind the soul, in some aspect?*

Answer: No, mind is always mind, soul is always soul. Mind is an instrument of the soul, as a machine is to an engineer.

Question: *If a person with closed heart has reflected that condition on another, how is this best remedied?*

Answer: If a person wishes to throw a glass of water upon you when walking under that person's window, what will you do? You will go away from there. You will escape, that is what one can do. It is a cold water, it will fall. Of course, that is an ordinary answer. The true answer is that you have to get the key of every heart. Once you have gotten the key, you are able to

1 Qur'an 24:19.

337

open it. And the question is: Where are we to find that key? Is that key love? Yes, certainly. With the power of love, that key is held. But the key itself is not love. That key is wisdom. There are many loving beings who cannot open the heart of another, because they have the power to hold the key, but they have not gotten the key. Love is a power, but the key is the tact, wisdom, that understanding of a person, that person's psychology.

* * *

Question: *Suppose two strong opposed personalities are in the presence of one another, but this* [text missing]

Answer: It must be a war.

Question: *But the stronger always throw reflection upon the weaker?*

Answer: Not at all. It is the one who happens to be for the moment negative who receives the reflection, the positive projecting it; and mostly it is then when both are unconscious. It is not always the stronger person who is positive at every moment, nor is it the weaker person who is always negative, for the phenomenon is always done unconsciously. One mind acts upon the other mind without the two persons knowing it, and sometimes the effect is felt afterward.

Question: *Then the depth of the human mind is unindividualized; must one try to individualize all that belongs to the mind to obtain wisdom?*

Answer: One need not try to individualize. It is already individualized. If one tried the other thing it would be better. Everything in life gives one the inclination to individualize. What one calls individuality comes from mind. It is not the individualizing mind, but the mind itself is the individual. But there is no necessity of doing anything in this respect to mind. What is necessary is the raising of the consciousness higher and higher, in order to widen the horizon of one's vision.

Question: *Can there be property spoken of individual souls?*

Answer: I do not know what is meant by *souls* here. But in my words, I call that a soul which owns no property. If it ever owns property, it is because it is caught by the property. But it is trying every moment to detach itself from the property it owns. It is the illusion that the soul gets of a certain property of mind or body, and as long that illusion remains, the soul is caught by that property. But in reality that property does not belong to the soul, nor does the soul belong to that property. It is this realization which is behind the thoughts of the ascetics. Nevertheless, if anyone came to me and said, "Is it good for the soul to hold the property?" I will say it is best for the soul to realize that all property is its own property. The larger the property it realizes to be its property, the better it is for the soul. The only thing that is harmful is to be owned by the property. There is a saying in the Qur'an, "We have made all that is in heaven and earth for humanity."[2] If that is so, there is nothing good or beautiful that is not for us. And it is no sin if we own it, as long as we are not owned by it.

---

2 Qur'an 22:65.

THE MIND WORLD 4

The impression that is made upon the mind has quite a different character from the impressions made upon objects. A human being is living, therefore creative. Whatever impression one's mind takes, it does not only hold—as a stone holds—an impression, but it produces the same several times in a moment and thus keeps it a living impression. And it is that life of the impression which is held in mind that becomes audible to the ears of the heart. It is therefore that we all, more or less, feel the thought or the feeling of another—the pleasure, the displeasure, the joy or disappointment—for it is continually repeated by the mind.

The impression in the mind does not stand still as a picture. The phenomenon of memory is such that one creates all that the memory holds, and not only the vibrations that the memory holds, but the vibrations or forms in answer to it. For instance, one has a deep impression of fear in one's mind. The consequence is that the mind is at work to produce an object for its fear. In the dream, in imagination, in a wakeful state, fear is created. One can easily understand that in the dream it is created, but how in the wakeful state? Everything that is around a person, one's friends, one's foes, conditions, environments, all take a form which will frighten the mind that is holding fear.

How wonderful then the phenomenon of mind is! The mind is its question, and it is itself its answer. Therefore, miseries are attracted especially by those who fear miseries. A disappointment is brought about by those who expect a disappointment. A failure is caused by holding the impression of a failure. I have often heard people saying, "Oh, I will never succeed, I will never succeed. Everything I do goes wrong." There is something wrong. It is very good that there are stars, that they can attribute their misery to the stars. But really speaking, it belongs to them, it is they who are holding it in their mind. When a person is continually thinking that, "Nothing right will happen, nothing good will come," failure is anticipated; and even if all the stars of heaven were in favor, even then that person will meet with failures. In this way one is the creator of one's conditions, of one's fate. Many there are who see no prospects before them in life. Does that mean that the world, the universe is so poor that it cannot provide for all they need? There is abundance. But by thinking continually that there is no way out of it, one becomes fixed in one's thought and brings about despair.

But whatever one is thinking or feeling, one is at the same time emanating it as a fragrance. One is creating around oneself an atmosphere which expresses what one says or what one feels. And it does not only convey to others one's thought and feeling, but it creates an answer. For instance, a person who, before leaving home, thinks that, "I may have an automobile accident," is preparing the accident and reflecting that thought perhaps upon some other driver of automobiles. That thought has struck the other driver, and when the person approaches that auto, there is an accident. And so it is with one's success. When one goes out in the world and says that, "In this, my business, I shall be successful," one attracts all that is necessary to make one successful.

Does it not prove to us that this is a mirror-land, a mirror-land with a living phenomenon because the mirrors are living? It is not only projecting and reflecting that takes place in the mirrors, but a phenomenon of creation that all that is projected and reflected is created at the same time, and materializes sooner or later. It is in this that the Sufi finds the mystery of mastery: that besides all the ideas of fate and worldly influences and heavenly influences, there is a creative power in mind which works. In one person perhaps the creative faculty of one's being is at work one degree, and ninety-nine degrees are the mechanical part of one's being at work. In another person perhaps, who is more evolved, ninety-nine degrees of creative power are at work and perhaps one degree of the mechanical part. It is the mechanical part of one's being which is subject to conditions and environments and which is helpless. And it is the creative part of one's being which is creative, which produces phenomena; and in this aspect, the divine essence is to be found.

* * *

Question: *Two-thirds of reflected thought would then be accountable for accidents which we feel not to have anticipated by thoughts.*

Answer: Yes, it is so.

Question: *Is it in this way that people get warning of accidents?*

Answer: Yes, sometimes. But sometimes also a fortune-teller tells you that such and such thing is going to happen to you—an accident in this year, a trouble, an illness in that month. In the life of one, it comes true; in the life of another, it does not come true. And you will also find that, in the life of the one who was impressionable, this comes true because that person had taken to heart that such a thing was going to happen. Therefore, in the East, especially in India, where the science of astrology is so advanced and for so many thousands of years the lives of the people depended upon it, you have a saying: "Never consult a foolish astrologer." One may be a good astrologer, but never consult that person; that person may say things that may impress you. When this is not taught, what happens? That a person easily says such things without thinking about it, in joke. For one person to say to another person, "Do not go there, you will be killed," it is an easy thing, a joke, but one does not know that it may make an impression upon that person and that impression may create a cause for death.

Question: *Will you please tell more about how one can wipe out all the innumerable pictures which hinder one?*

Answer: The whole process of the Sufi teaching is this: to make the plate of mind clear. Rumi begins his *Masnavi* by speaking on this question when he says, "The heart is like a mirror, and the first and the most important thing that one has to do with this mirror is to make it clean. Take away all the rust there is."[1] This can be done by the practice of concentration. The horses in the forest will not come if you call them to come to you, nor will they walk if you wish them to walk, because they are untrained horses. So are our thoughts and imaginations. They go about in the mind without harness, without the rein. When that is taken in hand, then it is just like the teacher of a circus, who tells the horse to come and the horse comes; and the teacher tells the horse "Go!" and the horse goes. The teacher tells the horse to run, and then says, "Stop!" and the horse stops. This is the first and most important lesson that you have to learn in the Sufi work. This is the foundation of the whole mysticism and practice of philosophy: that you are able to move your thoughts about as you want. When you wish to think of a rose, a lily must not come in your thought. When you think of a horse, an elephant must not appear before you. You must keep it away. This allows thoughts to come and be held, and expels every thought that you do not wish at the time. In this way, you become the master of your thoughts. You control them, and use them to your benefit.

Question: *If one has an impression before starting on a journey, one should not go with a thought of accident. One goes and an accident occurs. Is that the subconscious mind?*

Answer: This I do not call impression. This I call intuition, intuition that warns you—it is quite a different thing. Impression

1 See R. A. Nicholson, *Mathnavi* (Cambridge, 1930), book 2, p. 327.

is what one gets by one's own suggestion or the suggestion of another, and that materializes. That is the impression I am just now talking about. I have not yet touched that realm of intuition; that will follow.

Question: *If they fear warning of an accident, is this the result of another person's thought? Can we avoid the danger by using our own thought power to counteract it?*

Answer: Yes, we can, if we knew how to do it, because that is the practice of denial. We again come to the work that is done in the Sufi work. Self-denial apart, even denying the thoughts and impressions which we do not wish to come—it is not allowing our mind to be stained by those impressions with which we do not desire to impress our mind; that helps one to avoid it. The mystery of what we call an omen is to be found in the law of impressions. For they say that if you are going to do something, and if a cat crosses your way, you will meet with ill luck. It is easy to understand. In the first place, the swift action of a cat makes a great impression on a person. It forms a line before you, a line of action; and that line, impressed upon you, gives you the thought of a cross. You are intending to go straight and then your line is crossed by a horizontal action against your perpendicular action, which means that in action, your hands are nailed and feet tied. It gives the picture of the idea. Behind the whole mystery of omens, which used to be believed by the ancient people and are considered superstitions, there is this mystery of impression. Naturally, when a person is starting out to accomplish a certain work and happens to see beautiful flowers or fruits that give a promise of desire being fruitful, of its bearing flowers—these are the sign of success. A person going forward with this impression will certainly meet with success. Whereas, if a person sees burning wood or a sack of coal, which all show destruction, a fire which burns up, a person going to do something, impressed by this, certainly loses. Besides, there used to be a custom that when someone from the family was going out to accomplish something, no one must say any word that could hinder that person's success. They did not even ask the person, "Where are you going?" Because even asking raises a question. And the question stands before one: "Why? Where?" That means a stone on the way. Before "Why?" and "Where?" a person would be discouraged, even in answering. The strength of will with which the person is going may be exhausted in answering "Why?" and "Where?" and then one may not find that energy and power to accomplish what one is going to accomplish. This is the inner psychology of mind, the knowledge of which makes things easy. One must not become superstitious by holding beliefs, but one must know the science, the mystery, which is hidden behind all such things, which apparently seem small and little, but their result sometimes is most important.

Question: *Ought we not to get over impressions that cats and spiders make on people?*

Answer: I think we must get above all impressions, not only such as cats and spiders. Every impression that is against us, we must get above it. Only what is needed is to know the science, that we may act wisely toward others. Suppose we get above it or we do not care for it and believe in it, yet we may trouble others. For the sake of helping others, if we were thoughtful, that would make a great difference in our lives, in the lives of our friends.

Question: *How can one release the greater creative energy of a mind that has been accustomed merely to repeat automatically the same practices over and over?*

Answer: By giving the person quite the other direction, a direction which would interest that person most. In support of what I have said, I remember an incident. A maid had learned a new theatrical song, a song the words of which were, "How suddenly my fate has changed." She took such a liking to it that everywhere she was moving about in the house she hummed it and said the words. And what was the outcome? She was looking down from the balcony and suddenly dropped down and was found to be dead. And those who knew said she was especially happy three days before it, and was singing this song.

Then there is another example. The emperor Zafar of Delhi, in the Mughal dynasty, was a great poet, and a poet of highest order.[2] So delicate in his expression, such a great master of words, his imaginations so beautiful and refined—his poetry was nothing but a beautiful picture, a piece of art. And so was his person. But as it is natural that an artist, a poet, interests himself more in tragedy than in comedy, so this poet began to write the words of tragedy. What was the consequence? After the book was finished, his tragedy in life began. He came into decline, and his whole life was reflected in the same tragedy. His life repeated the same poetry which he had written.

2 Bahadur Shah Zafar (1775–1862) was the last of the Mughal emperors in India.

THE MIND WORLD 5

The phenomenon of reflection is such that every action, every thought is reflected in oneself, and there arises a production. It produces something, something which forms a direction in one's life and which becomes a battery behind everything one does, a battery of power and a battery of thought. There is a saying that one's real being speaks louder than what one says. It shows that, in this phenomenon of reflection, every person is exposed to all the mirrors, and there is nothing in the world that is hidden. What one does not say, one reflects, so therefore, there is no secret.

The words used by Solomon, "under the sun,"[1] are for night and day, both. The real sun is the intelligence, and in the light of that sun all mirrors, which are human hearts, reflect all that they are exposed to without any effort on the part of human beings. This is the reason why the desire of a person, if it is a real wish, becomes fulfilled sooner or later: because it is reflected, and through that reflection it becomes living. That reflection gives it life because it is not in a dead mirror. It is a living mirror, which is the human heart. It is not surprising that if the master of the house wished to eat fish, that the cook had the desire to bring it. It is natural. It is not surprising if you had just thought of a friend and the friend happens to come and meet you while you are going to do something else. It is unexpected

---

1 "There is nothing new under the sun." Ecclesiastes 1:9.

outwardly; it is arranged inwardly. It is arranged because your reflection, rising in the mind of your friend, has arranged your meeting.

Someone asked me if we shall meet in the hereafter those around us here. I answered, "Yes, we shall meet in the hereafter those whom we love and those whom we hate." This person was rather pleased with the first thing, but rather displeased with the next. I further explained that, "You think of two persons: the person whom you love most and the person whom you hate most. You cannot help thinking. Either one can be praying for the friend or cursing the enemy, but one will be thinking often of both." So naturally one is attracting them both. The most wonderful thing is that those whom you love or hate in life, you meet them unexpectedly. Without any intention on your part, you attract them. The person asked then, "What shall we do?" I said, "The best thing is not to hate anyone, only to love; that is the only way out of it." As soon as you have forgiven those you hate, you have got rid of them; then you have no reason to hate them, you just forget.

It is this reflection which we see in the success and failure of business. When a person goes to another person on some business, that person reflects. If one has failure in mind, one reflects failure in the other person. From all around, what comes is the condition of bringing about a failure. One, so to speak, causes one's own failure. If one goes with success in mind, one reflects success in the heart of everyone whom one meets, and nothing comes out of it but success. Therefore, it is those who are obsessed by failure who have failure. Those who have the impression of success, have success. We read in history there have been heroes, generals, kings who had success after success. And there are many examples to be found in everyday life of those who have failure after failure; there is no end of failure, everything they touch is shattered. Why? Because the destruction is there. They have it in themselves; only it is reflected in all things they touch.

Amir, who was a great Hindustani poet, says, "My eyes, you have the light of the Perfect One. And if you cannot see, it is not the lack of light in you; it is only because you keep covered."[2] We are seeking for a clear vision continually, wanting to see light continually, and yet we cover the very eyes, the sight which has divine light in it, by covering our hearts. No one can teach anyone, nor can anyone acquire that power of seeing clearly. A human being is naturally a seer. When we do not see it is a surprise. The seers do not only see an individual when an individual comes before them. They are capable of seeing, even if ten thousand persons are sitting before them, all as a multitude and each as an individual. The reason is that the larger a mirror becomes, the more reflections it accommodates in itself. And therefore, in one person a multitude can be reflected at one and the same time—their hearts and souls and minds and all. No doubt it begins by receiving the reflection from one, but as the heart expands, so it takes the reflection of the multitude.

It is in this that there is the mystery of spiritual hierarchy. It is only the expansion of heart. Do we not see in our everyday life that there is one person who says, "Yes, I can love a person whom I love, but then I cannot stand the others." It is only the limitation of the heart. There is another person who says, "Yes, I can love my friends, those with whom I feel at home and feel a contact, but not the strangers. I cannot love them, I am closed." And that person really is closed to strangers. One may be a loving person, but in the presence of strangers one's love is closed. And as the heart becomes more free of this limitation, naturally it becomes larger, because the length of the heart, as Nizam has said in his poetry, is unimaginably great.[3] Nizam says that if the human heart were expanded, it would accommodate the whole universe in it, just like a drop in the ocean.

2 Amir Minai, *Hindustani Lyrics*, trans. Inayat Khan and Jessie Duncan Westbrook (London, 1918).
3 Mir Mahboob Ali Khan, Asaf Jah VI (1869–1911), the Nizam of Hyderabad.

The heart can be large enough to hold the whole universe; it can hold all. And the heart that can hold all can receive the reflection from all. Therefore, the whole process of evolution is getting larger. Getting larger means getting freer from limitations; and the outcome of this condition is that the vision becomes clearer.

One might ask, "How can the minds of the multitude be reflected in the heart?" In answer to this I will say, "In the same way that the picture of their group is taken on the photographic plate." There may be a large crowd. The photographic plate will take them all. If it cannot take them all then it is not large enough. The heart is as capable as a photographic plate of taking reflection. If it cannot take it, it means it is limited, it is small. Once I asked my murshid[4] about the secret of telepathy. He said it is not a secret, it is the actual condition: we live in it, we move in it, we make our being in it.[5] The whole life is an absolute intelligence. It is a mirror-land in which all is reflected. When we think of it deeply, we feel that in the daylight we close our eyes and sleep.

* * *

Question: *When it is in our own hands to have success or have failure, wherefore is prayer used?*

Answer: It is in our own hands to say a prayer or not to say a prayer. It is doing our work, when we are doing it. When we are praying we are doing it, it is a work. Prayer is a certain kind of work. If we did not do it, it would not be.

Question: *But there are people who are unsuccessful, who have failure after failure and yet pray.*

Answer: Praying from the depth and praying from the surface are two different prayers. What Christ has called "vain repetitions,"[6]—one can do it, one can just repeat the prayer, and one

4 Muhammad Abu Hashim Madani.
5 See Acts 17:28.
6 See Matthew 6:7.

may not feel it. One may not fix the mind on the meaning of the prayer. If the depth of one's heart hears the prayer, God has heard it, because God hears through the ears of humanity. The one who prays, through one's own ears God hears it.

Question: *But the one is not open to praying so deeply; how will that one come to betterment?*

Answer: By practice. A person who is not able to draw a straight line, by drawing a thousand times, will learn to draw it, and so one will learn.

Question: *If there is only one mirror in each, does the heart reflect to the mind or the mind to the heart?*

Answer: In the first place it must be known that mind is the surface of the heart, and the heart is the depth of the mind. Therefore, heart and mind are one and the same thing. If you call [*text missing*], therefore, in the same mirror it is reflected. *Mirror* is a very good word, because it has both the mind and the heart.

Question: *Why is it for some so easy to love and difficult to hate; for others the reverse?*

Answer: It is a kind of attitude. A person who takes the right attitude or a harmonious attitude, naturally loves; at least that person's first desire is to love. And the one who takes a wrong attitude, which means an inharmonious attitude, then that person's first impulse is to hate. Very often such persons hate the best person, the most worthy person in the beginning. Then they may be won, then they may change, but their first impulse is to hate. These are the two different attitudes.

Question: *If we wish something ardently from another person do we not deprive that person of the freedom of choice by pulling that person into our direction?*

Answer: Unhappily so. And yet the whole mechanism of the world is such that it is done, either consciously or unconsciously. The whole mechanism is made like this. One does not know it, but behind all minds and therefore all these phenomena there is one mind. It is a kind of puppet show. Outwardly there are dolls dancing, fighting, killing, but behind it all there is one person. The one who is enjoying is the spectator. The one who enjoys it the most is the one who is making the play.

Question: *What is then the secret that the one who is behind all these dolls makes one a sinner and the other a saint?*

Answer: You may also blame a playwright who has written in that play a very nice part for one, and another part that is quite different from it, which is not very desirable. If the playwright had not written both parts, the drama would not be complete. What about a musician? If the composition, from beginning to end, were one note, what would it be? There are high and low notes, and all these make the picture complete.

Question: *But the one who is behind all must be obliged to both.*

Answer: Yes, there is no doubt about that: the one behind it all must be obliged to both. The one behind it all holds the strings of all the pictures, and is the one whose fingers, therefore, are testing the joy and sorrow of all. The one who is moving the dolls, in whose fingers are all the dolls, feels it while moving the hands. But this is just the outward picture. When we go from this picture to reality we see that the dolls are of the same essence as the player of the dolls. Therefore, the relationship is not the same as that between the player of the dolls and the puppet show. The relationship of the player of the dolls and the dolls is much closer; there is no distance here. I may, perhaps, give this example in another way. There are some persons in the East, sometimes a person finds them, who are qualified in moving their hands before a light and, by moving their hands, make pictures on the wall. And while doing it, they make all sorts of forms, and every form has a significance. The king and queen come. All is just done by the movement of the hands.

The whole story is performed by that one person. And after all, what is it? If something undesirable has been made, it is by that person's hand. If something desirable has been made, it is also by that person's hand. If the person had not created a variety, there would not be a complete story that gives the others amusement and a great satisfaction. In the end, that person's hands are not affected by it. The shadows are shadows, the hands remain that person's hands. It is momentary, it passed away.

Question: *Why must we try and become a saint then?*

Answer: Because it is our inner inclination to become a saint. If a person has an inclination to become a sinner, that person is not invited there. But it is not one's inclination to be a sinner. Even if a sinner had the greatest delight in being a sinner, I would never call that a sin, I would call it a virtue. But it is not so, it is not the sinner's delight or happiness. It is only a passion that comes within the sinner, and through that passion the sinner does wrong. After that the sinner is not happy. No soul can continually rejoice in something wrong, and if one did, if one continually rejoices in wrong, it is not wrong. What brings you joy and happiness cannot be wrong.

Question: *Why did Christ, who was nothing but love, attract so much hate?*

Answer: No, he did not attract hate. He only caused fear in their hearts, fear of losing their power, that is all. And through madness they did what they did. If hate is caused against a loving person, it is owing to the ignorance of the person who hates. If one were a little more wise, one would not hate.

Question: *What is the innermost nature of the five elements?*

Answer: The five elements are a process of development. The development of one essence, in each step of development, becomes a certain element. It is distinguished as such because of its distinct quality and it is recognized after it has manifested in a concrete physical form. For instance, if we would not have known earth, water, fire, air as we know them in the physical, concrete sphere, we would not have found out that it is the same element or the variety of elements which is to be found in the finer worlds, or the finer planes; that even in the mind such aspects as memory, thought, feeling, reason, retaining of thought—all this represents one particular element. Then we also find that not only the body, but even the breath, has five different elements, and according to what particular element is predominant at a certain time, we act. One is angry at the time when the fire element is going through one's breath. One is responsive and outgoing at the time when the water element is predominant in the breath. One is inclined to retire, or one feels heavy when the earth is predominant in the breath. One feels a desire to express oneself, one imagines or is active physically when the air element is predominant in the breath. It is especially most interesting to watch this in little children, the moods that come to them. Sometimes they get a kind of battery in them such that one child in the room is equal to one hundred children. That is their air element; they do not know what to do with themselves. And there are other times when they are as good as gold.

Question: *How do you change?*

Answer: Every person has one element which belongs to one's personality, one's individuality, which is predominant and upon which one's characteristic is based. But throughout the whole day it is necessary that the breath must go through all five elements. It is necessary for health, and so one has to go through these elements. If one only has control over oneself, then of course, one assimilates all these forces and turns them into one vital power, which is called magnetism. It is the assimilation of these forces which run through the blood and . . .

[*text missing*]. Ether produces melancholy, depression. It is not an active element, it is inertia.

Question: *When someone is ill, one has not the elements in equilibrium in one's body. How can we see which element fails, or which is too much in our breath? How can we control that?*

Answer: That is what we learn in Sufi culture. In practicing our meditations and silences, that is what we learn: how to govern life's subtle forces and how to use them to the best purpose.

THE MIND WORLD 6

The heart, which is called a mirror in Sufi terms, has two different actions which it performs. Whatever is reflected in the heart does not only remain a reflection, but a creative power productive of a phenomenon of a similar nature. For instance, a heart which is holding in itself and reflecting the rose will find roses everywhere. Roses will be attracted to that heart. Roses will be produced for it. As this reflection becomes stronger, so will it become creative of the phenomenon of roses. A heart that holds and reflects a wound will find wounds everywhere, will be attracting wounds, will be causing wounds. For that is the nature of the phenomenon of reflection.

Very often people have a superstition about a person, lucky or unlucky, coming to the house. A lucky person brings good luck, an unlucky person brings bad luck. What is it? It is only that the one who reflects bad luck creates bad luck wherever that person goes. That person produces bad luck in the environment. I have heard a matron saying that, "Since this maid has come in my house, every day glasses break and saucers break, and things become spoiled and destroyed." I could see the reason of it. I said, "As long as she lives in your house, this breaking will always be there."

There are many instances where one finds that a person joins a business or an industrial place. Perhaps the one joining doesn't have much means but has oneself. And since that person has joined it, a success has come to that business, that industry, every day greater and greater. This person has perhaps outwardly brought nothing, but inwardly has brought that re-flection which is a real phenomenon.

The more we think of this phenomenon, the more we find that if there is one thing that is reflected in our mind, we then reflect it on the outer life; and every sphere that our heart has touched has been charged with that reflection. One whose heart is reflecting joy everywhere, wherever one goes one will make people happy. The sorrowful, the troubled ones, the dis-appointed ones, those heartbroken will all begin to feel life; a food will be given to their souls because this person is reflecting joy. And the one who reflects pain and depression will spread the same in that one's environments, giving pain or sorrow to others. And life is such that there is no end of pain and sorrow and trouble, and what we need are the souls who will reflect joy in order to liberate those in trouble and sorrow and pain.

Now, there is another aspect of this reflection, and that is what one thinks, one becomes. One becomes identified with it. And therefore, the object which is in one's thought, that object becomes one's own property, one's own quality. A child who is impressed by soldiers from childhood, acts like a soldier. When the child is grown up, that person becomes a soldier; the quality of a soldier is developed in that person. The child who has thought of an artist and has been impressed by an artist, the artist's art, the artist's personality, that reflection has grown in the child. And as the child grows, so that quality of the artist becomes developed, and the child turns out to be an artist. And when you read the history of great poets, philosophers, and musicians, their rare merit has not only come by their practic-es, by their exercises, by the gift that is in them. Very often it has come by the impression that they have taken of someone. A reflection, which has developed gradually in their heart has produced in their soul the qualities which belonged to the ob-ject they were impressed by.

There are numberless examples of this to be found in the his-tory of the world, but especially in spiritual work, work which cannot be accomplished by a whole life's study, nor can be finished by the meditation of a hundred years in the solitude. And to attain to spiritual knowledge only by meditation or by learning is like saying, "I will make a language in my lifetime." But no one has been able to make a perfect language in one lifetime. It is tradition which makes a language; it has taken centuries for people to develop language. It cannot be made by one person alone; it is something that a person has inherited, acquired. And so it is in the reflection that a person develops the attribute belonging to that object which one holds in thought.

There are examples to be found in the world of people who have, by retaining a thought, created on the physical plane its manifestation, its phenomenon. The reason is that the reflection is not only a picture as is produced in a mirror, but that reflection in the heart is the most powerful thing. It is life itself, and it is creative. Therefore, the person who has understood the secret of reflection has understood the mystery of life.

* * *

Question: *You spoke about the person breaking many things in the house. If such a one who has a reflection in the heart able to make this person stop this breaking?*

Answer: The first problem that is before us is of ourselves; the next problem is about the other person. If we are able to clear reflections from our own heart, then the next thing is to clear the reflections from the heart of another. But what is accomplished first is clearing reflections from our own heart, reflections that hinder our path. For instance, a businessman came to me and said, "I cannot understand. There is some sort of bad luck with me that I always fail. Why do I fail? I cannot understand. I went to some spiritualists, some clairvoyants, people who make horoscopes. One says one thing, another says another thing. I cannot make out what is right." I said, "The right and wrong is in yourself. Listen to yourself. First find out what is going on in your mind. Is it not the memory of the loss you had? It is a kind of continual voice in your heart. The horoscope reader will say it is something that is around you, the spiritualist that some ghost is behind you. The real thing is that there may be this thing or not. But the real thing is that in your heart a voice is going on, that you have failed. Can you make this voice be silent? As soon as you get rid of this reflection all will be well." "What must I do?" he said. I said, "Determination." "And how to do it?" I said, "Promise me that from now on you will never give a thought to past failures. Past is past; present is before you. Pursue with hope and trust and courage. All will be well." You will always find those who say that "Everything is going wrong with me," hearing the voice inside; it is their own failure that is talking with them. As soon as you are able to make this voice silent, the failure is ended. A new page in the history of your life is turned, and then you can look forward in life with a greater courage and hope. I call the person brave who, in the face of a thousand failures, will say, "Now I am not going to fail. The failure was only a preparation for my success." That is the right spirit.

Question: *If all souls coming toward the earth are alike in the essence, why are some people good by nature, while others have to work and struggle for goodness during a whole lifetime?*

Answer: They all come from the same essence, but not from the same root. They come from the different paths. Their experience is different, and their path is their preparation. The explanation of this question is to be found in *The Soul, Whence and Whither*: that one has not only the past on the earth, but has the past of one's soul.[1]

Question: *Is not vanity a great hindrance to having a perfectly clear heart?*

---

1 See *The Soul, Whence and Whither* in volume 1 of the present series, *The Inner Life.*

Answer: Certainly, but I would call that vanity egotism, conceit, pride. *Vanity* is a very light word, for *vanity* is a poetic word, and according to the Eastern idea, *vanity* is a beautiful word. A poet says in Persian: "My vanity, have you not been the means for all good and bad I have done?" Because when we look at it from a different point of view, from that poetic point of view, we see that it is vanity which very often gives inclination to goodness, to chivalry. I will give you an example. Two children were fighting for one toy, wanting to snatch it from each other's hands, and both were crying. I said to the third one that, "This boy is a very good boy. He is a really good boy, and he does not mind if his brother takes away his toy because he is above it. He is a really good boy, he does not care. He is pleased to see his little brother play with his toy; he can even give up his own toy!" I did not say it to the child, but I said it to someone else. What did it touch? The ego: "I am a good boy, I must prove to be so." A kind of feeling of honor, of dignity that "I am considered so, I must prove to be so." But of course, there is another side of it, and that is pride and conceit that blinds a person's vision and keeps one back from the true progress and real attainment.

Question: *When God is to be found in every worm, plant, animals, bird, or stone, why has Muhammad commanded to remove idols?*

Answer: The answer is that it is not every soul who is developed enough to see God in the idol, in the stone, in all things. When one has come to this realization, one has come to a perfection. The prophet's work is not only pertaining to himself, but to humanity. He is the educator of the world and he has a certain responsibility toward his fellow human beings, to bring them gradually from that stage in which they are to spiritual realization. You read in the Qur'an where it is said, "Thou art in all objects, and in all conditions I see thee." Then nothing has he left; every name, every form, every condition he has considered as the being of God. But that was for himself. To elevate the multitude, who were just absorbed in the play with idols, the time had come when they must be lifted up. There is a childhood and there is youth. The works which are for a child are good for the child, while one is a child. When the child is grown up, its conception must be developed, its ideas must be raised, it must not be kept in the same condition. So it is with the multitude.

Question: *A reflection coming to us from without, from an ideal we see before us, must it enter the heart by means of the mind, which is the surface, or does it come directly to that heart through the one essence?*

Answer: It depends. If it comes from the surface of the heart, it touches the surface. If it comes from the depth of the heart, it reaches the depth. Just like the voice of an insincere person, it comes from the lips and it reaches the ears. The voice of a sincere person, it comes from the depth and it reaches the profound depth of those who hear it. What comes from the depth enters the depth, and what comes from the surface remains on the surface.

THE MIND WORLD 7

A clear vision depends upon a clear heart, open for reflection. Jalal ad-Din Rumi begins his *Masnavi* by speaking about the mirror quality of the heart, also by telling that this mirror quality sometimes disappears when a kind of rust takes a place upon the heart.[1] And then he goes on to tell us that by purifying the heart from this rust, one makes this mirror of the heart clear to take reflections. Once I asked my murshid about the science of telepathy. He said, "It is the reflection. If your heart is clear then you must know only how to focus it, and you need not do anything else; and all that is before it will be reflected in it." Therefore, it is not surprising if the seers see the soul of every person as clearly as an open letter, for it is the nature of the sight. If the sight is perfect, it must see whatever is before it. It cannot help seeing. It is not that one desires to see; it is natural. When the eyes are open, all that is before one is reflected in one.

So the seer cannot help seeing the soul of another, perceiving the thoughts and feelings that a person has. If the seer made an attempt to do this, it would not be right on the seer's part. No one must intrude upon another's privacy. No one has a right to try and find out the thoughts and feelings of another person. But as the eyes cannot help seeing what is before them, so the heart, once made clear and pure from the rust, sees as the eyes see. But the eyes can see so far and no farther. The dimension which is before the eyes is different; before the heart there is

1 *Masnavi*, 1:34.

another dimension, and that is the human heart. When the eyes see the surface, the heart sees the depth of a person. Never, therefore, think that a real mystic does not see into a person's life. Never think that a mystic is unable to see a certain side of a person's nature. No, the mystic sees all, but only if the mystic's heart is clear.

Now the question is: What is the rust? What is it made of? The rust is made of the dense outcome of the mind itself. It does not come from outside, it comes of its own self. It is its dense part. It comes from the surface and thereby covers at the same time its mirror quality. The heart becomes covered by confusion, by fear, by depression, by all manner of excitement that disturbs the rhythm of its mechanism. As the health of body depends upon its tone and rhythm, so the health of the heart depends upon the regularity of its tone and rhythm. A person may be virtuous in actions, pure in thoughts, kind in feelings; at the same time, if that person has ups and downs, then the rhythm is not kept aright. Then that person cannot see the mirror's reflection clearly, for the mirror is clear, but when the mirror is continually moving, the reflection is blurred, the reflection does not show itself clearly.

Once we think of it, we begin to think what a wonderful instrument this human personality is for perceiving life and experiencing life fully. If there were a mirror sold for a million dollars which showed the conditions of thought and feeling of every person, there would be a great demand for it. You would collect numberless orders, even for a million dollars, for such a machine. And here one has it and is unaware of it. One does not believe in it; therefore, one neglects it. And as one does not believe in it, one would rather spend that much money and buy that mirror than try to cultivate something in which one does not believe. And as one does not believe in it, one does not believe in oneself. And as one does not believe oneself, one does not believe in God. One's belief in God is most superfluous.

Numberless souls believe in God, and yet they know not if God really exists. They only believe because others believe in God. They have no proof and live their whole life without a proof of the being of God. And there is no other way of getting the proof of God's existence except the one way by which to get that proof, and that is to become acquainted with oneself, to experience the phenomenon which is within oneself. And the greatest phenomenon that one can experience is the phenomenon of one's heart. Could there be anything more interesting in life, more precious to give life to, than the thought that you could be an instrument of knowing all that is in the person who is before you: that person's nature, character, condition, past, present, future, that person's weakness, and strong points? Nothing in the world could be more interesting and more precious than arriving at this stage, than experiencing this, more precious than wealth or power or position or anything in the world. And this is something which is attained without cost, even without the hard work which human beings do for their everyday livelihood. When we think of this, we find that we thirst for water while standing near the stream. What we thirst after is within ourselves, and what keeps us from it is the lack of belief in ourselves, in truth, in God.

People try to study the outer life, but for the study the sight must be the first thing. This outer sight can show the surface of things; it is the inner sight that is the seeking of the soul. Science as we know it is built on the study that one has made of the things which are visible, which are on the surface, and therefore that study is incomplete. That study can be completed by seeing the inside of things. The beginning of science can even be traced as the outcome of intuition. The ancient physicians used to follow the wild animals, such as the bear and others animals, who sought for different herbs when they were in need of curing themselves of some illness, because their intuition was clear pertaining to the things they must take for their cure. Physicians used to live a life of solitude, a life of meditation. They used to live a pure life, and from that they used to get their inspiration; and from that inspiration they knew what to give in order to cure different diseases. The science which we know today is borrowed from what was known to them, although it was not called science at that time. It is a heritage of the ancient people which we now have and name it science. But its beginning was in intuition, and if ever a scientist today discovers something new, something wonderful, that scientist is again indebted, not to that scientist's outer studies, but to intuition. If this is true, then the faculty of intuition must be developed. The heart must be made clear; then, even if a person were not a spiritual person, not a scientist, that person could be completed, be benefited by this study and practice in life.

* * *

Question: *Is love to our fellow human beings the means to clear the heart, and contemplation or love of God the means to focus it?*

Answer: Love is the original quality of the heart. One need not love in order to cultivate the heart, but the cultivated heart is always full of love. For love is something which one cannot learn, which one cannot force oneself to learn; love must rise itself. If the heart is in its natural condition, it rises of itself. It is not something to be taught or acquired, it is something which springs naturally. And then the question is how to clear the heart. It must be clear from all impressions, good or bad. One must erase anything from it in contemplation. It is by that way that the heart is made clear; therefore zikr is taught.

Question: *Is heart in this lecture the same as soul?*

Answer: No, the heart is heart, and soul is soul. For the soul cannot be rusted, it is always pure from rust. Both can be master in their turns. If the soul allows the heart to be master, the heart is master. But when the soul is master of the heart, it is better. The outcome is quite different. One may be called from God and the other from a person. When the body masters the mind and the mind the soul, then it is from the other soul.

Question: *When by kindness the mirror of the heart gets disturbed by working and helping others, perhaps people who behave stupidly, should we give up helping?*

Answer: We must help, but we must help ourselves first. If we are not quiet and say, "I shall calm down another person," instead of calming down we shall disturb the other person. We must first become quiet in order to calm the other person. Besides that, if we have not earned and acquired that means by which to help others, with all our kindness and goodwill, we shall not be able to help. So first we must gain and acquire what is needed and then share with the others.

Question: *If a seer can read the future of another person, can the seer also see the seer's own future?*

Answer: Certainly, it is only a matter of turning that instrument: instead of turning it to the person, to turn it to oneself, and there one sees. When once a person learns this and understands it, one rises above all things such as palmistry or horoscopes or crystal reading or anything. It does not mean that one thinks that those things are of no use. One sees that for those to whom they are of use, they may use them, but for oneself there is no use for these things.

Question: *Is the future settled forever?*

Answer: Yes. It is settled. But this principle must not be taken as a hindrance to one's action, because one's own action against things that one does not wish in one's life includes that settled future. Besides this, destiny, or the way to destiny, can be changed. But the outcome cannot be changed; the depth remains the same; the surface changes. The outline remains the same, the details change. For instance, a great healer went to a person who was ill, and all the power the healer had was used to cure this person. But it is possible that this person was not meant to be cured, did not respond to this healer. There was something that kept the healer back, and therefore, the healing could not be accomplished. There is a wonderful experience. I knew a person who said, "Every time I am called to get some post for my living, I am refused. Can you do something to avert this misfortune?" I said, "Yes, certainly. Now this next time you are going to get that post, I am sure, quite certain." "What shall I do?" "There is only one thing: every day you will do your exercises for a certain length of time." "Yes," he said. He went, and perhaps he did his exercises for four or five days, and when three days were left before he was called, he slept during his exercises, did not feel like doing them. Then his chance was lost. He came to me and said, "I have lost only two days; I could not do it, because I slept." "Why did you sleep?" Again a call came, and I said, "Now do it." He did it for some time and then he caught cold and did not do it. In the end he went to that place, but was refused. And I asked, "Did you continue your practices?" He said, "No, I caught a cold." A third time he came to me, and he said, "Now I am going to do it, even if I shall be taken to my grave." He went on and, in spite of the cold or grave, he continued; and in the end when he continued it, there was a success. Is it because it was meant to be done not at that time, but at this time? Or was it because of his practices? There is equal truth in both. It was meant to be that he must change his mental attitude in order to get it; and it was meant to be that he was to get it after two failures. If he would not have done his practices, he would not have got it. No, it would not have happened. It was meant that he should come to me and that I should tell him, and, after two times, that it should happen on the third time. But if the destiny is fixed, why must we do the work? Because it is also a part of destiny to do the work. That must be included in the destiny. "But if I did not work, what then?" That also is included in destiny.

THE MIND WORLD 8

The soul is likened to a caterpillar. As a caterpillar reflects all the beauty of the colors that it sees and out of them turns itself into a butterfly, so does the soul. When in the angelic world it reflects angelic beauty, manifesting itself in the form of an angel. When in the world of genius it reflects the jinn qualities, thereby covering itself with the form of a jinn. When in the human world it reflects human qualities, therefore manifesting itself in human form. If the caterpillar is impressed by one form only or by a number of forms of leaves and flowers and colors, it reflects them and becomes them. Very often you will see that a caterpillar has the color of its surroundings, in the leaves or the flowers or whatever is before it—it becomes that. It does not partake of the color and the form of trees and flowers which are at a distance and which it has not contacted. The same is the condition of the soul: all that it comes in contact with, it partakes of its quality, of its color, and perfume, reflecting it in time. It becomes that which it reflects.

This shows us that the mirror quality which the heart shows, does not show only when the soul is on the earth, but it shows from the beginning of the soul's adventure toward manifestation. Therefore, the soul's captivity and freedom both come from itself. Qudsi, the great Persian,[1] has said, "It is thou thyself who becomest a captive, and again thyself becomest free

---

1 Haji Jan Muhammad Qudsi (seventeenth century), poet laureate in the court of the Mughal Shah Jahan.

from this captivity." Both these things—captivity in this body of clay and liberation from this dense earth—both things the soul does itself and does it by one law, and that is the law of reflection. There may be different ideas, as dogmas or speculations, expressed by different wise people as to the soul's coming on earth, as to the soul's return from here. But the thoughtful souls, however different they may be in their conception of the divine law of nature, cannot deny for one single moment this principal law, working as the most powerful factor in the soul's journey toward manifestation and in the soul's return to the goal.

Therefore, naturally a mystic thinks, "What is past is past; what is done is done; I do not trouble about it. What I am concerned with is to make the present moment as I wish it to be, and to make the path which leads to my destination in the future easy for me." It is on this principle that the whole of mysticism has been based. The Sufis concern themselves little with what happened yesterday. Yes, if the knowledge of yesterday has a relation with the things of today, if that knowledge can help one to make life better, in that case alone they consult with the past, but not for the sake of the past. As Omar Khayyam says, "Tomorrow, why tomorrow I should be myself with yesterday's seven thousand years,"[2] which means: If I lived for seven thousand years in the past, what is it to me just now? The greatest problem that faces humanity is today, just now: How can I make my life best for myself, for others? If the Sufis occupy themselves with this science, there is not one single moment that they can spare. It will occupy a whole life to make the best of *just now*. And after all it is *just now* which repeats, and it is *now* that makes the future.

Besides, it is the science of reflection, the study and practice of which brings a person to that attainment which is the seeking

2 "Why tomorrow I may be / Myself with yesterday's sev'n thousand years." *The Rubaiyat of Omar Khayyam*, trans. Edward FitzGerald, quatrain 20.

of every soul. As Zeb-un-Nisa,[3] the Persian poetess, says, "If thou thinkest of the blooming rose, thou wilt become a rose; and if thou thinkest of the crying nightingale, thou wilt become a nightingale. Such is the mystery of life. If thou thinkest of the divine spirit, thou wilt reflect it and thou wilt be it."

One might ask the question: Why does not a mosquito turn into a butterfly, for a mosquito also sometimes lives among beautiful plants and flowers?" And the answer is that a mosquito is not interested in listening, it is interested in speaking. It does not learn, it teaches; so it remains what it is. The caterpillar, on the contrary, is silent. It silently meditates, gently moves, quietly sits and meditates. That is why in the end it turns into the beautiful butterfly.

* * *

Question: *Are there not two ways to live in the present: the belief in the physical and the contemplative eternal? How can we balance them?*

Answer: By being conscious of both. Neither to dive deep in the eternal so much that one does not know what time it is, nor to be involved in the physical so that one is unaware of immortality. As there is night and day, so there is the change of consciousness from physical to spiritual, from spiritual to physical, just like action and repose. By keeping such a balance between these two conditions, a person lives a complete life.

Question: *Why is it that one soul reflects the properties of a murderer and another soul those of a saint, both being souls, equally divine. What law covers that phenomenon?*

Answer: As I have already said, the soul is likened to a caterpillar who first reflects and then becomes what it reflects, and so it is with the murderer and the saint. But one thinks: Did a murderer reflect on a murderer? Yes, the murderer gradually tuned to that reflection by trying to do a little harm here and there,

3 Zeb-un-Nisa (1637–1702), eldest daughter of Mughal emperor Aurangzeb and Sufi poet.

by trying to erase from the heart that sympathy, that kindness, that tenderness, by trying to be blind to that aspect of the murderer's own being, and by trying to cause harm and hurt to others without feeling anything—the murderer has developed that way. And very often, a young murderer is reflecting somebody's thought, either on this side or on the other side. Very often there are arrested from among the anarchists people who are most innocent, who had no enmity for the person whom they have killed; it has only come as a reflection on their mind, projected by someone who was really bitter toward that person. This person who killed only became an instrument. But someone might say, "Is that one not responsible for it?" Yes, for one prepared one's mind for that reflection.

Question: *Last time you said that the fire element was destructive, fear-giving, revengeful. But is there not a good side to the fire element? Is there not a fire element in love?*

Answer: What was not completed last time, I wish to complete this time. I say yes, love, devotion, affection—they all come from the fire element; but you must see how different aspects of fire have their different influences. There is a glow, there is a flame, and there is smoke. The glow produces warmth, the smoke produces confusion and darkness, and the flame illuminates and gives light. And so it is with love: love in the form of affection is a glow, in the form of devotion is a flame, in the form of a blind passion is smoke.

Question: *Why are some very musical people always disappointed even by the best music? Is it because their soul remembers the music of the spheres?*

Answer: I do not think they can be disappointed with the best music. The question is: Was it the best music? If it was the best music to them, they would not be disappointed; if it was the best music for someone else, that person would not be disappointed. Somebody's best music cannot be another person's best music.

Question: *But what about the innocent child reared in a bad environment or in a murderer's family?*

Answer: It is all reflection, as I have said. Certainly, associations from childhood make a great impression upon a person. Therefore, it is a great responsibility for the parents to become the example and impression for the child, that the child may be rightly guided in life. It is the parents' great responsibility. But if we said what is just and what is unjust, it will be very difficult to judge for ourselves the whole scheme of nature. As Mme. Goodenough[4] has said in her lecture this afternoon, if in the play there were only good things and there were not murderers and comedians who make the play complete, it would be a very uninteresting play. If this world were full of pious and good people, this world would be uninteresting, too. It is just as well that people are of various kinds, and we all evolve in the end, slowly but surely. With all our faults and weaknesses and infirmities, there is one desire: to evolve. So therefore, there is a hope for every person.

4 Murshida Lucy Sherifa Goodenough (1876–1937), an English murid of Inayat Khan.

THE MIND WORLD 9

There are many teachings, doctrines, speculations, and ideas to be found as to the hereafter. But if there was anything that could explain the nature and the character of the hereafter, it is one word, and that is reflection. From whatever point of view one looks at it, it is one thing and that is reflection, either from the point of view of the one who believes in heaven and hell after death, or from the point of view of the one who believes in reincarnation which follows after death. For there is not one place made like a town for the ones who have done good deeds, that all the good people would be in a town which is called heaven or paradise, and another town for the ones who have been sentenced to the other place. In the first place, each one has one's own way of looking at life, and according to one's attitude toward life, according to one's outlook on life, there is one's hereafter. And therefore, the heaven of one person cannot be the heaven of another person, neither can the hell of one person be the hell of another person.

As there are different ideals for different people, so there is a peculiar world for every person. And what is that world? That world is one's soul. And what does that world contain? That world contains all that the soul contains. The soul is therefore like a photographic plate. A photographic plate might contain the reflection of one person or it may contain the reflection of a group or of the view of thousands of souls. It is capable of accommodating in itself the reflection of a world before it. So is the soul. What is the hereafter? The hereafter of each one is what one's soul contains. If one's soul contains a heaven, the hereafter is heaven. If one's soul contains something else, then the hereafter is that.

But then one might say, "Is it not the soul which comes as the reincarnation?" Yes, a soul; certainly, a soul comes. But what soul, which soul? A soul which has a reflection in it. It is that reflection which is its reincarnation. Then one might ask a question, "Does it not make everything so unreal, just like the play of shadows?" But is it not that? If it is not the play of shadows, then what is it? If one finds reality in the unreal, if that is consoling, then one may console oneself for some few days. But unreality is unreality. Unreality will not prove satisfactory to the end, because satisfaction lies in the knowledge of truth. For the time being, if unreality satisfies one that this is real, one may continue to think in the same way. But it must be said that, in the end, this will not prove to be real. In order to avoid future disappointment, one must find it out sooner in life, if one is capable of grasping and then assimilating the main truth.

Now the question comes: What is the nature of the soul that experiences the conditions of heaven or hell in the hereafter? The nature of the soul is that it is surrounded by what it has collected. As Christ has said, "Where your treasure is, there your heart will be also."[1] So whatever the soul has treasured in this life, it is that which is the future of that soul.

One might ask what difference there is between these two distinct ideas: that one says that the soul goes on in reincarnation, going from one thing to another; there is another person who says after death the soul experiences heaven or hell, and so it goes on toward God. It is only the difference of two different ways of looking at this one particular soul. The one who calls personality the soul sees that personality continuing from one condition to another; that the personality which one has once

1 Matthew 6:21.

seen has not ceased to exist in the world, but it is going on with its reflections, repeatedly, one after another. And if one considers that personality as soul, that one calls it the chain of incarnations, one after the other.

The other person, who sees the soul as independent of personality, who considers personality as the garb of the soul but not soul itself, then sees the actual condition of that ray of divine intelligence which has come into the world of a soul, sees it as projecting outward and withdrawing inward, and understands this projecting as manifestation and withdrawing as returning to the goal.

But one might say, "Is there not anything of that soul left to go on?" The soul which has journeyed to the goal certainly left something behind when the body was left in the earth. There is something that has become of that body; either that body has been eaten by an animal, and the animal's being has become at one with the body; or several insects have eaten it, and through them it has manifested some result that this body has reached just the same. But at the same time we do not consider that body as that person. We say that it was the body of that person; that person has gone away, and therefore, we do not take account what has become of that body. But if we study and analyze the different conditions that the body has gone through, we shall find that it has been able to give a form to different creatures and different objects, to the trees and plants and flowers perhaps, or to little insects or germs or worms, and directly or indirectly it has reached the birds. Besides, the little lives, blown by the wind, have reached far and have been breathed by many and have been absorbed in the breath or food or water by many beings. If we look at it that way, we shall find that nothing that has been once created has been entirely lost. It has just been changed, and that change has put it to a new life. And therefore, death has been nothing but a kind of illusion to our eyes. And behind this illusion, something has been accomplished toward the maintenance of life. And then we come to what we call the world of mind, of personality. This is another garb upon the soul; this also goes on. Just as the body goes on journeying into a thousand things, the personality does also, either swallowed by one or partaken of by many wayfarers coming from the source and arriving at manifestation, proving at the same time the same personality, for it is the same personality.

The caterpillar is a representative of the flower, of the tree, of the plant that it has absorbed in itself; the caterpillar is a reincarnation of them. Yet the caterpillar is itself an entity, which is known by us as it appears to be. A personality, representing a finished person, certainly has absorbed in it that which it is reflecting; in other words, that which it has taken in itself, which has been projected upon it, which it has borrowed. And it is of that personality that it may claim to be the reincarnation.

But when we come to the soul, around which the body was a cover and the personality was a cover, it is just a divine ray. Recognizing the ray as a soul—that is difficult for every mind to grasp. But when inspiration and intuition permit us to grasp it clearly, then we see a soul—not a personality, not a body, but a soul: an independent entity by itself, originally an angel, a jinn; and passing through those conditions, even something that is arriving at its origin, which is the only purpose that is at the bottom of its heart. As the seer says, "This whole manifestation before me is the play of shadows. It continues for the night, and in the morning all is over."

One might ask, "If that is the condition, then what are we supposed to do?" By considering it unreal we do not arrive at anything. But at the same time, by not considering it unreal we stay in the unreal, and we do not open our eyes to the real. The idea, therefore, is to make the . . . [*missing word*] of this world which is unreal, and at the same time to hold fast with both hands to the knowledge of reality, which alone is the savior, and in which we find our liberation. Verily, truth is inspiring, and truth alone will save.

* * *

Question: *How do you explain the mummifying of people?*

Answer: Well, I do not see any particular aim in it. On the other hand, I think people use artificial ways in order to deprive nature of playing its own part. Humankind has come from nature . . . it is just paying the debt back.

Question: *In regard to mind, what connection has the mind with the mummy?*

Answer: Mind has, to a certain extent, attachment to the body, too—even after having passed from here. It somehow or other feels attracted to it, but the higher the soul, the less it is attracted. And therefore it is better for that reason to get above the earthly things in one's own life during one's lifetime.

Question: *Is each soul an individual ray or has one ray more than one soul in it, like a group soul?*

Answer: Even the word *individual* has a certain illusion in it. For instance, one thinks one's body separate from everybody else. One sees the body as the sign that one is an individual. And at the same time each atom of one's body has an individual, an exclusive life. Every blood cell has its exclusive life. It has its illness. It has its death, it has its birth. And once I had an interesting talk with a physician who used to go into blood research. And I was very interested to see how every blood cell is a living being and that it can die, that it can be ill, and that it can also cause death to the other blood cells. Of course, this cover of the body hides it from our eyes. And so far as we can see, we see that this is individual. But how many individuals are in us? Besides, a family also has a kind of individual significance; a country, a nation has a kind of individual significance; a world, a planet also has a kind of individual appearance. And yet as every cell of the body makes a part of the body, so we all make a part of a city, and all cities make a part of the world, and a plane [of being] makes a part of the world, and all planets make a part of the cosmos. Which is the individual? There is one individual. And then all else which we can see for the moment we may call it individual. When we no longer see it, we may no longer call it that. It is as we see it. When we see an entity standing remote, exclusive, separate, we call it an individual. It is according to our eyes that we see it as separate, but there is a time when we do not see it as a separate entity. We see it linked up with all else that exists. Therefore, naturally a Sufi, after absorbing life keenly, arrives at seeing one individual, and sees the whole being reflected in one individual. It is toward that idea that we have to develop.

Question: *Can personality be regarded as a picture which the soul projects in order to manifest to the outer world?*

Answer: I would not say personality is a picture which the soul reflects in order to manifest on that design; it is something of which the soul partakes. For instance, a person was going on a journey, and on the way there found the snow and was covered with snow. Then that person comes to a place where it is dry, but at the same time the person has brought snow there. And so it is with the manifesting soul. The soul which is manifesting has brought with it a personality. It is that personality which is now guiding one's destiny in the physical world, which is now building one's form in the physical world, designing one's destiny in the physical world, and is therefore something which the soul has already brought. If one has to give it a name, one can give it. But the soul originally does not start as a personality. It starts as a divine ray.

Question: *The soul as a separate divine ray, does it remain separate during the vivifying of different ray incarnations, or does a new ray have* [text missing]?

Answer: A new ray vivifies in each incarnation. For the action of the soul is not going out and then coming half back and then going forward. Neither is the action of the breath like that. The action of the soul is the same as the action of breath. It goes out fully and then comes back fully. Each breath must touch the innermost of one's being in order to exist; that life is impossible without being charged every moment by the innermost spirit, that with every breath according to the verse of Sa'di, which you will read in *The Message of the Spiritual Liberty*,[2] that every breath that a person takes touches the very depth of one's spirit, and that it would be impossible for anyone to live if the breath did not touch the depth of life. Therefore, really speaking, we think that it is nourishment or food or outward things that keep us alive. But if there is really anything that maintains us it is the life of God which we take at every moment with our inhaling and exhaling.

Question: *Does destruction by fire bring almost annihilation? For instance, a body burnt to ashes, and ashes flying into the water?*

Answer: No, even that does not end. In India the chemists make ashes of pearls and of gold and of copper and of sulphur and of silver. And these ashes, as burnt as they are, still retain the essential property of which they are the ashes; and the power that they have is so great sometimes that they really work wonders by the people who use them. The human body is more radiant, more wonderful, more powerful in every way, and more living than any other substance in the world. If that body is burnt to ashes, has it lost all its properties? No, it will reach the fishes if it is put in the water. It will reach plants, germs, and worms and the little living beings who live in the earth; and so it will go on through a process of regeneration, and be utilized to their advantage.

Question: *Is the personality you speak of the same as the deeds and thoughts? As continuing in the hereafter?*

---

2 See *The Message of Spirity Liberty*, the forthcoming volume 5 of the present series.

Answer: Certainly it is. But at the same time, you can look at it from a different point of view. There are two points of view for looking at it. One point of view is that a body remains with one as one goes on in life, and the other point of view is that by cutting one's nails a part of the body is separated from it. By cutting the hair, that part which is separated is not lost, not destroyed; but one does not think about it, what has become of it. But something has become of it. And so every thought and every feeling, as I have said in my lecture during these days, that sometimes the thoughts become elementals. They become living beings. They become as alive as living creatures. They work for you or against you. And if that is true, then different parts of one's body—sometimes people without hands from the war or hands cut or fingers gone—that part which is gone, that person does not think about it. But that part is used by nature, too, that part is existing somewhere. The world is a place where nothing is lost; it is continuing its work. The finger, the leg, has not been lost, it is going on. And so, perhaps, is every thought that has become separated from one's mind; it has gone in the sphere. It is still continuing its life. And as parents find that their children live after them, so a thought is also continuing its own life in the mind-sphere. But at the same time, by losing one finger, a leg, one has not lost one's body. And so with the feeling going out, one has not lost one's personality. One is making one's hereafter.

Question: *Then the expression "an old soul" is not true, as every soul is a new soul, a new ray of God?*

Answer: What really happens is that, instead of calling it an old personality, we call it an old soul. But we must always understand it as an old personality because it is the soul as we know it, only we know it garbed under a personality. And therefore, in its ordinary sense, it is its personality which generally we call soul. In that sense we may say "old soul." But really speaking it is old personality.

Question: *A person may live in a hideous and wicked environ-ment and reflect it unwillingly. Does this one not have to make oneself negative, so as to hinder reflection?*

Answer: One must run away from there if one can. One must not choose hideous or wicked environments. One must always avoid such things, but at the same time, the one who will find fault will find fault with everything. Even good things become bad for that person. But the one who is appreciative and wants to turn bad things into good things will do so. Everything falls short of our ideal. What we can do to retain our progress in the path to the ideal is to add what it lacks. For instance, what we see lacking in a person, we must add to that person, thus making the perfect vision of the divine, which is the aim of our life's observation and study.

Question: *Does it not depend upon the evolution of consciousness of the soul on all planes in how far it can reincarnate?*

Answer: Certainly it does.

THE MIND WORLD 10

There is little consideration given at this time of the world's evolution to what may be called inherited qualities. It is partly because the individual's progress is lacking, and partly because of materialism growing more and more every day. If there is a question of buying a dog, purchasing a horse, one gives a thought to its ancestors because one attaches value to the dog or horse according to its origin. But in the human being one is apt to forget it. As days pass, so less and less consideration is given to this. No doubt, it has its advantages. Nevertheless, there remains the fact that the qualities of both parents and the qualities of ancestors on both sides are manifested in the child. Therefore, the building of its life and of its life's career is placed upon what the child inherits from its parents and from its forefathers. That is the foundation of its life. And if upon a weak foundation a large building is erected, that foundation proves in the end to be not strong enough to hold the building. And if upon a good foundation a building is erected, you can always be sure that it is secure.

One might ask: How does this come? Yes, if a child is liked by one of its parents or its relations on its mother's side or father's side, one sees the reason of it. But in the mind of the child one is apt to forget it; one is apt to neglect the question of how a mental quality can come in a child. But it must be understood that the body is the expression of the soul, and if the body represents the parents and the ancestors, the mind also represents them, for the body is the outcome of the essence of the mind. Besides, the image that a child shows of its parents or of its ancestors is not physical, it is mental. If the mental image is outwardly manifested in the visage of the child, certainly the qualities of the parents and of ancestors are also reflected in the mind of the child.

Now, the question is, "What about the qualities a soul shows which are quite different from the qualities possessed by its parents or ancestors?" The answer is that in the first place one knows so little about one's genealogy; as far as one can trace back is hardly five generations. Few people know more than four or five generations of their family. And a child may inherit qualities of an ancestor six or seven generations back which are not known to its family, and those may manifest in quite a concrete form. One might ask, is there no other way of a soul's inheriting qualities which did not belong to its parents or ancestors? Yes, and that way is a reflection that the soul has brought with it from before it has come to this physical plane.

Those qualities may be even more clear in the life of a soul than the qualities the child has inherited from its parents or ancestors. It is therefore that sometimes one finds a hero, a king, a poet, a general, a great politician having been born in a most ordinary family, and that there is no trace of that knowledge to be found among ancestors or in parents. Nevertheless, one may be a representative of Shakespeare or of Alexander the Great from the higher spheres; but still one has some properties in one's body and in one's mind which are inherited from one's parents and ancestors and which also remain as a reflection fallen upon one's soul.

One might ask a question, "Which quality is greater in a soul, the quality of the ancestors and of the parents, or the quality that the soul has brought with it from the higher spheres? And the answer is that in the depth of the soul there is that quality which it has brought with it; on the surface there is that quality which the ancestors have given. If the innate quality is greater, then it may also manifest on the surface, covering the qualities which the parents have given, which the ancestors have given. But if that quality is not powerful enough, then the outer qualities which manifest on the surface will be the principal qualities, shining as the characteristics of a person.

*   *   *

Question: *How is it to be understood in the Old Testament that the sins of the parents will be punished on the children down to the seventh generation?*[1]

Answer: This only supports my argument. Sins as well as virtues, both the quality of mind as well as the elements of the body—it is both that manifest for generations. It is natural from the scientific point of view, so naturally it is from the metaphysical point of view. Only according to science you would say a person has perhaps inherited a bodily illness or deficiency from the parents. But at the same time it must be understood that mind is the principal thing. Does the child not get a share of its parents' minds? Certainly. The child inherits the spirit of its parents, and even if it be for seven or ten generations, the qualities that they have held. It is not always a sin, but the virtues and merits they have held are to be found in the child.

There are many instances in the old stories that we find, when there was no communication between countries and nations, and there were not so many ships going about and trains, and it was a great difficulty to travel from one country to another. At that time the children of great heroes or kings or learned people happened to leave their country; they were exiled perhaps, or they renounced their country. They happened to arrive in a country where there was no penny with them, no one knew where they came from, what family, at a time that genealogy was thought of very much. We find that such a young man married a princess or arrived at the stage of attainment, even if it be of an earthly or worldly attainment, which another per-

---

1 Deuteronomy 5:9.

son might perhaps have worked for many years and not have arrived at. The reason is, though the person perhaps had no money or outward sign to show that he was so brought up or cultivated or cultured, but that he was himself a written letter of recommendation. Wherever he went, among whom he stayed, by his own qualities he showed what he was. For instance, you take a rose of Persia to China, or a jasmine of Japan to Siam, where perhaps they have never known about the shape or color or perfume; nevertheless, perfume will attract and will prove that it is a rose. It need not say or have a paper attached to it. So the perfume of a person is the qualities that person has, innate qualities: it will never hide, it will always rise. In these old legends we read that in the end that prince or person came to be known as such. But really speaking, it is the test and trial through which a soul has gone, it is that which brings out its qualities to fullness.

And a person who has once passed that examination proves more princely than that person ever could have been. What is princeliness? It is the nobleness of soul and has nothing to do with title or money or anything else. It is inherent; it is the soul itself which has a noble way, attitude, a noble manner. It will prove at every moment, it will prove at the end of every test and trial what it is. For instance, take real gold and imitation gold: while it is not tested, it is just the same, but when once it has gone through tests, the imitation will prove to be imitation; the real gold will prove to be real.

Question: *What causes one soul to become impressed by a Shakespeare or a great genius? Where is the justice in that?*

Answer: Of course, if one wants to get an immediate answer, one must come to consult with the law of karma. It immediately answers and satisfies one, that the personality is naturally attracted to that personality and takes it, because the personality itself is such. And if one wants an answer which a mystic gives, that answer is that it is just the effect, not the cause.

Question: *Does the soul consciously choose its parents?*

Answer: Yes, according to its consciousness at that time. One might ask: Does a child consciously catch a burning fire? Yes, it consciously does it, but it is not conscious of its result yet. That consciousness comes afterwards.

Question: *How is it that often a child has a visage more like the mother and a character like the father?*

Answer: There are many psychological reasons for it. In short, it may be said, a child is an outcome of reflections of both the mother and the father. It is the greater or smaller degree of concreteness of this reflection, and also the greater or smaller degree of conceiving these reflections upon which the visage of the child depends. But are the children responsible for sins of their parents? Not at all. But suppose a child is entitled to inherit the wealth of its parents, of its father; if that is so, it is entitled also to pay back the debts that the father has incurred.

Question: *Children who are living apart from their parents and by their adoptive parents, who are spiritually strong persons, will they be free from the influence of their not good natural mother?*

Answer: Spiritual influence is unlimited. It can bring about any desired results. It can turn out of a thorn, a flower, for all these influences—parents or ancestors or inner influences—which a soul has brought with it, are reflections, shadows just the same. The real is in the depth of every soul, however high or low. And if a real soul meets or if it is brought into contact with a real soul, that real soul will sooner or later penetrate through all reflections which cover the real which exists in every soul. That is the meaning of Christ pointing out to humanity, all the time, the parenthood of God, to see in God a parent, and so to inherit the qualities of God which are great and superior and kingly and noble, and which are divine, and which no one in the world, parents or ancestors or those whom one has met on one's way, possesses. The Sufi calls these qualities *akhlak*

Allah, which means the "manner of God," or "divine manner." A seeker after truth or a worshipper of God need only believe in one parent, which is God. Not only believe in it, but know it, be conscious of it, and inherit from that perfect source, perfecting one's life with it. And it is that heritage which is called divine.

THE MIND WORLD II

A soul inherits qualities from its parents and ancestors, also qualities which it has brought with it from the higher spheres. But a soul also inherits the qualities of its teachers, especially in spiritual culture, but also in all different teachings. When a child goes to an elementary school, even there the child is learning something from the teacher which is not only taught by the books the teacher is teaching, but from the spirit of the teacher. It is very often to be found in schools where children go to learn that the influence of a certain teacher has an impression upon their character and upon their progress.

Since spiritual guidance is not necessarily a study, the teaching which reaches from a teacher to a pupil reaches in the form of reflection. This teaching is called in Sufi terms *tawajjeh*. What one learns is learned from books, but what one learns from a spirit, from a soul, is learned from a living source. For instance, the same thing read in a book does not reach so deeply as when it is spoken. And when it is spoken by the teacher it goes still further. I have had most interesting experiences with this question. A murid who had read a certain idea, a teaching, in a book, had read it four times or five times, but only understood it more fully when I told him. Telling him once was more helpful for him than if he had read the same idea fifty times over. The letters on the paper sometimes reach as far as the eyes, but the word coming from the soul reaches the soul. Therefore, that which is learned by the phenomenon of reflection is of a

388

greater value than the learning in any other form, especially in the spiritual line.

There was once a meeting of religions in Calcutta, and representatives of all mystical schools, of all occult schools were invited to this congress. Shankaracharya[1] was the leading representative of Brahmanism present there. After a most impressive lecture Shankaracharya gave before the meeting, he wished to sit silent. But there was a desire on the part of the audience that some of their questions may be answered. Shankaracharya looked here and there to his disciples and asked a disciple to answer the questions. Which disciple was this? This was someone who was not even known to Shankaracharya's pupils, for he was mostly busy looking after Shankaracharya's dinner or dusting his room and keeping it in order. So the people who were known to be something were not asked; this man was asked. They did not know him, that he existed. And he gave the answer to every question—a thing which he never did in his whole life. It was only because he was asked that he stood, without thinking if he will be able to give the answer or not; and every answer was as if it was given by Shankaracharya himself. The pupils of Shankaracharya were filled with admiration and bewildered at the same time, not having seen this man among them. It is this which is recognized by Sufis as *tawajjeh*, reflection. It was not that pupil, it was the teacher himself who was speaking there.

Besides, what is called the chain of murshids—which means from one soul another soul has received and from another soul another soul has received, and so it goes on—it is also a reflection. A treasure which cannot be gained by meditation or by study is gained by reflection. No doubt study makes one understand it, and meditation prepares the heart to take reflection better, but the wonder that reflection of mind produces is far greater than any attainment made in the spiritual line

---

1 Adi Shankaracharya (788–820), leading exponent of Advaita (non-dualistic) Vedanta.

by studies. There are wonderful examples to be found in the ancient schools of mystics, among Sufis, among Yogis, among Buddhists also, that the knowledge which has been given, perhaps four thousand years ago, is put in clearer language and explained better, and yet it keeps the beauty and characteristic of the whole tradition. And the beauty of mystical knowledge is that whatever school it may be, and from whichever part of the world, the central theme of the knowledge of truth is one and the same. People who have attained knowledge of different aspects of life may differ in their experiences, they may dispute over them, they may not agree upon certain things, but those who have touched the ultimate truth, they cannot but agree, they cannot but understand the same thing. The reason is that the truth remains the same, evolution or involution—nothing diminishes it or adds to it. It is what it is, and it is best attained by the way of reflection.

* * *

Question: *Is it possible that someone by reflection speaks great wisdom without oneself understanding what one is saying?*

Answer: Yes, certainly. At the same time a reflection of mind is not as a reflection on a photographic plate. A reflection on a photographic plate remains but does not live; but reflection upon a mind lives, and therefore it is creative. Yes, it is true that it does not all live, but it helps one to create within oneself the same thing. Now, this brings us to the mediumistic question. I have heard people singing songs which do not belong to them, which they never learned, which they are not supposed to know. I have heard of a young girl in Bombay who never knew Persian, but there used to be times when she would speak Persian. And the Persian was so nice that the learned Persian scholars used to come and discuss with her. And she used to discuss points of metaphysics and would always stand firm on her arguments. And they were so impressed by it. And then at other times she would not know it. But it is mostly seen with poets, especially mystical poets. They write things sometimes which they themselves do not know. Sometimes they can interpret or can understand their poetry better after ten years. I have seen a friend of mine writing a poem, using in it terms which are known to high initiates. I was very astonished, and I asked this friend, "What do you mean by this?" It was then that he knew that he did not know. That particular point, he did not know what it meant. He never knew that he was a mediumistic poet, but no poet can be a great poet who was not by nature mediumistic; for the perfect source is within, and reflection that comes from within is more perfect than what one has learned here.

Question: *Does not the spoken word transcend the written, because the voice carries the soul vibration?*

Answer: Certainly so. There is a soul behind it. In spoken word its impression is greater, because a spoken word is enlightening, it inspires one. The same word read in a book does not have that influence. I remember having heard first thing in my life a sentence which made such a living impression upon me that I could not forget it for weeks altogether. And every day I reflected upon this sentence, it brought a new light. And when I heard that sentence, it seemed as if it was spoken by my own soul, that my soul knew it, that it never was new but it was most dear and near to me. And that sentence was a verse, a couplet. It says, "Though I am a bubble and thou art the sea, still I and thou are not different." It is a simple sentence, but it went in my heart just like a seed thrown in the ground. From that time it always grew; and every time I thought about it, it brought to me a new reflection.

Question: *Is there a fundamental difference between reflection through a master and reading? Or is study in a book only an indirect reflection?*

Answer: Hearing from a teacher is a direct reflection. It is not only the word that a teacher speaks, but even the silence, which is a still greater reflection. Sometimes the words by the same teacher written on paper, if they have come from the depth, then they also make a reflection. But if the same words were spoken by the teacher, that reflection is greater still. When Tagore[2] recites his poetry himself, it is twenty times more delicious. For instance, the words of Rumi from his *Masnavi* have still a living charm. It is long ago that the master passed away, but the words had risen from his soul. And their effect is so great that when one reads the words of Rumi they just penetrate through the soul. It is therefore that mystics used to give names to their pupils. A dervish gave a name to a young man, hearing him sing, and said, "You're going to be the greatest singer of this land." What was it? It was reflection. That reflection was materialized in time; and so it was with a poor man lying in the forest. A mystic met him and said, "You are going to be the emperor of this land," to a man who had left the world because of the ill luck he had experienced all his life, and was awaiting his death. And there he hears from this man, "You are going to be the king of this land," and so it happened. It is not only a reflection just like a moving picture on a curtain, it is reflection from a soul upon a soul, which is creative, which is productive, which is living.

Question: *Does not the reflection come from the teacher from a distance?*

Answer: Certainly it does. Distance makes no difference. The pupil who is near to the teacher may be at the other side of the world, but is closer than a person who is not near and all the time by the teacher's side. Although in the path of spiritual progress, a meeting on the physical plane is often necessary, a contact is valuable. It is just like a winding of a clock.

Question: *Would you kindly give a good interpretation of the word reflection? In ordinary use it means thinking, if I am right; and I do not think it is your meaning.*

2 Rabindranath Tagore (1861–1941), Bengali poet, musician, and artist.

Answer: The best example of the word *reflection* I would give in the projection of a picture upon a magic lantern upon a curtain, that the curtain reflects the picture which the magic lantern has thrown upon it. And so the whole life is full of reflections; from morning till evening we are under reflections. The association with the restless gives us restlessness. That person may not speak to us, but because that person is restless, our heart reflects it. And so contact with a joyous person makes us reflect joy. But an amusing experience I had, when once I went to see a king's waiter. And when I went in the house of the king's waiter, I was so surprised to see that it was the miniature of the palace, the miniature of the court. The way that he came, how he spoke, how he made me sit, and every manner and every word he spoke—it was kingly. What is it? Being the whole day in the presence of the king, he was reflecting the king. The whole day it goes on with us. We do not know it. And sometimes the person whom we reflect has gone from our sight, but we are still reflecting that person. That is the reason that we can give for some tendencies to hum or some tendencies to laugh or some tendencies to cry without reason, it is all from reflection.

Question: *Is the reflection cast by the conscious volition of the reflector, or does it pass unconsciously between souls in tune?*

Answer: It works in both ways. It works sometimes by a conscious action on the part of the reflector, and it sometimes works in a subconscious way. Now, for instance, with a pious mind, good thoughts, peaceful spirit—that person's spirit is, without one trying to reflect, reflected by those who come in contact with it, and they take it with them. Some absorb it and keep it, and the others lose it. But the idea is this, that when a person is not conscious which reflection to keep and which reflection to give away, one will perhaps take the reflection of sadness or sorrow or all undesirable reflections and keep them within, because one receives them. And therefore, one must know that the whole of life is a life of reflection. From morning till evening we receive reflections from those near and dear to us, from those who dislike and hate us, and those from the other side who have passed. We are always exposed. One might ask if it is a good thing to receive them, but one cannot help receiving them. One may call it a good thing or a bad thing, but it is there. We all receive it. If our heart is clear we receive it consciously, the reflection is distinct. If it is not clear we receive it unconsciously, and the reflection is not clear. But we cannot help receiving it. For instance, if there is a gong and a piece of wood, both will receive vibrations. But one is sonorous and will resound, the other will not resound. But at the same time, both are affected by it just the same. If the heart is clear enough to receive reflections fully and more clearly, one can choose for oneself which to retain and which to repel.

THE MIND WORLD 12

Everything that one learns and expresses in one's everyday life has been learned by the way of reflection. And this can be well studied if one observes the lives of growing youths, for the way of walking, the way of sitting, the way of speaking that a youth shows is always from a reflection, an impression which has fallen upon the heart of the youth, and the youth has caught it and expresses it as the youth's own manner, movement, and way of expression. It is not difficult for careful parents to realize how youths suddenly change the manner of their movements, suddenly take a fancy to a certain word that they have picked up from somewhere, suddenly change the way of bearing themselves. And there are youths in whose lives you will see every day a new change—a change in their voice, word, and movement. Even the youths do not know where it has come from, and yet it has come from somewhere. The voice, word, or movement, a manner or attitude which has impressed the heart, is now manifest in their everyday lives. Of course, as a person grows older, so there is less change because then there is a time for the collected impressions to appear in all that one says or does. But especially a child, a youth, is impressionable, and all that it expresses is what it has caught from others.

It has been a custom in the East that no one was allowed to see a newborn infant for three days except those esteemed in the family and whose impression was considered allowable, inspiring a good influence. It has been experienced very often that a child has inherited its foster-mother's qualities, not only physical elements but also mental qualities. And it has often been proved that sometimes the foster-mother's qualities are more pronounced in the child than even the qualities of its own mother. It does not mean that the infant does not possess the qualities of its mother more than the foster-mother's. The only thing is that the foster-mother's qualities are on the surface and they are more pronounced. Very few know or think about this question of what great influence a nurse, a governess, has upon a growing child. It is the nurse's faculties which develop in the child unknowingly, and at this time of artificial life, the parents who neglect their children so much that they give it absolutely into the hands of another person, they do not know of what they deprive that child. They deprive the child of the influence of its own parents, which perhaps would be more advisable. No doubt, in some cases the influence of the governess is better than the influence of the parents. In those cases it is just as well that the child should be in the care of the governess. Nevertheless, the child deeply impresses and reflects, whether it is from an impression which first falls in its infancy, whether it comes from the foster-mother, or whether it has been gained from the nurse or the governess who has taken care of it.

And now coming to the lives of the great personalities of the world, most of the great souls, poets, musicians, writers, composers, inventors, have had a reflection of some personality upon them. They maintained it consciously or unconsciously, till it grew so that it culminated in a great personality, for that reflection becomes just like a seed, and it brings the flowers and fruits according to its nature and character. Roses grow in the environment of roses, and thistles in the place of thistles. The shadows of great personalities produce great personalities. For what is it all? It is all a reflection. The whole phenomenon is a reflection, and therefore, the reflection which is worthwhile will bring forth worthwhile results.

The sages of India, known as Krishna and Rama and Mahadeva, and known as avatars or incarnations of divine personalities, what was it? The divine personality reflected in them. The numberless great avatars of whom we read in the traditions of the Hindus were the manifestations of that reflection. The Christlike personalities which we find in the saints of ancient times, what was it? It was Christ manifested in their hearts. The inspiration of the twelve apostles, the Holy Spirit descending upon them, what was it? Was it not the reflection of Christ himself?

We need not go far to find support for this argument. The khalifs after the Prophet Muhammad—Umar, Siddiq, 'Ali, Usman—showed in their character, in their nature, the fragrance of the Prophet's life. And then we come to the line of the great murshids in the Sufi line, and we see the reflection of Shams-i Tabriz in his murid, Jalal ad-Din Rumi, the author of the *Masnavi*. And especially in the school of Chishtis, which is the best-known school of the Sufis of ancient times, we find perhaps more than ten great personalities at different times who prove to be the examples of souls who won the world by the divine manner of their personality.

And now coming to our everyday experience. Every little change we find in ourselves, in our thought and feeling, in our word and movement, is also caught by us unconsciously from someone else. The more intelligent person, the person who is more alive, is more susceptible to reflections. And if that person happens to be more spiritual, then that person has reflections from both sides, from the earth and from the other side. You will find a change that person every day and every moment, a certain change which is again the phenomenon of reflection.

* * *

Question: *Can it only be in the case if we love or admire someone that we can get reflections?*

Answer: We get reflection from both whom we admire and whom we hate, but then we can repulse it. But the repulse comes after we have already got the reflection. The moment before we see ugliness, the ugliness has been reflected in our eyes already. It is the condition; the mind is just like the eye. We say this is ugly, but before we say it is ugly, we have received the impression of the ugliness. Effect comes more by allowing it to interest one. What one likes more, one catches.

Question: *Does it always mean spirituality if a person gets reflections from the inner worlds, or is it sometimes due to an abnormal negative state?*

Answer: It can be also due to an abnormal negative state. For there are many cases in the insane asylum you will find of mediums; they are mediumistic. The physicians may not acknowledge it, and name it hallucination or some other name. But it is really a mediumistic soul which is open to any reflection from the other side. But, as Omar Khayyam says, a hair's breadth divides the false from true. Such is the condition between normal and abnormal. It is just a hair's breadth. It is the same faculty, the same condition of spirit that could make one illuminated, and just a little difference can make a person insane.

Question: *Can we say that a soul has chosen that, when it came back?*

Answer: That is a very good question. However high a person rises or evolves, and yet without control one has no credit for one's evolution. The credit for evolution is to one who evolves intentionally, one who evolves because one wishes to evolve; one is the master of oneself. Therefore, the credit is in the mastery. Now, for instance, an adept was sitting in the ship with an ordinary person, and this person said, "Oh, how terrible this noise is, continually going on; it breaks my nerves to pieces. Terrible, terrible, terrible! Day and night, day and night to hear this going on; it almost drives me mad." The adept said, "I did

398

not hear it till you reminded me of it. I hear it when I want to hear it. I do not hear it when I do not want to hear it." That is the idea. Both have the sense of hearing; but one has the power to close it and to open it. The other has the doors of the sense open and cannot close them.

Question: *Is there not next to the passive attitude, the active attitude, to open ourselves to be good and beautiful? How to do this?*

Answer: To be one's own master in everything one does. To master one's life, and that comes by self-discipline.

Question: *Can a reflection of a great personality reach a person through that personality's works? For instance, a poet through poems, a painter through art?*

Answer: Certainly. If I were to say, it is at such times that one does the greatest work one has ever done in one's life, a work which one marvels at; one cannot understand how it has been done.

Question: *Is there a certain characteristic alive in every person's character which one keeps throughout one's life, in spite of all reflections which change one continually?*

Answer: Well, nobody has one's own peculiar characteristic, although everyone thinks, "I have my particular characteristic." Although everyone likes to think, "I like this, I believe this, I . . . ," to no one does this belong. The soul comes pure of all these things; it takes them as it comes. But what belonged to one yesterday is one's own characteristic as we know, and what one shows today, we think one partakes of it from somewhere else. Therefore, the best way of knowing what belongs to us is that all we have belongs to us.

THE MIND WORLD 13

We see that our life is full of impressions which we receive consciously or unconsciously, and thereby we derive benefit, or we have the disadvantage of it. We learn from this that if it were in our hand to receive or to reject reflections, we should become the masters of life.

And now the question is how to learn it. How can we manage to receive impressions which are beneficial and reject those that we do not wish to receive? The first thing and the most essential thing is to make the heart a living heart by purifying it from all undesirable impressions, by making it clear from set thought and beliefs, and then by giving it a life. And that life, which is love, is within itself. When the heart is so prepared, then by the way of concentration, learn how to focus it. For it is not everyone who knows how to focus the heart to receive a certain reflection. Yes, unconsciously a poet, a musician, a writer, a thinker focuses the mind on the work of someone who has lived before, and by focusing the mind on the work of the great personality, one comes in contact with the spirit of that personality, and derives benefit out of it, very often not knowing the secret. I have very often seen young musicians or poets thinking of Bach or Beethoven or Wagner. By putting the mind to that particular work they derive, without knowing, that reflection of the spirit of Wagner or Beethoven which is a great help in their work; and they express in their work the reflection which they receive. But then this teaches us that as we go on in the path of spiritual attainment, we arrive at a stage when we are able to focus our mind, our heart to God. And there we do not only receive the reflection of one personality, but the reflections of all personalities. Then we do not see water in the form of a drop, but in the form of an ocean. There we have the perfect reflection, if we could only focus our heart to God.

Why is it that among the simple and illiterate people there is a belief in God to be found, and among the most intelligent there seems to be a lack of that belief? The answer is that the intelligent ones have their reason. They will not believe in what they do not see; and if the method, such as in the old faiths and beliefs, were prescribed of worshiping God by worshiping the sun or a sacred tree or a sacred animal, or worshiping God before a shrine, an altar, or an image of some ideal, the intelligent one today would say that, "This is something that I have made. This is something which I know. It is an object. It is not a person." And in this way the intelligent seem to be lost. The unintelligent ones have their belief in God, and they stay there; they do not go any further, nor are they fully benefitted by that belief for the very reason of ignorance of their belief.

But the process that the wise thought as best for the seeker after truth to adopt is the process of first idealizing God, next realizing God. In other words, first make God and God will make you. As you read in the *Gayan*, "Make God a reality and God will make you the truth."[1] And this may be understood by a little story I will tell you now. There was an artist; this artist was devoted to her art. Nothing else in the world had attraction for her. She had a little studio, and whenever she had a moment to spare, her first thought was to go into that studio and to work on a statue she was making. People could not understand her very well, for not everybody is devoted to one thing like this. For a time people interest themselves in art, at other

1 Hazrat Inayat Khan, *Gayan, Vadan Nirtan* (New Lebanon, NY, Sulūk Press, 2015), p. 16.

times something else, at other times at home, at other times in the theater. Yet she did not mind. She went every day to her studio and spent most of her time in making this piece of art; the only piece of art that she made in her life. And the more the work was finished, the more she began to feel delighted with it, attracted by that beauty to which she was devoting her time. And her thought began to manifest to her eyes, and she began to communicate with that beauty. It was no longer a statue for her, it was a living being.

The moment the statue was finished she could not believe her eyes that it had been made by her. She forgot the work that she had put in that statue, the time that this statue had taken, the thought, the enthusiasm. It made her absorbed in its beauty. The world did not exist for her. It was this beauty which was produced before her. She could not believe for one moment that this could be a dead statue. She saw there a living beauty, more living than anything else in the world, inspiring, revealing. She felt exalted in the beauty of this statue. And she was so overwhelmed by the impression that this statue made on her, that she knelt down before this perfect vision of beauty, with all humility, and asked the statue to speak, forgetting entirely that this was her work, that this was a statue she had made. And as God is in all things and in all beings, as God is all beauty that there is, and as God answers from everywhere if the heart is ready to listen to God's answer, and as God is ready to communicate with the soul who is wakened to the being of God, there came a voice from the statue: "If you love me, there is only one condition, and that is to take this bowl of poison from my hand. If you wish me to be living, you no more will live. Is it acceptable?" "Yes," she said, "you are the beauty, you are the beloved, you are the one to whom I have given all my thought, my admiration, my worship; even my life I will give to you." "Then take this bowl of poison that you may no longer be." For her it was nectar to feel, "I shall now be free from being. That beauty will be. The beauty that I have worshiped and adorned

402

will remain. I no longer need be." She took the bowl of poison and fell dead. The statue lifted her and kissed her, giving her its own life, the life of beauty and sacredness, the life which is everlasting and eternal.

This story is an analogy of the worship of God. God is made first. And the artists who have made God were the prophets, the teachers who have come from time to time. They have been the artists who have made God. When the world was not evolved enough, they made God of rock. Then, when the world was a little more advanced, they gave God words. In the praise of God they pictured the image of God, and they gave to humanity a higher conception of God by making a throne for God. Instead of making it in stone, they made it in the human heart. When this reflection of God, who is all beauty, majesty, and excellence, is fully reflected in a person, then naturally that person is focused to God. And from this phenomenon what arises out of the heart of the worshipper is the love and light, the beauty and power which belong to God. It is therefore that one seeks God in the godly.

* * *

Question: *Can a philosophical conception of God do the same thing when the heart is exalted by the beauty of that conception?*

Answer: In order for the heart to be exalted, the heart must be wakened with a beauty, and the beauty of the conception of God is so high and so great that it cannot be appreciated by an ordinary mind. Therefore, it is better that the heart was first wakened in love or in devotion to a limited being, and from there it was elevated to conceive the thought of God. There is a well-known story of Jami, the great poet of Persia. A young man had a fancy to go to Jami and asked him to teach him the love of God. Jami said, "Have you in your life loved anyone, my little fellow?" He said, "No, not yet." Jami said, "You better go and love someone and know what it is like. Then you will be prepared to understand what the love of God is."

Question: *In one of your books we read, "Nowadays no medium of a priest is required for the communication of humanity and God as it was in former days." How are we to understand this change? How was this change effected?*

Answer: If I were to read my words I could give the answer to this to a greater satisfaction. But now that I have not my words and cannot remember what I have said in connection with this, I will only say that there was a time when it was right to claim, to profess the spiritual service which had been given to a human being from above. But this time is different. At this time it is not right for the servant of God to claim any office, and the best way of serving God is to serve God in the humble, unassuming service of humanity. For it is not necessary for a servant of humanity to say, "I am this" or "I am that"; if one can serve humanity in the path of God, that is quite enough. It is this idea, if I have ever expressed it in a book.

Question: *What is the way to become noticed and favorable to the godly person?*

Answer: The more a person is godly, the more noticed that person is. So no effort may be made for the person to be noticed. Before the person makes an effort, the person is already noticed by the godly. For as everyone has two eyes, the godly one has three eyes, and therefore, the godly sees further. And in order to be favorable, the best way of being favorable is a response with open heart, with appreciation of the God-ideal. For very often a person may seek in the path of God and yet may have preconceived ideas. One may not want to part with them. One would like to go on in the path, and yet may have to carry a burden on one's shoulders which would not enable one to go as quickly as the godly one is going, for the very reason that one is carrying a burden.

There is a story that a great Yogi was going on a journey with his *chela* (pupil). When a Yogi is traveling, his work is that when in a town he will beg and get some food; and when not in a town, then in the forest, if he can get some fruits or vegetables, he will take them for food. And so this *chela* had to adapt himself to this condition, which was rather hard. He had come from a comfortable family and was a young man and quite new in his enterprise. As he went on in the forest, he saw that the town was left far away and there were no houses and villages to be found on the way, and they were quite in the midst of the wilderness. This *chela* began to feel uneasy. And he said to his guru, "Guru, I feel a kind of fear coming to me." "Fear," the guru said, "throw away your fear." The *chela* could not understand. What does it mean to throw away fear? They went a little further. "Guru," said the *chela*, "I feel very afraid." The guru said, "If you are afraid, what are you afraid of? There is wilderness, there is dark, there is no house to live in, is that what you are afraid of? Throw away your fear." The *chela* said, "I cannot understand, what do you mean, throw it away?" The guru said, "Have you put something in your pocket when leaving home?" He said, "Yes." "What is it?" He said, "Some few bricks of gold." "That is what I am saying to throw away. That is the fear. Therefore, I say throw it away and there will be no more fear."

Question: *How can we prolong, during daily life, the perfect stillness of being felt in the contemplation of unity with God?*

Answer: If the contemplation is perfect it will have a winding effect. After winding the clock, it goes on for the whole day, for twenty-four hours. And if one winds one's spirit with contemplation, then it must go on night and day with everything you do. As a king was asked why did he pray most part of the night and work most part of the day, he answered, "At night I pursue God; during the day God follows me."

Glossary

ab-i hayat (Persian): water of life.

Abu Bakr: Abdallah ibn Abi Quhafah, al Siddiq (573–634), companion and father-in-law of the Prophet Muhammad.

Abu Hashim Madani: (d. 1907) Sufi murshid of Hazrat Inayat Khan.

Abu'l-Qasim Firdausi: (d.1020) Persian poet, author of *Shahnameh*.

a'ina khana (Persian): house of mirrors

akhlaq Allah (Arabic): divine manner.

'Ali: 'Ali ibn Abi Talib (d. 661), cousin and son-in-law of the Prophet Muhammad.

Amir Minai: (1829–1900), nineteenth-century Indian poet.

atma (Sanskrit): breath, life, soul.

avatar (Sanskrit): descended deity.

Avicenna: Ibn Sina (980–1037), Persian physician, polymath, philosopher.

Babur: Zahir ad-Dīn Muhammad (1483–1530) First ruler of the Mughal empire.

Bahadur Shah Zafar: (1775–1862), last of the Mughal emperors in India.

balakush: one who drinks all difficulties.

Bayazid: Abu Yazid Bistami (804–740), Persian Sufi.

Brahma (Sanskrit): in Hinduism, the Creator.

Brahmin (Sanskrit): Hindu priestly caste.

chaitanya (Sanskrit): intelligence, the spirit or the light of God.

chela (Sanskrit): student of a guru.

Coué de la Châtaigneraie, Émile: (1857–1926) French psycho-therapist who used positive autosuggestion in his practice.

dervish: Sufi practitioner.

du'a: invocation of benefaction.

Goodenough, Lucy M. (Murshida Sharifa): (1876–1937)

hadith (Arabic): "tradition," a saying attributed to the Prophet Muhammad.

hahut (Arabic): the transcendent plane.

Hafiz: Khwaja Shams ad-Din Muhammad Hafiz Shirazi (d. 1326), Persian Sufi poet.

huffaz (Arabic): those who have memorized the Qur'an.

iman (Arabic): faith.

jabarut (Arabic): the spiritual plane.

jagrat (Sanskrit): the physical plane.

Jami: Nur ad-Din 'Abd ar-Rahman Jami (d. 1492), Persian Sufi poet.

jinn (Arabic): genie, inhabitant of the plane of the mind.

khalif (Arabic: khalifa): successor or representative.

khamush (Persian): silence.

Krishna: Hindu avatar of Vishnu.

kun bismillah (Arabic): "awake in the name of God."

kun bismi (Arabic): "awake at my command."

mahatma (Sanskrit): "great soul."

majzub (Persian; Arabic: majdhub): God-intoxicated dervish.

malakut (Arabic): the mental plane.

mana (Sanskrit): mind.

mantra shastra (Sanskrit): science of the psychic phenomenon of words.

murid (Arabic): "willing," a Sufi initiate.

murshid(a) (Arabic): "the guide," senior Sufi teacher.

Nada Brahma (Sanskirt):" Sound, the Creator."

nafs (Arabic): self, ego.

nasut (Arabic): the physical plane.

nirvana (Sanskrit): transcendent state.

Nizam of Hyderabad: Mir Mahbub 'Ali Khan, Asaf Jah IV (1869–1911), ruler of the princely state of Hyderabad.

nur (Arabic): light.

Omar Khayyam: Ghiys ad-Din Abu'l-Fath 'Umar al-Khayyam Nishapuri (d. 1131), Persian scientist and poet.

paramatma (Sanskrit): "Supreme soul."

prana (Sanskrit): breath, vitality, light.

qadr (Arabic): divine power.

qaza' (Arabic): individual power.

Qudsi: Haji Jan Muhammad Qudsi (seventeenth century), poet laureate in the court of the Mughal Shah Jahan.

quwwat-i maknatis (Arabic): magnetism.

rajas (Sanskrit): stimulating type of food.

Rama: avatar of Vishnu in Hinduism.

ruh (Persian): spirit, soul.

Rumi: Jalal ad-Din Muhammad Balkhi Rumi (d. 1273), famed Persian Sufi poet of Konya and founder of the Mawlawi (Mevlevi) Order.

Sa'di of Shiraz: Abu Muhammad Musharaff al-Din Muslih Shirazi (d. 1291), Persian Sufi poet.

saheb-i-dil (Persian): "master of the heart," master mind.

samadhi (Sanskrit): meditative absorption, the last state in Yoga.

sattva or sant (Sanskrit): calming type of food.

Shams ad-Din Muhammad Hafiz: (1315–90) Persian Sufi poet from Shiraz.

Shams-i Tabriz: Shams ad-Din Muhammad Tabrizi: (d. 1248), spiritual mentor of Jalal ad-Din Rumi.

Shankaracharya: Adi Shankaracharya: (788–820), leading exponent of Advaita (non-dualistic) Vedanta.

Shiva (Sanskrit): Hindu deity of destruction.

Singh, Ranjit (1780–1839): ruler of Sikh empire.

sushupti (Sanskrit): the spiritual plane.

sura (Arabic): chapter of the Qur'an.

Tagore, Rabindranath: (1861–1941), Bengali poet, musician and artist.

tamas: type of food that causes laziness and confusion.

Tansen: (1506–1589) Indian singer, musician, and composer at the court of the Emperor Akbar.

taviz (Arabic): amulet of protection.

tawajjeh (Arabic): reflection of the teacher.

Umar: (584–694) khalif of the Prophet Muhammad.

Usman: Uthman ibn Affan: (577–656), khalif of the Prophet Muhammad.

Vedanta (Sanskrit): the philosophy of the Upanishads.

Vishnu (Sanskrit): in Hinduism, the Preserver.

Vivekananda, Swami: born Narendranath Datta: (1863–1902), Hindu monk and philosopher.

wahm (Arabic): imagination.

yad-i baiza: having a light in the hand.

Zeb-un-Nisa: (1637–1702) eldest daughter of Mughal emperor Aurangzeb and Sufi poet.

zikr (Persian; Arabic: dhikr): "remembrance," Sufi ritual of divine remembrance.

Sources

Below are listed sources of the text within the volumes of *The Complete Works of Pir-o-Murshid Hazrat Inayat Khan, Source Edition* series.[1] Sources of other text from *Sufi* magazine and esoteric papers are cited within those sections.

Health

Health 1	1924 Vol. II, 27–35
Health 2	1924 Vol. II, 76–87
Health 3	1924 Vol. II, 129–34
Health 4	1924 Vol. II, 185–92
Health 5	1924 Vol. II, 227–33
Health 6	1924 Vol. II, 326–37
Health 7	1924 Vol. II, 377–84
Health 8	1924 Vol. II, 432–42
Health 9	1924 Vol. II, 501–9
Health 10	1924 Vol. II, 556–65
Health 11	1924 Vol. II, 603–11
Health 12	1924 Vol. II, 660–67

Mental Purification

Mental Purification	1926 Vol. I, 353–65
Unlearning	1926 Vol. I, 395–406
The Distinction between the Subtle and the Gross	1926. Vol. I, 431–42
Mastery	1926 Vol. I, 467–77
The Control of the Body	1926 Vol. II, 313–20
The Control of the Mind 1	1926 Vol. I, 306–15
The Control of the Mind 2	1926 Vol. II, 185–93
The Power of Thought	1925 Vol. I, 147–53
Concentration	1925 Vol. I, 134–38
The Will	1925 Vol. II, 728–34
Mystic Relaxation 1	1926 Vol. II, 517–27
Mystic Relaxation 2	1926 Vol. I, 322–31
Magnetism	1925 Vol. I, 154–63
The Power Within Us	1926 Vol. II, 468–78
The Secret of Breath	1926 Vol. I, 484–95

---

1 Omega Publications, New Lebanon, NY, www.omegapub.com. Free download available at www.nekbakhtfoundation.org.

Sources

Silence 1	1925 Vol. I, 115–19
Silence 2	1924 Vol. II, 733–40
Dreams and Revelations 1	1924 Vol. I, 185–91
Dreams and Revelations 2	1924 Vol. I, 262–69
Insight 1	1926 Vol. I, 421–30
Insight 2	1926 Vol. II, 507–16
The Expansion of Consciousness	1926 Vol. III (forthcoming)

The Mind World

The Mind World 1	1924 Vol. II, 49–57
The Mind World 2	1924 Vol. II, 103–10
The Mind World 3	1924 Vol. II, 156–62
The Mind World 4	1924 Vol. II, 205–14
The Mind World 5	1924 Vol. II, 250–63
The Mind World 6	1924 Vol. II, 296–304
The Mind World 7	1924 Vol. II, 345–54
The Mind World 8	1924 Vol. II, 400–06
The Mind World 9	1924 Vol. II, 460–71
The Mind World 10	1924 Vol. II, 526–33
The Mind World 11	1924 Vol. II, 575–82
The Mind World 12	1924 Vol. II, 626–32
The Mind World 13	1924 Vol. II, 674–82

BIOGRAPHICAL NOTE

Hazrat Inayat Khan was born in Baroda, India, in 1882. Trained in Hindustani classical music from childhood, he became a professor of music at an early age. In the course of extensive travels in the Indian subcontinent, he won high acclaim at the courts of the maharajas and received the title of Tansen-uz-Zaman from the Nizam of Hyderabad.

In Hyderabad Hazrat Inayat Khan became the disciple of Sayyid Abu Hashim Madani, who trained him in the traditions of the Chishti, Suhrawardi, Qadiri, and Naqshbandi lineages of Sufism, and at last blessed him to "Fare forth into the world."

In 1910, accompanied by his brother Maheboob Khan and cousin Mohammed Ali Khan, Hazrat Inayat Khan sailed for the United States. Over the next sixteen years he traveled and taught widely throughout the United States and Europe, building up the first Sufi order ever established in the West.

In London Hazrat Inayat Khan married Ora Ray Baker. Four children were born to them, whom they raised in London during the First World War and afterward in Suresnes, France, where a little Sufi village sprung up around their home, Fazal Manzil.

The doors of Hazrat Inayat Khan's Sufi Order[1] were open to people of all faiths. Appealing to experience rather than belief, Hazrat Inayat Khan's discourses and spiritual instructions illuminated the twin themes of the presence of God in the depths of the human soul and the interconnectedness of all people. Numerous books were compiled from Hazrat Inayat Khan's teachings during his lifetime and posthumously. In September 1926 Hazrat Inayat Khan bade farewell to his family and disciples and returned to India. On February 5, 1927, he died and was buried in New Delhi.

---

1 Known today as The Inayati Order.

Index

A

48–49, 51, 62, 140; culmination of belief 70; false
belief 23, 73; lack of belief
72, 240, 252, 284, 325,
363, 401–402; power of
belief 46. *See also* believers,
dogma, faith, religion.
believers 17, 72, 106, 114, 136,
177; mind of the believer
71. *See also* belief, devotion,
superstitions.
bells 11–13
benediction 107. *See also* blessing.
Bible 43, 47, 61, 63, 147, 203,
205, 221, 270, 279, 293,
311. *See also* Christianity,
Hebrew.
biology 44
bird 50, 55, 115, 148, 162, 188–
189, 201, 219, 250, 261,
300, 308, 321, 323–324,
360, 375; bird fighting
188. *See also* eagle.
blessing 13, 35, 71, 74, 102, 113,
117, 121–122, 132, 150,
156, 167, 173, 222, 260,
333. *See also* benediction.
bliss 60, 173, 225, 239, 261, 288,
331. *See also* ecstasy, exaltation, joy, nirvana, samadhi.
blood 3, 16, 37, 52, 54, 83, 101,
214, 354, 377; blood relationship 228; divine blood
47. *See also* circulation,
pulse, veins.
Brahma 196, 204, 407
Brahmin 94, 107, 226, 407. *See
also* Brahmanism.
Brahmanism 389. *See also* Hinduism.
brain 15, 22, 35, 69, 142, 174–
176, 178, 279, 286, 318,
330; atoms of the brain

174; brain of the poet 69;
cavity in the brain 15, 67;
power of brain 195. *See
also* insanity, intelligence,
memory.
breath 9–11, 17, 22, 27–28, 60,
88, 90–91, 95, 97–100,
102, 107–108, 117–118,
127, 201, 210, 214, 245–
252, 266, 314, 354–355,
375, 407–408; action of
breath 379; capacity of
breath 28; current of breath
114; exercises of the breath
80; kinds of rhythm in the
breath 99; manifestations
of the breath 97; mystery
of breath 245–246; power
of breath 80, 97, 100, 107,
117, 121; science of breath
245–246; weak breath
100. *See also* air, breathing,
prana.
breathing 10, 28–29, 41, 70, 90,
99, 107–108, 126–127,
132, 142, 214, 230, 246–
247, 250–251, 375; breathing practices 80; mastering
the breath 97, 99; perfect
way of breathing 29. *See
also* breath, exhalation,
inhalation, lungs, prana,
rhythm.
Buddha 24, 162, 234. *See also*
Buddhists.
Buddhists 253, 314, 390. *See also*
Buddha.
butter 81, 95, 180
butterfly 368, 370

C

caterpillar 368, 370, 376

Index

fears 10–12, 14–15, 22, 27–28,
    34, 65, 84, 86, 88, 92, 142,
    156–157, 174, 178, 188,
    190, 278, 340, 344, 353,
    363, 371, 405
feelings 6, 11, 25, 33–35, 45, 47,
    49, 51, 59, 84, 88, 91,
    109–112, 119–120, 145,
    149, 151, 161–162, 164,
    171, 176, 180, 183–185,
    188, 190, 194–195, 197,
    214–215, 239–240, 249–
    250, 259–261, 268, 275,
    284–285, 289, 292–293,
    296, 299–300, 311,
    322–323, 325, 328, 334,
    336–337, 340–341, 354,
    360, 362–363, 371, 380,
    397; control of the feelings
    293; feeling of an animal
    323; moods 9, 354. *See also*
    emotions, passion.
fikr 114
fingers 80–81, 90, 97, 99, 103,
    107, 109–110, 113, 119,
    121, 236, 380; power of the
    fingertips 102, 117
Firdausi *See* Abu'l-Qasim Firdausi.
fire 18, 28, 53–54, 56, 83, 101–
    102, 108, 110–111, 119,
    175, 274, 300, 344, 354,
    371, 379, 386, 407; fire of
    devotion 121, 196; fire of
    illness 29; fire of insanity
    92; fire of the heart of the
    Messiah 112; flame 101,
    108, 182, 208, 371; soul on
    fire 221, 257.
flower 42, 90, 94, 108, 183, 185,
    191, 193, 207, 330, 344,
    368, 370, 375–376, 386,
    396. *See also* rose.

food 4, 17, 33, 35, 60, 68, 82,
    94–95, 107, 119, 121, 160,
    169, 177–178, 212, 249,
    316–317, 321, 357, 375,
    379, 404–405; food of the
    believers 72; kinds of foods
    94. *See also* butter, diet,
    eating, rajas, sattva, tamas.
forgetfulness 113, 8, 59, 68, 73,
    104, 129, 134, 136, 149,
    258, 348, 382, 391, 402;
    self-forgetting 113, 141,
    150, 221
forgiveness 7, 150, 232, 297, 348.
    See also compassion, kind-
    ness, mercy.
fortune-teller 32, 193, 342. *See
    also* astrologer, occultist,
    psychism, seer.
fragrance 149, 169, 183, 341;
    fragrance of the Prophet's
    life 397. *See also* incense,
    perfume.
freedom 187, 277, 295, 331,
    351, 368. *See also* free will,
    liberation.
free will 62, 85, 182, 217, 305. *See
    also* freedom, willpower.
friendship 82, 109, 162, 229,
    234, 271–272, 296, 299,
    302, 304, 311–312, 321,
    340, 345, 348; friendliness
    232–233, 306; friendly
    attitude 303
fulfillment 13, 154, 166, 197,
    202, 3221, 257, 47. *See
    also* attainment, happiness,
    success.

G

Ganges 150
genius 231, 287, 368, 385

425

gentleness 11, 220, 233, 285, 294,
313. *See also* compassion,
kindness, mercy, sympathy.
Germany 247
germs 6, 21–22, 25, 27–29, 49,
98, 110, 119, 212, 321,
375, 379; germ of insanity
92; spirit of the germ 21.
See also microbes.
ghost 279, 359. *See also* séances
spirits.
glance 6, 23, 51, 80, 90, 97,
110–112, 145, 273, 282,
290, 291, 335; control of
the glance 293; kind glance
121; penetrating glance
110. *See also* eyes.
God 6, 10, 18, 23–24, 35, 48,
56–58, 60–61, 63, 70, 85,
96, 105, 111, 136, 138–
140, 150, 166, 186–187,
202–204, 215–217, 221,
226–227, 239, 243, 257,
261–262, 268, 270, 273,
275, 283, 288, 307,
310–311, 333, 351, 360,
363–365, 374, 379–380,
387, 401–405, 407–408,
471; atoms of God's being
236; at-one-ment with God
118; command of God
216; conception of God
84, 170, 403; devotion to
God 98; God manifested
24; God-consciousness 85,
114, 242–243; God-evolu-
tion 25; God-ideal 401,
404; God of rock 403;
God-realization 23–24, 63,
401; God's intelligence 56;
grace of God 73–75, 288;
image of God 248, 403;

kingdom of God 22, 38,
66, 139, 144, 187, 216,
250, 293; light of God 96,
166; love of God 74, 113,
243, 403; parenthood of
God 216, 311, 386–387;
pleasure of God 233, 236,
265; power of God 24,
102, 113, 118, 182, 222,
236. 403; presence of God
113; 177, 262; proof of
God's existence 364; qualities of God 386; names of
God 132, 202; reflection
of God 403; servant of God
56, 196, 404; service to
God 60, 252; spirit of God
56, 248, 315; thought of
God 112–113, 403; union
with God 223, 226, 240,
405; will of God 74, 217,
236, 237; worship of God
401, 403. *See also* Creator.
gold 106, 129, 222, 281, 354,
379, 385, 405; golden age
147
gong 394
Goodenough, Lucy M. (Murshida
Sharifa) 372, 408
Greece, mystical symbology of 307
grown-up 14, 67, 195, 280
Gruner, Dr. Otto C. 38
guidance 121, 136, 145, 171–172,
207, 231, 260, 262,
273–274, 293, 296, 304.
313, 372, 378, 388
guru 187, 241, 313, 405, 407. *See
also* master, teacher.

H

habit 11, 17, 49, 62, 88, 91–92,
120, 138, 151, 237, 300,

Q

repetition 113, 132, 200, 223–
224, 335–336, 350; repetition of a sacred word 106
repose 11, 17, 29, 35, 41, 52,
69–70, 79–80, 99, 126,
142, 172–173, 214–215,
218, 230–231, 250, 370;
repose of the senses 79. *See
also* quietism, relaxation,
rest, sleep, tranquility.
rest 28, 33, 35, 41, 81, 85, 93,
101, 142, 175, 192, 210,
214–215, 231, 249–250,
267, 309. *See also* relaxation, repose, sleep.
revelation 171, 174, 210, 282–
283, 286–288, 292, 299,
302–303; degrees of reve-
lation 284; highest aspect
of revelation 287. *See also*
prophecy, vision.
rhythm 3, 9–14, 16, 29, 67, 69,
80, 83, 85, 88, 98–100,
132, 187, 209–214, 216–
217, 250–251, 258, 266,
285, 330, 363; rhythm of
mind 12, 67, 285; three
rhythms 99, 209–216. *See
also* breathing, circulation,
movement, pulse, rajas, regularity, sant, sattva, tamas.
river 56, 188, 330
rock 15, 44, 56, 148–149, 171,
188, 221, 277, 282, 290,
309–310; God of rock 403.
See also stone.
rose 220, 335, 343, 356, 370, 385,
396; rose water 81. *See also*
flower.
ruh 255, 409. *See also* spirit.
Rumi *See* Jalal ad-Din Rumi.
Russia 11

rust 239, 365; rust upon the heart
343, 362–365

S

sacrament 107, 119
sacrifice 62, 115, 120, 132, 156,
162, 167, 169, 189, 195,
225, 252, 269, 288. *See also*
self-denial.
Sa'di *See* Abu Muhammad Musharaff al-Din Muslih Shirazi
Muslih Sa'di.
sage 117, 138, 150, 156, 185,
213–214, 222, 232,
237–238, 243, 273, 288,
290, 302, 397; power of the
sage 209, 242; sagely spirit
165. *See also* philosopher,
teacher, wisdom.
saheb-i-dil 292, 409
saint 32, 211, 232, 273, 324,
352–353, 370, 397. *See also*
Holy Ones, mystic.
samadhi 262, 409. *See also* bliss.
Sanskrit 90, 147, 175, 183,
196, 210, 239, 256, 260,
407–410. *See also* Hindu,
Vedanta.
sant 211, 409
sattva 94–95, 210, 409
science 18, 34, 37, 126, 154, 172,
206, 219, 222, 240–241,
247–248, 251, 277, 283,
304, 316, 345, 364, 365,
369, 384, 408; medical science 32–33, 38, 245–246;
science of numbers 153;
scientific knowledge 304;
See also biology, electricity,
medicine, scientist.
scientist 37, 83, 109, 115–116,
126, 153, *(cont. overleaf)*

Sulūk Press/Omega Publications is an independent publisher dedicated to issuing works of spirituality and cultural moment, with a focus on Sufism and, in particular, on the works of Hazrat Inayat Khan, his successors, and followers. For more information on the legacy of Hazrat Inayat Khan, please contact the Inayati order at 112 East Cary Street, Richmond, Virginia, 23219. www.inayatiorder.org.

Sulūk Press/Omega Publications

www.omegapub.com